Lymphedema Management
The Comprehensive Guide for Practioners

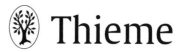

Lymphedema Management

The Comprehensive Guide for Practioners

Joachim E. Zuther, C.I., M.L.D./C.D.T., C.L.T.
Founder
Academy of Lymphatic Studies

Thieme
New York · Stuttgart

Library of Congress Cataloging-in-Publication Data
Zuther, Joachim E.
Comprehensive lymphedema management/
Joachim E. Zuther.
p. ; cm.
Includes bibliographical references and index.
ISBN 1-58890-284-G (alk. paper) —
ISBN 3-13-139481-1 (alk. paper) 1. Lymphedema.
[DNLM: 1. Lymphedema—physiopathology.
2. Lymphedema—therapy. WH 700 Z96c 2005]
I. Title.
RC646.3.Z88 2005
616.4'2—dc22   2004012694

Important note: Medical knowledge is ever-changing. As new research and clinical experience broaden our knowledge, changes in treatment and drug therapy may be required. The authors and editors of the material herein have consulted sources believed to be reliable in their efforts to provide information that is complete and in accord with the standards accepted at the time of publication. However, in the view of the possibility of human error by the authors, editors, or publisher of the work herein or changes in medical knowledge, neither the authors, editors, or publisher nor any other party who has been involved in the preparation of this work warrants that the information contained herein is in every respect accurate or complete, and they are not responsible for any errors or omissions or for the results obtained from use of such information. Readers are encouraged to confirm the information contained herein with other sources. For example, readers are advised to check the product information sheet included in the package of each drug they plan to administer to be certain that the information contained in this publication is accurate and that changes have not been made in the recommended dose or in the contraindications for administration. This recommendation is of particular importance in connection with new or infrequently used drugs.

Copyright © 2005 by Thieme Medical Publishers, Inc.
Thieme Medical Publishers, Inc.
333 Seventh Ave.
New York, NY 10001

Assistant Editor: Jennifer Berger
Editor: Melissa Von Rohr
Vice-President, Production and Electronic
Publishing: Anne T. Vinnicombe
Production Editor: Becky Dille
Marketing Director: Phyllis Gold
Sales Director: Ross Lumpkin
Chief Financial Officer: Peter van Woerden
President: Brian D. Scanlan
Compositor: primustype Hurler GmbH, Notzingen
Printer: Gulde Druck, Tübingen

Printed in Germany

TMP ISBN 1–58890-284–6
GTV ISBN 3 13 139481 1   5 4 3 2 1

Contents in Brief

List of Contributors

Teresa Conner-Kerr, Ph.D., P.T., C.W.S., C.L.T.
Associate Professor and Coordinator
Anatomy Laboratory
Department of Physical Therapy Education
Elon University
Elon, North Carolina

Michael J. King, M.D., F.A.C.P., F.A.C.C.
Board Certified Cardiologist
Lymphedema Specialist
Physician In-Chief
Medical Director
Lymphedema Treatment Service
Lauderhill, Florida

Kimberly D. Leaird, M. Ed., P.T., C.L.T.
Instructor for Complete Decongestive Therapy
Academy of Lymphatic Studies
Sebastian, Florida

Joachim E. Zuther, C.I., M.L.D./C.D.T., C.L.T.
Founder
Academy of Lymphatic Studies
Sebastian, Florida

Contents

Foreword

I am a board-certified internist and cardiologist who became interested in lymphedema ten years ago. I have been involved with the clinical aspects of lymphology since that time. Initially, I knew very little about the pathology of the lymphatic system. The subject was not taught to me in medical school. Lymphedema is a real medical problem that has been ignored in this country. As a result, I found that most of my peers looked upon lymphedema treatment as an alternative form of therapy, outside the mainstream of conventional medicine. I, being academically oriented, with teaching experience, at first felt the same way. In Europe, the basic principles for the treatment of lymphedema were described decades ago.

As medicine advances, people are living longer, and more patients are presenting with edema and lymphedema. The need for proper evaluation and diagnosis of the edematous patient has become increasingly important. The pathophysiology of edema varies depending on the etiology, and an understanding of this is essential to choose the appropriate course of intervention. In all cases, a thorough evaluation of the patient's overall medical condition is necessary.

Several articles and books have been written on this subject. The book written in the format Mr. Zuther has chosen is needed. It is not, for the most part, written in prose, and the reader does not have to pour through entire paragraphs and chapters to find the desired information. The book is a complete and comprehensive discussion of lymphedema, and is presented and organized in a way so that facts are readily obtainable. It serves as a reference source and text both to individuals who know little about lymphedema and to those knowledgeable about the condition who want to review specific topics. It is a valuable source of information and instruction to lay persons, students, therapists, and physicians. Unlike many other books on the subject, this book is not a "cookbook" or "how to" manual. It contains the complete anatomy and physiology of the lymphatic system, discusses treatment options, and also covers patient education and administrative issues.

This textbook is a valuable addition to the literature dealing with the field of lymphedema.

Michael J. King, M.D., F.A.C.P., F.A.C.C.
Lauderhill, Florida

Preface

Closely associated with the cardiovascular system, the lymphatic system represents a drainage system primarily responsible for immune defense and the return of substances from the interstitial spaces back into the blood circulatory system.

The lymphatic system functions like a "sweeper" to clear the interstitial spaces of excess fluids, protein molecules, cellular debris, and long-chain fatty acids (found only in the intestines). It is the responsibility of the lymphatic system to facilitate the movement of those substances that are not reabsorbed by the venous end of the blood capillaries from the tissues back into the bloodstream.

Contrary to the cardiovascular system, the lymphatic system does not represent a closed circulatory system but works according to the one-way principle. It starts with blind or dead-end vessels in the connective tissue and ends in the venous system in the area of the venous angles.

There is a continual shift of fluids at the microcirculatory level of the blood capillaries, and to maintain fluid balance within the body, it is essential that the lymphatic system function properly. Disturbances within the lymph transport often lead to edema or lymphedema, which in most cases has a significant impact on the patient's life.

The focus of this text is on the insufficiencies of the lymphatic system and discusses lymphedema as well as related conditions and currently available intervention techniques. Chapters cover the anatomy, physiology, and pathology of the lymphatic system, which should give the reader a clear understanding of how the lymphatic system works and why certain treatment approaches may be more effective than others in case of an insufficient lymphatic system. Additional chapters on diagnosis, evaluation, therapeutic interventions, and administrative issues, as well as an appendix covering patient education and sample forms for lymphedema treatment centers, are intended to make this text a comprehensive resource.

Illustrations and tables are included to clarify the anatomic and functional basis of the lymphatic system and treatment interventions. To help the nonmedical reader, I have done my best to use simple terms in the figure legends when feasible. Most of these terms are also listed in the glossary at the end of this textbook.

I hope that the first edition of the textbook for *Lymphedema Management: The Comprehensive Guide for Practioners* will prove to be a valuable tool for physicians, therapists, students, and patients.

All royalties and proceeds generated by sales of this textbook are donated to charitable organizations and research projects.

Joachim E. Zuther, C.I., M.L.D./C.D.T., C.L.T.
Sebastian, Florida

Acknowledgments

Heartfelt thanks to my wife, Susanne, who posed as a model for most of the photographs depicting therapeutic interventions, and to my children, Mona, Christoph, and Michael, for enduring all the late hours while writing this textbook.

Thank you to Dr. Michael J. King, M.D., F.A.C.P., F.A.C.C., a pioneer in the treatment of lymphedema in the United States and my long-time friend, for writing the foreword to this textbook and for his contribution of the section Diagnosis and Evaluation of Lymphedema in Chapter 3.

Great appreciation to Kim Leaird, M.Ed., P.T., C.L.T., for her excellent contributions of the Evaluation section of Chapter 3, the Exercise section of Chapter 4, and for her welcome feedback throughout the writing of this textbook.

My gratitude to Teresa Conner-Kerr, Ph.D., P.T., C.W.S., C.L.T., for her valuable contribution of Wounds and Skin Lesions, in Chapter 3.

I am very grateful to Heather Hettrick, P.T., Ph.D., C.W.S., C.L.T., Clinical Assistant Professor at New York University Department of Physical Therapy, for reviewing this text. Her many astute comments and suggestions greatly enhanced the quality of this textbook.

I would like to acknowledge JUZO, Inc., which provided funds enabling us to produce this book in full color.

Thanks to Tony Pazos for providing many of the excellent illustrations throughout the textbook.

Many thanks to my colleagues and staff at the Academy of Lymphatic Studies for their valuable contributions and feedback.

Finally, I wish to thank Melissa Von Rohr, Editor at Thieme Medical Publishers, New York, for suggesting that I write this textbook. Her collaboration and understanding were valuable assets throughout the production of this first edition.

Joachim E. Zuther, C.I., M.L.D./C.D.T., C.L.T.
Sebastian, Florida

1

Anatomy

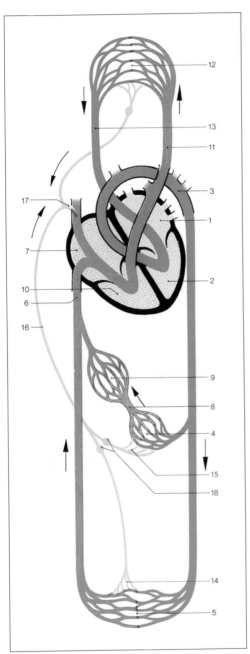

Figure 1–1 Organs of circulation. 1. Left atrium; 2. Left ventricle; 3. Aorta; 4. Blood capillary network of the intestines; 5. Blood capillary network of other organs; 6. Inferior vena cava; 7. Right atrium; 8. Portal vein; 9. Blood capillary network of the liver; 10. Right ventricle; 11. Pulmonary artery; 12. Blood capillary network of the lungs; 13. Pulmonary vein; 14. Vessels of the superficial and deep lymphatic system; 15. Lymphatic vessels draining the intestinal system; 16. Lymphatic trunks; 17. Venous angles; 18. Lymph nodes.

The lymphatic system represents an accessory route by which lymph fluid can flow from the tissue spaces into the bloodstream. En route to the venous circulation, lymph travels through successive lymph nodes, thereby filtering the impurities from the lymph fluid (Fig. 1–1).

The cardiovascular system is closely associated with the lymphatic system. The commonalities between the two systems include

- Superficial, deep, and organ systems
- Similar vessel structure
- Leukocytes (both systems contain monocytes and lymphocytes)
- Blood plasma (the lymphatic system returns percolated or filtered blood plasma to the bloodstream)
- Serum proteins (lower concentration in the lymphatic system)
- Common pathways to the heart
- Protection of the body from infection and disease

The main differences between the two systems include

- The lymphatic system is not a closed circulatory system. It is therefore more appropriate to speak of lymph transport rather than of lymph circulation
- There is no central pump in the lymphatic system
- The lymph transport is interrupted by lymph nodes

◆ Topography

The lymphatic system is divided into the superficial and deep layers and is separated by the fascia (connecting the skin to the underlying tissue). The superficial (suprafascial) layer is responsible for the drainage of skin and subcutaneous tissue, whereas the deep (subfascial) lymphatic system drains the lymph from muscle tissue, tendon sheaths, nervous tissues, the periosteum, and joint structures (some distal joints on the extremities drain via the superficial layer). The transport vessels of the superficial system are embedded in the subcutaneous fatty tissue; deep transport vessels generally accompany blood vessels and are grouped together with them in the same membrane. Perforating vessels connect the deep with the superficial system.

The lymphatic system of the internal organs represents a subcategory of the deep system.

◆ Components

The lymphatic system consists of lymph vessels, which absorb and transport lymph fluid, and lymphatic tissues (see Lymphatic Tissues on page 11).

Lymph Fluid

Once the interstitial fluid enters the lymphatic system, it is called *lymph*. Lymph fluid is a clear and transparent semifluid medium, with the exception of the cloudy chylous fluid found in lymph vessels draining the intestinal system (fatty acids absorbed by intestinal lymphatics produce a cloudy or milky appearance of the lymph fluid).

Lymph fluid is composed of *lymphatic loads*. This term was coined by Földi and summarizes all those substances that leave the interstitial areas via the lymphatic system.

Lymphatic Loads

Lymphatic loads include protein, water, cellular components and particles, and fat.

◆ **Protein.** In 24 hours at least half of the proteins circulating in the blood will leave the blood capillaries (and the postcapillary venules) and travel into the interstitial spaces. Given this fact, the protein concentration in the interstitium continues to remain lower than that of the blood. Proteins in the interstitium perform such important tasks as cell nutrition, immune defense, and blood coagulation (fibrinogen). They are also responsible for the transport of fats, minerals, hormones, and waste products. Proteins play a vital role in fluid balance; for example, maintenance of the colloid-osmotic pressure difference (see also Chapter 2, Filtration and Reabsorption).

Proteins are unable to reenter the bloodstream via the blood capillaries.

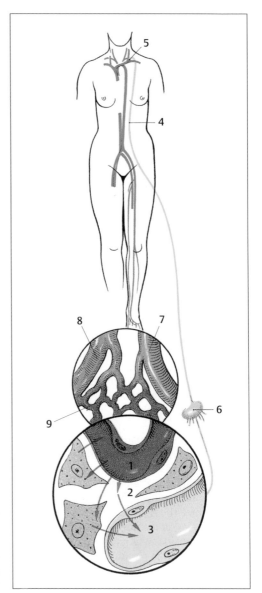

Figure 1–2 Lymphatic return. 1. Blood capillary; 2. Interstitial tissues; 3. Lymph capillary; 4. Larger lymph vessels (collectors and trunks); 5. Venous angle; 6. Lymph nodes; 7. Precapillary artery; 8. Postcapillary vein; 9. Blood capillaries.

The return of the proteins circulating in the interstitium back into the bloodstream is facilitated by the lymphatic system. Intercellular openings (Figs. 1–2, 1–3) in the lymph capillary level allow the large protein molecules to be absorbed.

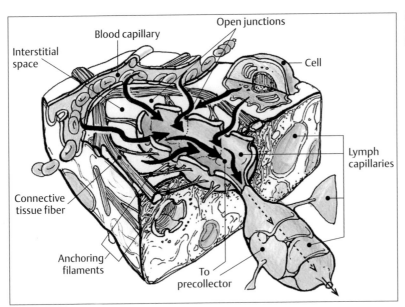

Figure 1-3 Lymph capillary and anchoring filaments.

Foreign proteins such as those resulting from the breakdown of bacteria also constitute a lymphatic load.

The implications resulting from insufficient protein return in case of lymphedema will be discussed in Chapter 3.

◆ **Water.** Approximately 10 to 20% of the water leaving the blood capillary system by way of filtration comprises the lymphatic load of water. This remaining fraction of filtrate is returned to the blood circulation via the thoracic duct, the right lymphatic duct, and the venous angles, and amounts to ~2–3 L per day. However, considerably larger volumes of lymphatic load of water than the roughly 3 L returned by the thoracic duct and the right lymphatic duct are produced throughout the body during the course of a day. The blood capillaries in the lymph node level reabsorb most of the remaining filtrate (see Lymph Nodes on page 11).

> The lymphatic load of water plays an essential role in the body's fluid management and serves as a solvent for other lymphatic loads.

◆ **Cells and Particles.** White blood cells (as well as some red blood cells) leave the blood capillaries continuously and are absorbed by the lymphatics. The circulation of lymphocytes back into the bloodstream plays an essential role in the immune response of the body.

Cell fractions resulting from trauma or tissue neoformation as well as bacteria and cancer cells are also transported by the lymphatic system. Cancer cells use the lymphatic system to form metastases in lymph nodes and other tissues.

Other particles entering the body by way of inhalation, digestion, or injury (dust of various sources, dirt, fungal spores, and other cellular components) are also absorbed by the lymphatic vessels and transported to the lymph nodes, where immune response mechanisms are activated.

◆ **Fatty Acids.** Certain fat compounds cannot be reabsorbed by the blood vessels of the small intestines and are absorbed by the intestinal lymph vessels, also referred to in the literature as chylus vessels. In addition to the lymphatic loads described previously, chylus vessels return fatty acids and fat compounds back to the bloodstream. If fat is part of the lymph, the normally transparent lymph fluid takes on a milky color.

Lymphatic Vessels

Lymphatic vessels, also referred to as lymphatics, are found in all areas with a blood supply. Exceptions to this include the central nervous system (CNS). No lymph vessels are present in nail tissue, cornea, and hair.

Lymphatic vessels can be differentiated between lymph capillaries, precollectors, lymph collectors, and lymphatic trunks. The following section discusses the different characteristics of each vessel.

Lymph Capillaries

Lymph capillaries are also referred to in the literature as initial lymph vessels and represent the beginning of the lymphatic drainage system. They originate in close proximity to blood capillaries as closed or dead-end tubes in the interstitial spaces of the subendothelial layers of the skin and in mucous membranes (Figs. 1–2, 1–3). The lymph capillaries of the superficial lymphatic system are connected to each other and form a unit covering the entire surface of the body like a network, also known as the *initial lymph vessel plexus*. The meshes of this plexus are finer in the areas of the fingers (flexor aspect), palms, and soles of the feet.

Lymph capillaries resemble blood capillaries but have distinct differences. The lymph capillaries are slightly larger, have a more irregular lumen, and are more permeable than blood capillaries. Because of their unique structure, lymph capillaries are able to absorb macromolecules (e.g., proteins). The flat endothelial cells of lymph capillaries are arranged in a single layer. Cell junctions may have a continuous connection (*tight junction*), lay adjacent to each other, or overlap each other. The overlapping structures of the endothelial cells create inlet valves (*open junctions*). This structural adaptation ensures the return of protein, water, and other macromolecular substances to the cardiovascular system.

Semi-elastic fibers, also referred to in the literature as *anchoring filaments*, connect the microfiber network located in the subendothelial layer of the lymph capillaries with the surrounding connective tissue (Fig. 1–3). This enables the lymph capillaries to stay open even under high tissue pressure.

> The main purpose of lymph capillaries is *lymph formation*, that is, the absorption of lymphatic loads into the lymphatic system.

As discussed earlier, ~20% of the blood capillary filtrate remains in the interstitium, causing an increase in the volume and pressure of interstitial fluid. The more fluid accumulates, the more the connective tissue fibers are stretched away from each other, subsequently causing a pull on the anchoring filaments that connect the lymph capillaries with the surrounding fiber network.

The anchoring filaments transfer this force to the lymph capillary, which in turn will dilate and cause the open junctions of the endothelial cells to open like inlet valves. The difference in pressure between the inner lumen of the lymph capillary (lower pressure) and the surrounding tissue (higher pressure) creates a suction effect, facilitating the movement of tissue fluid and other components from the interstitial space into the lymphatic system.

This directional flow of lymphatic loads ends when the lymph capillary is filled to capacity. In this phase, the pressure inside the lymph capillary is actually greater than the pressure in the surrounding interstitial tissues. This pressure difference causes the open junctions (or inlet valves) to close. The opening and closing mechanism of the lymph capillaries adapts to the volume of fluid in the interstitial spaces. This repetitive process will continue in those areas with blood supply and ultrafiltration of fluid from the blood capillaries.

Mobilization of connective tissue from the outside (see also Chapter 4, Manual Lymph Drainage) can also manipulate anchoring filaments with subsequent opening of lymph capillaries, thereby increasing the uptake of lymphatic loads into the lymphatic system.

Lymph capillaries do not contain valves; thus lymph fluid is able to move freely in all directions throughout the initial lymph vessel plexus. Under physiological conditions, lymph fluid moves from the capillaries into the precollectors because the resistance in the slightly bigger precollectors is lower than in the lymph capillaries.

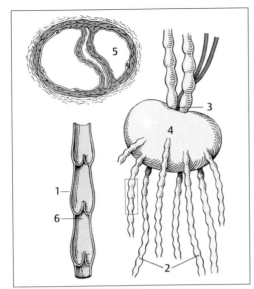

Figure 1–4 Lymph collectors. 1. Lymph collector; 2. Afferent lymph collector to lymph node; 3. Efferent lymph collector from lymph node; 4. Lymph node; 5. Cross section through a lymph collector in the area of the valves; 6. Lymph angion.

Precollectors

Precollectors represent the connection between lymph capillaries and collectors. Precollectors of the superficial lymphatic system generally connect the lymph capillaries with the superficial collectors embedded in the subcutaneous fatty layer of the tissue. Some of these precollectors perforate the fascia and create a connection between the superficial and deep lymphatic system (*perforating precollectors*).

The wall structure of precollectors varies. Endothelial cells have predominantly tight junctions, and smooth musculature is present in some areas in the wall. There are also areas with open junctions between endothelial cells as in lymph capillaries. Precollectors may also contain valves, although in fewer numbers than those found in collectors.

> It is postulated that the main purpose of precollectors is the transport of lymph fluid from the capillaries to lymph collectors. Due to the capillary-like wall structure in some areas, precollectors are able to absorb lymphatic loads. This is why these vessels are also referred to in some literature as part of the initial lymphatics.

Lymph Collectors

Lymph collectors transport lymph fluid to the lymph nodes and the lymphatic trunks. The diameter of collectors varies between 0.1 and 0.6 mm; their walls are structured similarly to those of veins and consist of three distinct layers. The inner layer (intima) consists of endothelial cells and a basal membrane, the medium layer (media) contains a network of smooth musculature, and collagen tissue is present in the outer layer (adventitia).

Collectors contain valves, which, as in venous vessels, allow the flow of fluid in one direction only (proximal). The interval between the valves is irregular and varies between 6 and 20 mm (up to 10 cm in larger trunks). The segment of a collector located between a proximal and a distal pair of valves is called *lymph angion* (Fig. 1–4). The media in valvular areas of lymph collectors contains less smooth musculature than the angion area. Lymph angions have an autonomic contraction frequency of ~10 to 12 contractions per minute at rest (*lymphangiomotoricity*).

In healthy lymph collectors, the proximal valve is open during the systole, whereas the distal valve is closed; in the diastole, the opposite is the case. This permits directional flow of lymph fluid from distal to proximal angions. In lymphangiectasia (dilation) with valvular insufficiency, the lymph flow may reverse into distal lymph angions (*lymphatic reflux*).

Lymph collectors have the ability to react to an increase in lymph formation with an increase in contraction frequency. The increase in lymph fluid entering the lymph angion will cause a stretch on the wall of the angion, which in turn results in an increase in lymphangiomotoricity (*lymphatic safety factor*; see also Chapter 2, Safety Factor of the Lymphatic System).

Other factors that may influence lymphangiomotoricity are external stretch on the lymph angion wall (e.g., manual lymph drainage), temperature, activity of muscle and joint pumps, diaphragmatic breathing, pulsation of adjacent arteries, and certain tissue hormones. Stimulation of the local sympathetic tone may also increase the pulsation frequency of lymph collectors.

As stated earlier, the superficial and deep lymph collectors can be differentiated. The

Figure 1-5 The pattern of lymphatic return to the venous system.

transport vessels of the superficial lymphatic system are embedded in the subcutaneous fatty layer of the skin and follow a fairly straight path within their drainage areas toward the lymph nodes, whereas the collectors belonging to the deep and organ systems follow the anatomy of larger blood vessels and organ vessels, respectively.

Lymph collectors are responsible for draining lymphatic loads from certain body areas, called *tributary or drainage areas*. Most drainage areas of the superficial lymphatic system are subdivided into *lymphatic territories*.

Lymphatic territories consist of several collectors that are responsible for the drainage of the same body area. All collectors in a lymphatic territory transport lymph fluid into the same group of lymph nodes (regional lymph nodes). Lymphatic territories are separated by *lymphatic watersheds* (see discussion later in this chapter). Traversing toward the lymph nodes, collectors on the extremities parallel the watersheds, whereas collectors on the trunk tend to originate at the watersheds.

Connections between lymph collectors belonging to the same territory (*intraterritorial lympho-lymphatic anastomoses*) are frequent and important to ensure sufficient return of the lymph fluid from peripheral areas. Connections between lymph collectors of adjacent territories are much less frequent. These interterritorial anastomoses vary depending on location (see discussion later in this chapter).

Lymphatic Trunks

These vessels show the same wall structure as lymph collectors, but generally they contain a more developed muscle structure in the media. Lymphatic trunks, as lymph collectors, are innervated by the sympathetic nervous system. Intralymphatic valves have the same structure and passive function as in collectors.

Lymph collectors transport the lymph fluid from the superficial, deep, and organ systems to the lymphatic trunks, which then forward the lymph to the venous angles (Fig. 1-5).

◆ **Lumbar Trunks.** The left and right lumbar trunks are responsible for the drainage of the lower extremities, the lower body quadrants, and the external genitalia (Figs. 1-6, 1-7, 1-8). Both lumbar trunks, together with the gastrointestinal trunk (which brings lymph fluid from the stomach and digestive system, the liver, and the pancreas), form the *cisterna*

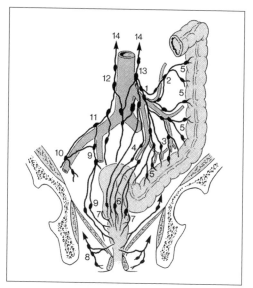

Figure 1-6 Lymphatic drainage of distal colon and rectum (anterior view). 1. Inferior mesenteric lymph nodes; 2. Left colic lymph nodes; 3. Sigmoid lymph nodes; 4. Superior rectal lymph nodes; 5. Paracolic lymph nodes; 6. Pararectal lymph nodes; 7. Lymphatic vessels draining to sacral lymph nodes; 8. Lymph nodes in the ischioanal fossa with drainage to the superficial inguinal lymph nodes; 9. Internal pelvic lymph nodes; 10. External pelvic lymph nodes; 11. Common pelvic lymph nodes; 12. Right lumbar lymph nodes; 13. Left lumbar lymph nodes; 14. Left and right lumbar trunks.

Components

7

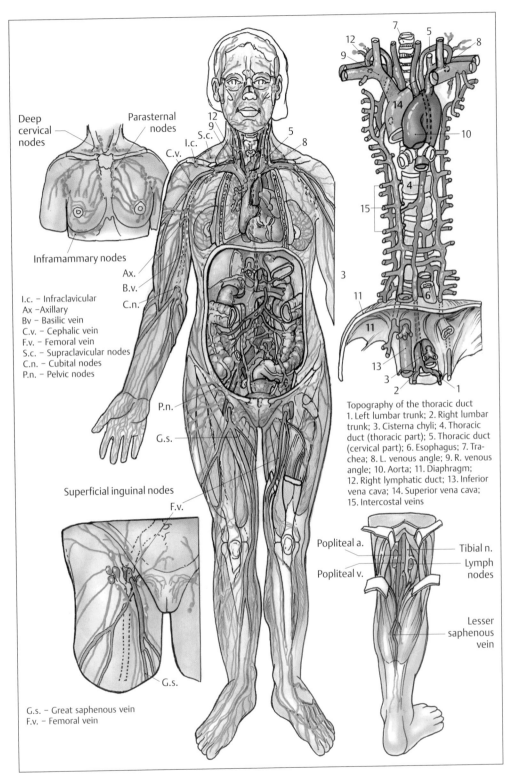

Deep cervical nodes

Parasternal nodes

Inframammary nodes

I.c. – Infraclavicular
Ax –Axillary
Bv – Basilic vein
C.v. – Cephalic vein
F.v. – Femoral vein
S.c. – Supraclavicular nodes
C.n. – Cubital nodes
P.n. – Pelvic nodes

S.c.
I.c.
C.v.
Ax.
B.v.
C.n.
P.n.
G.s.

Superficial inguinal nodes

F.v.
G.s.

G.s. – Great saphenous vein
F.v. – Femoral vein

Topography of the thoracic duct
1. Left lumbar trunk; 2. Right lumbar trunk; 3. Cisterna chyli; 4. Thoracic duct (thoracic part); 5. Thoracic duct (cervical part); 6. Esophagus; 7. Trachea; 8. L. venous angle; 9. R. venous angle; 10. Aorta; 11. Diaphragm; 12. Right lymphatic duct; 13. Inferior vena cava; 14. Superior vena cava; 15. Intercostal veins

Popliteal a.
Popliteal v.
Tibial n.
Lymph nodes
Lesser saphenous vein

Figure 1–7 Lymphatic system: overview.

chyli (Figs. 1–7, 1–8). Chylous lymph fluid from the digestive system is mixed with the transparent lymph fluid from various other tissues (described in Superfical Layer and Deep Layer, later) in the cisterna chyli. The location of this saclike reservoir varies but is usually between the vertebral levels T11 and L2 (anterior); it is between 3 and 8 cm long, and its width varies between 0.5 and 1.5 cm.

◆ **Thoracic Duct.** The thoracic duct originates together with the cisterna chyli and represents the largest lymph trunk in the body. The length varies between 36 and 45 cm, its width between 1 and 5 mm. Its origin is located between the peritoneum and the vertebral column and varies, as with the cisterna chyli, between T11 and L2 (Figs. 1–7, 1–8). On its way to the venous angle, the thoracic duct perforates the diaphragm together with the aorta at the aortic hiatus and runs in the posterior mediastinum in the cranial direction. In the majority of cases, the thoracic duct empties the lymph fluid (average 3 L per day, representing approximately three fourths of the total body lymph fluid) into the left venous angle. The left venous angle is composed of the left internal jugular and left subclavian vein (Fig. 1–7). Valves at the junction between the venous angle and the thoracic duct prevent reflux of venous blood into the lymphatic system.

◆ **Right Lymphatic Duct.** This 1- to 1.5-cm-long trunk is generally formed by the confluence of the right jugular, supraclavicular, subclavian, and parasternal trunks and connects with the venous system in the area of the right venous angle (formed by the right internal jugular and subclavian veins). Approximately one fourth of the lymph fluid passing through the body in the course of a day returns to the venous system via the right lymphatic duct (Figs. 1–7, 1–8).
  The jugular, supraclavicular, subclavian, and parasternal trunks are bilateral and located in the upper half of the body. They connect either separately or together with the thoracic duct or the right lymphatic duct with the respective venous angle (additional trunks in that area, which are not primarily relevant to the management of lymphedema, are omitted).

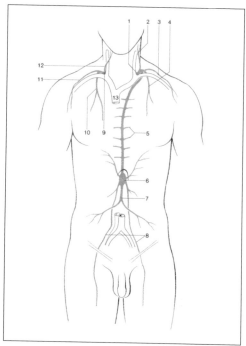

Figure 1–8 Lymphatic trunks. 1. Thoracic duct; 2. Left jugular trunk; 3. Left subclavian trunk; 4. Left bronchomediastinal trunk; 5. Intercostal lymph collectors; 6. Cisterna chyli; 7. Gastrointestinal trunk; 8. Lumbar trunks; 9. Right lymphatic duct; 10. Right bronchomediastinal trunk; 11. Right subclavian trunk; 12. Right jugular trunk; 13. Vena cava.

◆ **Jugular Trunk.** The jugular trunk is formed by the confluence of the efferent lymph vessels coming from the internal jugular lymph nodes, which filter the lymph originating in the head and neck (Figs. 1–8, 1–9).

◆ **Supraclavicular Trunk.** The supraclavicular trunk is formed by efferent lymph vessels of the supraclavicular lymph nodes, which filter the lymph coming from the head and neck areas, the shoulder region, and parts of the mammary gland (Fig. 1–9).

◆ **Subclavian Trunk.** This trunk (~3 cm long) drains the lymph originating from the axillary lymph nodes, which are responsible for filtering lymph from the upper extremities, the upper quadrants (anterior and posterior), the majority of the mammary gland, and the shoulder region (Figs. 1–8, 1–9).

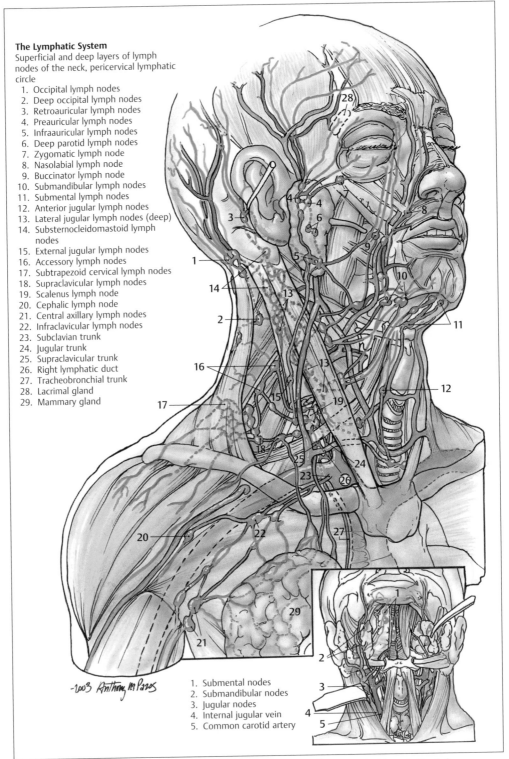

The Lymphatic System
Superficial and deep layers of lymph
nodes of the neck, pericervical lymphatic
circle
1. Occipital lymph nodes
2. Deep occipital lymph nodes
3. Retroauricular lymph nodes
4. Preauricular lymph nodes
5. Infraauricular lymph nodes
6. Deep parotid lymph nodes
7. Zygomatic lymph node
8. Nasolabial lymph node
9. Buccinator lymph node
10. Submandibular lymph nodes
11. Submental lymph nodes
12. Anterior jugular lymph nodes
13. Lateral jugular lymph nodes (deep)
14. Substernocleidomastoid lymph
    nodes
15. External jugular lymph nodes
16. Accessory lymph nodes
17. Subtrapezoid cervical lymph nodes
18. Supraclavicular lymph nodes
19. Scalenus lymph node
20. Cephalic lymph node
21. Central axillary lymph nodes
22. Infraclavicular lymph nodes
23. Subclavian trunk
24. Jugular trunk
25. Supraclavicular trunk
26. Right lymphatic duct
27. Tracheobronchial trunk
28. Lacrimal gland
29. Mammary gland

1. Submental nodes
2. Submandibular nodes
3. Jugular nodes
4. Internal jugular vein
5. Common carotid artery

–2003 Anthony M Pazos

Figure 1–9 Superficial and deep layers of lymph nodes on the neck; pericervical lymphatic circle.

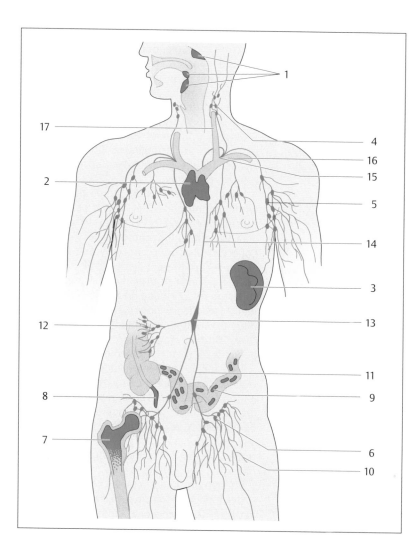

Figure 1–10 Lymphatic tissue, lymph vessels, and regional lymph nodes. 1. Tonsils; 2. Thymus; 3. Spleen; 4. Cervical nodes; 5. Axillary nodes; 6. Inguinal nodes; 7. Bone marrow; 8. Appendix; 9. Peyer's patches in the intestinal system; 10. Afferent lymph collectors to the inguinal nodes; 11. Lumbar trunks; 12. Intestinal nodes; 13. Cisterna chyli; 14. Thoracic duct; 15. Left venous angle; 16. Subclavian vein; 17. Internal jugular vein.

◆ **Parasternal Trunk.** Coming from the parasternal lymph nodes, this trunk drains part of the mammary gland as well as parts of the pleura, diaphragm, liver, pericardium, and striated musculature in the chest and abdominal areas (see Drainage of the Mammary Gland later in this chapter).

Lymphatic Tissues

Lymphatic tissue is made up of a framework of reticular fibers, which are produced by reticular cells. Lymphatic tissue may be found either as scattered foci of cells, as dense nodules within connective tissue (especially in the intestines as tonsils or Peyer's patches), or as ag-

gregations of lymphoid cells enclosed within a capsule such as the lymph nodes, spleen, and thymus (Fig. 1–10). Generally, it can be said that lymphatic tissues are dedicated to produce and distribute lymphocytes.

Lymph Nodes

Lymph nodes have three main functions.

◆ **Protective Function.** Lymph nodes serve as filters for harmful material (e.g., cancer cells, pathogens, dust, and dirt) in the lymph fluid.

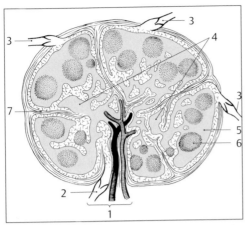

Figure 1–11 Cross section of a lymph node. 1. Hilus area (blood vessels enter and blood and lymph vessels leave the lymph node); 2. Efferent lymph collector from lymph node; 3. Afferent lymph collector to lymph node perforating the capsular area; 4. Lymphoreticular tissue between the outer layer of the lymph node and the hilus; 5. Sinus system; 6. Lymphatic follicles; 7. Trabeculae.

◆ **Immune Function.** Lymph nodes are responsible for the production of antigen-stimulated lymphocytes (antibodies). Lymphocytes are white blood cells, which circulate in the blood and the lymphatic system. They harbor in the lymph nodes and spleen and are part of the immune system responsible for both directly (T cells and macrophages) and indirectly (B cells producing antibodies) attacking foreign invaders. The antibodies produced in the lymph nodes leave via efferent lymph collectors and travel within the lymph fluid to the blood for distribution throughout the body. The number of lymphocytes in efferent lymph vessels is greater than in afferent vessels.

◆ **Thickening of the Lymph Fluid.** Blood capillaries inside the lymph nodes reabsorb a large portion of the water content in the lymph fluid, thereby reducing the amount of lymph returning via the thoracic duct (and the right lymphatic duct) into the venous system.

The number of these round, kidney-, or bean-shaped encapsulated lymphatic organs in an average human varies between 600 and 700, with most of the nodes located strategically in the intestines and the head-neck areas (place of entry for pathogens).

Their size in adults varies between 0.2 and 0.3 cm. The shape, number, and size of lymph nodes depend on factors such as age, sex, and constitution. A set number of lymph nodes is present at birth; although lymph nodes increase and decrease in size during the course of life, they do not regenerate or vanish.

Most lymph nodes are embedded in fatty tissue and are arranged in either groups or chains. Their capsular area consists of dense connective tissue.

Lymph fluid enters the lymph nodes via afferent lymph collectors, which perforate the capsular area, and leaves the nodes at the hilus area via efferent lymph collectors (Fig. 1–11). Collectors also interconnect lymph nodes; for example, an efferent lymph collector of one node may also represent an afferent lymph collector for the node situated further proximally (secondary node). To ensure sufficient filter function, lymph fluid will pass in most cases through more than one lymph node before it reenters the blood circulation.

The inside of lymph nodes consists of trabeculae, which compartmentalize the lymph node lumen. Those trabeculae originating at the hilus area contain the intranodal blood vessels. A large number of lymphocytes and macrophages are located between the trabeculae and are connected by a loose net of fibers.

The lymph fluid circulates within the sinus system, which is located between the capsular area, the trabeculae, and the clusters of defense cells. Upon entering the intranodal sinus system via afferent lymph collectors, the lymph flow is considerably slower than in collectors, which enables macrophages to better identify and phagocytose harmful substances.

In many cases, regional lymph nodes represent the first line of defense in the lymph transport. The drainage or tributary area of a group of regional lymph nodes may include several lymphatic territories. For example, the tributary area for the lymph nodes located in the groin (inguinal lymph nodes) consists of the lower extremities, gluteal area, external genitalia (skin), perineum, and lower body quadrants (abdominal and lumbar areas).

◆ Lymphatic Watersheds

Watersheds represent linear areas on the skin that separate territories from each other and contain relatively few lymph collectors (Figs. 1–12, 1–13). Although collectors within the same territory anastomose frequently, connections between collectors of adjacent territories are much less frequent.

Watersheds located on the trunk and between the trunk and extremities are discussed in the following section.

Sagittal Watershed

The sagittal watershed, also referred to as the median watershed, connects the vertex with the perineum (anterior and posterior). It divides the lymphatic drainage of the head, neck, trunk, and external genitalia into equal halves.

Horizontal Watershed

The upper horizontal watershed separates the neck and shoulder territory from the territories of the arm and thorax. It forms a line from the jugular notch (manubrium), running laterally to the acromion, and continues posterior to the vertebral levels between C7 and T2.

The lower horizontal (or transverse) watershed starts at the umbilicus and follows the caudal limitation of the rib cage to the vertebral column. This watershed separates the upper from the lower territories on the trunk.

The sagittal and horizontal watersheds create four territories on the trunk; these territories are also known as quadrants (see also Lymphatic Drainage of the Trunk later in this chapter).

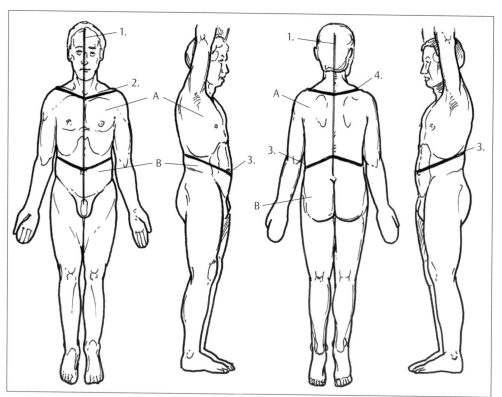

Figure 1–12 Lymphatic watersheds. 1. Sagittal (median) watershed (anterior and posterior); 2. Upper horizontal watershed (anterior); 3. Horizontal (transverse) watershed (anterior and posterior); 4. Upper horizontal watershed (posterior): A. Upper quadrants (anterior and posterior); B. Lower quadrants (anterior and posterior).

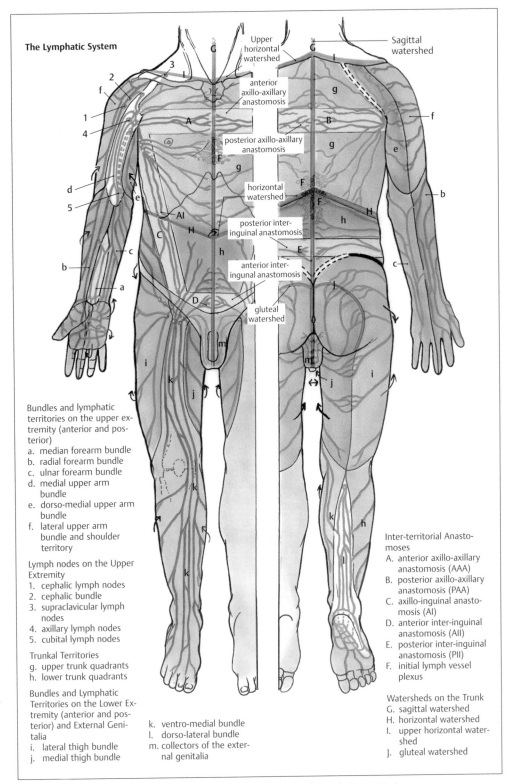

The Lymphatic System

Upper horizontal watershed

Sagittal watershed

anterior axillo-axillary anastomosis

posterior axillo-axillary anastomosis

horizontal watershed

posterior inter-inguinal anastomosis

anterior inter-inguinal anastomosis

gluteal watershed

Bundles and lymphatic territories on the upper extremity (anterior and posterior)
a. median forearm bundle
b. radial forearm bundle
c. ulnar forearm bundle
d. medial upper arm bundle
e. dorso-medial upper arm bundle
f. lateral upper arm bundle and shoulder territory

Lymph nodes on the Upper Extremity
1. cephalic lymph nodes
2. cephalic bundle
3. supraclavicular lymph nodes
4. axillary lymph nodes
5. cubital lymph nodes

Trunkal Territories
g. upper trunk quadrants
h. lower trunk quadrants

Bundles and Lymphatic Territories on the Lower Extremity (anterior and posterior) and External Genitalia
i. lateral thigh bundle
j. medial thigh bundle
k. ventro-medial bundle
l. dorso-lateral bundle
m. collectors of the external genitalia

Inter-territorial Anastomoses
A. anterior axillo-axillary anastomosis (AAA)
B. posterior axillo-axillary anastomosis (PAA)
C. axillo-inguinal anastomosis (AI)
D. anterior inter-inguinal anastomosis (AII)
E. posterior inter-inguinal anastomosis (PII)
F. initial lymph vessel plexus

Watersheds on the Trunk
G. sagittal watershed
H. horizontal watershed
I. upper horizontal watershed
J. gluteal watershed

Figure 1–13 Lymphatic watersheds, lymphatic anastomoses, and lymphatic territories.

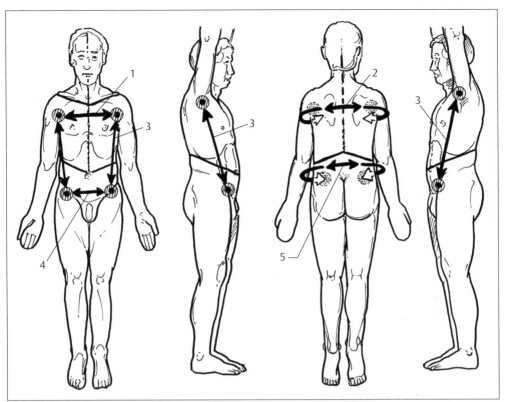

Figure 1–14 Lymphatic anastomoses. 1. Anterior axillo-axillary (AAA) anastomosis; 2. Posterior axillo-axillary (PAA) anastomosis; 3. Axillo-inguinal (AI) anastomosis, also known as inguinal-axillary (IA) anastomosis; 4. Anterior inter-inguinal (AII) anastomosis; 5. Posterior inter-inguinal (PII) anastomosis.

Watersheds between the Trunk and the Extremities

The watershed separating the lower extremities from the trunk (inguinal watershed) starts at the pubic symphysis and follows the iliac crest to the apex of the sacrum. A line starting at the coracoid process traveling along the axillary fold, then continuing posterior to roughly the midpoint of the spine of the scapula, separates the arm from the trunk (axillary watershed).

The location and direction of the valves inside lymph collectors inhibit the flow of lymph between adjacent territories under normal conditions. Some lymph fluid may cross the watershed via lymph capillaries (initial lymphatic plexus).

In case of lymph stasis, lymph fluid is able to move against the normal flow, over the watershed, and through alternative routes:

◆ Dilated capillaries of the initial lymph vessel plexus (Fig. 1–13). Congested lymph fluid causes the lymphatics in the affected area to dilate. The subsequent greater resistance in these dilated collectors and precollectors forces the lymph back into the lymph capillaries (dermal backflow) and across the watershed.

◆ Abnormal dilation of lymph collectors may eventually result in valvular insufficiency. The valvular insufficiency leads to a retrograde flow of lymph from the congested territory to an adjacent territory free from edema. These pathways are known as *interterritorial anastomoses* (Figs. 1–13, 1–14).

◆ Interterritorial Anastomoses

If normal lymph flow within a territory is interrupted, activation of interterritorial anastomoses may prevent the onset of swelling as part of the body's own avoidance mechanisms to lymph stasis (see also Chapter 3, Avoidance Mechanisms). If swelling is present, accumulated lymph fluid can be re-routed manually by use of these anastomoses. For example, if lymphedema is present in the right upper extremity, the axillo-axillary anastomoses on the anterior and posterior thorax as well as the axillo-inguinal anastomosis on the right side can be utilized to reroute lymph fluid into adjacent tributary areas. (Refer to Chapter 5 for a more in-depth discussion of anastomoses in the treatment of lymphedema.)

Lymph collectors on the trunk generally originate at the watersheds and run in a straight line toward their regional lymph nodes. Some of these collectors originate "in line" or horizontal to the collectors of an adjacent territory. These collectors seem to anastomose more frequently than others in the same territory.

◆ **Anterior Axillo-Axillary (AAA) Anastomosis.** This connection is found between the right and left upper quadrants. Collectors of this anastomosis create a connection between the contralateral axillary lymph node groups on the anterior side of the trunk.

◆ **Posterior Axillo-Axillary (PAA) Anastomosis.** This is the connection between the contralateral axillary lymph nodes on the posterior side of the upper quadrants.

◆ **Axillo-Inguinal (AI) Anastomosis.** In axilloinguinal anastomosis, also known as inguinal axillary (IA) anastomosis. Collectors of the ipsilateral upper and lower quadrants connect and form a connection between the axillary and inguinal lymph node groups of the same sides.

◆ **Anterior Inter-Inguinal (AII) Anastomosis.** This anastomosis is located over the mons pubis area and connects the contralateral inguinal lymph nodes on the anterior lower body quadrants.

◆ **Posterior Inter-Inguinal (PII) Anastomosis.** Collectors forming this anastomosis are found on the sacrum and connect the contralateral inguinal lymph node groups on the posterior lower body quadrants.

◆ Lymphatic Drainage and Regional Lymph Node Groups of Different Body Parts

Lymphedema manifests itself almost exclusively in the skin and subcutis. This section concentrates on the superficial lymphatic system in different body sections and will only occasionally remark on the lymphatic drainage of the deep lymphatic and organ systems (Table 1–1). In the discussion that follows, the number of lymph nodes is noted in parentheses.

Lymphatic Drainage of the Scalp, Face, and Neck

◆ **Scalp and Face.** Most of the collectors in this area drain toward lymph nodes that are arranged in a circular pattern along the head-neck border. Most of the efferent collectors of the circle pass to the deep cervical lymph nodes (see Lateral Group later in this chapter). The following regional lymph nodes are collectively referred to as the *pericervical lymphatic circle.*

◆ **Submental Lymph Nodes (2–3)**

Location: beneath the platysma, embedded in fatty tissue between the anterior bellies of the digastric muscles (Figs. 1–9, 1–15, 1–16)

Tributaries: central portion of the lower lip and the chin

◆ **Submandibular Lymph Nodes (3–6)**

Location: the superficial surface of the submandibular saliva gland behind the mandible (Figs. 1–9, 1–15, 1–16)

Tributaries: medial portion of the lower lid, cheek, nose, upper lid, and lateral part of the lower lip and chin

Table 1–1 Tributaries and Efferent Drainage of Regional Lymph Nodes

	Lymph Nodes	Superficial Tributaries (Skin)	Efferent Vessels
1	Submental	Central portion of the lower lip; chin and cheek	to 6 → VA
2	Submandibular	Medial portion of the lower lid; cheek; nose; upper lid; lateral part of lower lip and chin	to 6 → VA
3	Parotid	Temporoparietal of scalp; forehead; upper lid; lateral part of lower lid; anterior auricle	to 6 → VA
4	Posterior auricular	Parietal portion of scalp; posterior auricle	to 6 and 7 → VA
5	Occipital	Occipital portion of scalp, upper part of neck	to 7 → VA
6	Internal jugular	Receives lymph fluid from 1 to 5	Jugular trunk → VA
7	Accessory	Receives lymph fluid from 4 and 5	8 → VA
8	Supraclavicular	Receives lymph fluid from 7 and intercostal lymph nodes; skin of anterolateral neck; portions of lateral upper arm; portions of mammary gland	Supraclavicular trunk → VA
9	Parasternal	Mammary gland (~25%)	Parasternal trunk → VA
10	Axillary	Upper extremity; mammary gland (~75%); upper quadrants (anterior/posterior)	Subclavian trunk → VA
11	Inguinal	Skin of penis and scrotum; lower vagina; perineum; anus; buttocks; lower quadrants (anterior/posterior)	Pelvic lymph nodes → Lumbar lymph nodes → Lumbar trunk → Cisterna chyli → Thoracic duct → VA

VA, venous angle.

◆ **Parotid Lymph Nodes**

(~8 in the deep and 9 in the superficial group; number varies greatly in the literature)

Location: the superficial group is embedded in the subcutaneous fatty tissue around the parotid gland and directly anterior of the ear; the deep group is embedded in the parotid gland (Figs. 1–9, 1–15).

Tributaries: temporoparietal scalp, forehead, upper eyelid, lateral portion of the lower eyelid, and skin of the anterior auricle

◆ **Posterior Auricular Lymph Nodes (2–3)**

Location: at the mastoid insertion of the sternocleidomastoid muscle, beneath the auricularis posterior muscle (Figs. 1–9, 1–15)

Tributaries: parietal portion of the scalp and posterior auricle

◆ **Occipital Lymph Nodes (1–3)**

Location: insertion of the semispinalis capitis muscle (Figs. 1–9, 1–15)

Tributaries: occipital portion of the scalp and the upper part of the skin on the neck

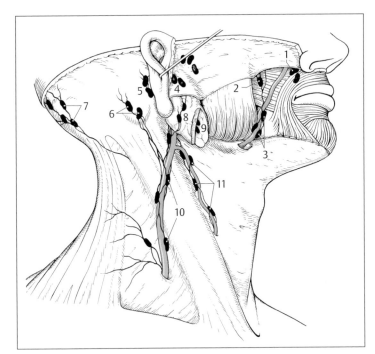

Figure 1–15 Superficial lymph nodes of the neck and head. 1. Nasolabial node (below the nasolabial fold); 2. Buccinator node (deep within the buccinator muscle); 3. Mandibular nodes (located on the mandible); 4. Parotid nodes (preauricular); 5. Infra-auricular nodes (posterior auricular); 6. Mastoid nodes (posterior auricular); 7. Occipital nodes; 8. Deep parotid nodes (beneath the parotid fascia); 9. Intraglandular nodes (embedded within the parotid gland); 10. Lateral superficial nodes (external jugular lymph nodes); 11. Anterior superficial nodes (anterior jugular lymph nodes).

Lymphatic Drainage of the Neck

An anterior and lateral group of lymph nodes can be differentiated in the neck region. These groups are further divided into deep and superficial nodes.

Anterior Group

The nodes belonging to this group are irregular and inconsistent. The superficial nodes (anterior jugular lymph nodes) are grouped around the anterior jugular vein; its tributary areas include portions of the skin and musculature of the anterior neck (Fig. 1–15).

The deep nodes of this group are arranged anterior and lateral to the larynx, the trachea, and the thyroid gland. This deeper set drains the lower part of the larynx, the thyroid gland, and the upper part of the trachea. The efferent collectors of the superficial and deep group drain into the deep cervical lymph nodes, which are part of the lateral group (Figs. 1–9, 1–16).

Lateral Group

The nodes belonging to the superficial portion (external jugular lymph nodes) are grouped along the exterior jugular vein between the parotid gland and the supraclavicular lymph nodes. The deep portion of this group is embedded in fatty tissue, which extends from the base of the skull to the venous angle area. The nodes form chains and follow the borders of the lateral neck triangle, which is outlined by the sternocleidomastoid (anterior), the upper trapezius (posterior) muscles, and the clavicle (inferior). Numerous connections are present between the chains of the deep lateral lymph node chains (Figs. 1–9, 1–16).

◆ **Internal Jugular Lymph Nodes (10–20)**

Location: posterior to the sternocleidomastoid muscle and along the internal jugular vein

Tributaries: scalp and face (pericervical lymphatic circle), nasal cavities, palate (hard and soft), tongue, tonsils, auris media, pharynx, and larynx (including vocal cords)

The efferent vessels converge into the jugular trunk (see Lymphatic Trunks previously in this

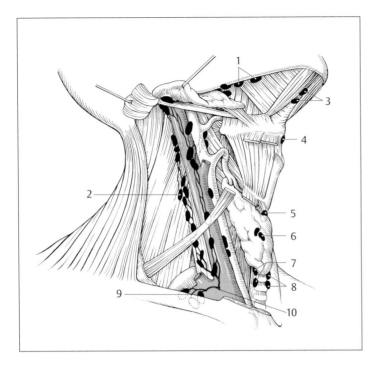

Figure 1–16 Deep lymph nodes of the neck and head. 1. Submandibular nodes; 2. Internal jugular nodes; 3. Submental nodes; 4. Infrahyoid nodes; 5. Prelaryngeal nodes; 6. Thyroid nodes; 7. Paratracheal nodes; 8. Pretracheal nodes; 9. Supraclavicular nodes; 10. Right venous angle.

chapter), which connects to the venous angle either directly or via the thoracic duct, or to the right lymphatic duct, respectively (Figs. 1–9, 1–16).

◆ Accessory Lymph Nodes (5–20)

Location: along the upper trapezius and anterior to the accessory nerve

Tributaries: receive lymph fluid from the occipital and posterior auricular lymph nodes

Additional tributaries: occipital portion of the scalp, skin of the lateral neck, and portions of the neck musculature

The efferent vessels from the accessory lymph nodes connect with the supraclavicular lymph nodes (Fig. 1–9).

◆ Supraclavicular Lymph Nodes (4–12)

Location: between the inferior belly of the omohyoid muscle and the sternohyoid muscle (venous angle area), behind the clavicle

Tributaries: transport lymph coming from the accessory lymph nodes

Additional tributaries: skin of the anterolateral neck, intercostal lymph nodes, lateral upper arm, and portions of the glandular tissue of the breast

Efferent vessels from the supraclavicular nodes converge into the supraclavicular trunk (see Lymphatic Trunks previously in this chapter), which connects to the venous angle either directly or via the thoracic duct or right lymphatic duct, respectively (Fig. 1–9).

> The proximity and possible connections of the supraclavicular trunk with the thoracic duct and other trunks terminating in the venous angle area explain why metastatic tumors from the mammary gland, lung, and esophagus, as well as from reproductive and intestinal organs, can be found in the supraclavicular lymph nodes.

Lymphatic Drainage of the Trunk

Four territories or quadrants can be differentiated on the trunk (Figs. 1–12, 1–13). The upper territories (anterior and posterior) are

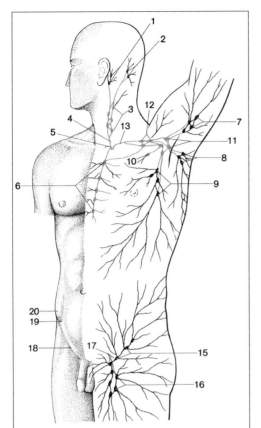

Figure 1–17 Lymphatic drainage of the trunk. 1. Mastoid nodes; 2. Occipital nodes; 3. Deep cervical nodes; 4. Jugular trunk; 5. Thoracic duct; 6. Parasternal nodes; 7. Lateral (infraclavicular) group of axillary nodes; 8. Posterior (subscapular) group of axillary nodes; 9. Anterior (pectoral) group of axillary nodes; 10. Interpectoral axillary nodes; 11. Central axillary nodes; 12. Apical axillary nodes; 13. Subclavian trunk; 15. Inguinal nodes (horizontal group); 16. Inguinal nodes (vertical group); 17. Lymph drainage via deep inguinal nodes to pelvic nodes; 18. Inguinal ligament; 19. Origin of sartorius muscle; 20. Antero-superior iliac spine.

located between the upper and lower horizontal watersheds (see separate section in this chapter) and the axillary watershed, which separates the trunk from the upper extremity (see Watersheds between the Trunk and the Extremities previously in this chapter). Regional lymph nodes for the upper territories are the axillary lymph nodes. The lower horizontal watershed and the watershed separating the lower extremity from the trunk outline

the lower territories (anterior and posterior); regional nodes are the inguinal lymph nodes. Upper and lower territories are separated by the sagittal watershed (see discussion earlier in this chapter) into right and left upper and lower quadrants.

The collectors of all four quadrants are arranged like spokes on a wheel, with the origin emanating from the watersheds and the center in the regional lymph node groups (Figs. 1–13, 1–17). Some of the collectors form connections with collectors of adjacent territories, allowing interterritorial lymph flow (see Interterritorial Anastomoses previously in this chapter).

The structure of the initial lymphatic system corresponds with the conditions described in Lymph Capillaries previously in this chapter. The initial lymph vessel plexus covers the entire surface of the anterior and posterior trunk, including the watershed areas (Fig. 1–13).

> Lymph fluid may use the plexus vessels to move from the extremities to the trunk, bypassing the regional lymph nodes, or to move between quadrants.

Drainage of the Mammary Gland

Regional lymph nodes: axillary (and indirectly supraclavicular) and parasternal nodes

◆ **Axillary Lymph Nodes (10–24)**

Location: In a triangular outline, where the apex is the axilla, the anterior border is the pectoralis minor and the posterior border the subscapularis muscle. Most nodes are embedded in fatty tissue; others are arranged around blood vessels (lateral thoracic and subscapular arteries, axillary vein) and nerves (subscapular nerve). Axillary nodes can be found in the epi- and subfascial systems and are divided into five groups (Figs. 1–7, 1–17, 1–18):

◆ Anterior (pectoral) group
◆ Posterior (subscapular) group
◆ Central group
◆ Lateral (infraclavicular) group
◆ Apical group

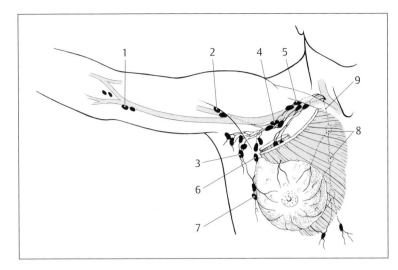

Figure 1–18
Drainage of the mammary gland. 1. Cubital nodes; 2. Lateral (infraclavicular) group of axillary nodes; 3. Posterior (subscapular) group of axillary nodes; 4. Central axillary nodes; 5. Apical axillary nodes; 6. Anterior (pectoral) group of axillary nodes; 7. Paramammary nodes (on the lateral margin of the mammary gland); 8. Parasternal nodes; 9. Parasternal trunk.

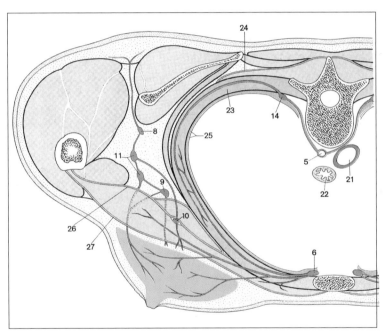

Figure 1–19
Drainage of the trunk wall and the mammary gland.
5. Thoracic duct; 6. Parasternal nodes; 8. Posterior (subscapular) group of axillary nodes; 9. Anterior (pectoral) group of axillary nodes; 10. Interpectoral group of axillary nodes; 11. Central axillary nodes; 14. Intercostal nodes; 21. Aorta; 22. Esophagus; 23. Deep layer of thoracic wall (ribs and intercostal musculature); 24. Thoracolumbar fascia; 25. Parietal pleura and endothoracic fascia; 26. Clavicopectoral fascia; 27. Pectoral fascia.

Tributaries: axillary lymph nodes receive lymph from the ipsilateral upper quadrant (anterior and posterior), the ipsilateral mammary gland (~75%). and the ipsilateral upper extremity.

The efferent vessels from the axillary lymph nodes converge into the subclavian trunk (see Lymphatic Trunks previously in this chapter), which connects to the venous angle area either directly or via the thoracic duct or right lymphatic duct, respectively.

◆ **Parasternal (Internal Mammary) Lymph Nodes (4–6)**

Location: at the anterior border of the intercostal spaces and parallel to the internal mammary artery (Figs. 1–17, 1–18, 1–19, 1–20)

Tributaries: mammary gland (~25%), parts of the liver and pleura, diaphragm, pericardium, and striated musculature in the chest and abdominal areas. The efferent vessels pass via

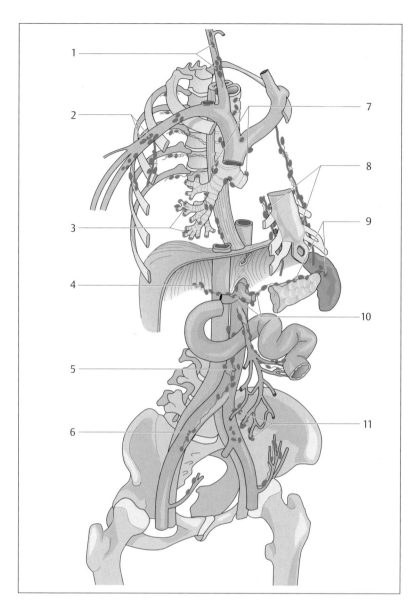

Figure 1–20
Regional lymph nodes of the trunk. 1. Deep cervical nodes; 2. Axillary nodes; 3. Bronchopulmonary nodes; 4. Hepatic nodes; 5. Common pelvic nodes; 6. Pelvic nodes; 7. Tracheobronchial nodes; 8. Parasternal nodes; 9. Nodes of the spleen and pancreas; 10. Colic (abdominal) nodes; 11. Mesenteric nodes (100–150).

the parasternal trunk to the venous angle area.

The lymphatic vessels of the mammary gland originate in a plexus in the interlobular spaces and on the walls of the lactiferous ducts. Those vessels from the central part of the glandular tissue pass to an intricate plexus situated beneath the areola. This plexus also receives the lymphatics from the skin over the central part of the mammary gland and those from the areola and nipple. About four efferent vessels leave this area and drain roughly three quarters (preferably the lateral quadrants) of the breast to the axillary nodes. The vessels draining the medial part of the mammary gland originate in the same intraglandular plexus and pierce the thoracic wall to connect with the parasternal lymph nodes, which drain approximately one third (preferably the medial quadrants) of the glandular tissue.

The intraglandular plexus interconnects all drainage areas of the breast. With this connection, the lateral quadrants may also drain into the parasternal nodes and the medial quadrants into the axillary lymph nodes.

Metastases in breast cancer are most often found in the central axillary lymph nodes.

Lymphatic Drainage of the Upper Extremity

Lymph vessels of the upper extremity are divided into a superficial and a deep layer. Connections between the two layers are found in both directions. In the area of the hand, the connection from deep to superficial dominates. Perforating precollectors (see earlier discussion in this chapter) create connections from superficial to deep in other areas of the arm.

The regional lymph nodes for both layers are the axillary lymph nodes.

Superficial Layer

The meshes of the initial lymph vessel plexus, which pervades the skin everywhere, are finer in the palm and the flexor aspects of the fingers. Territories on the upper extremity (and the lower extremity) are also referred to as *bundles* (Figs. 1–13, 1–21).

◆ **Collectors on the Hand**

A pair of collectors, which run on the sides of each digit (originating on the second digit) and incline backward to reach the dorsum of the hand, drains the digital plexuses. From the dense plexus of the palm, collectors traverse in different directions. Collectors belonging to the *mesothenar territory* drain the central palmar plexus and run on the volar side between the thenar and hypothenar eminence upward to form the medial forearm territory. The *radial hand territory* drains the radial border of the palm, the web space between the index and the thumb, and the thenar eminence. The *ulnar hand territory* drains the ulnar border of the palm, the hand, and the hypothenar eminence. Collectors belonging to the *descending hand territory* are responsible for the drainage of the web spaces as well as the adjacent skin covering the palmar metacarpophalangeal joints. The collectors belonging to the radial, ulnar, and descending territories pass around the hand to join the collectors on the dorsum of the hand, which are also responsible for the

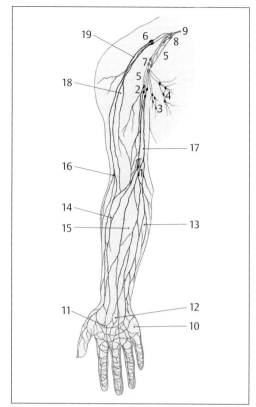

Figure 1–21 Drainage of the upper extremity. 1. Cubital nodes; 2. Lateral (infraclavicular) group of axillary nodes; 3. Posterior (subscapular) group of axillary nodes; 4. Anterior (pectoral) group of axillary nodes; 5. Plexus of lymph collectors in the axilla; 6. Deltoideopectoral nodes; 7. Central axillary nodes; 8. Apical axillary nodes; 9. Subclavian trunk; 10. Ulnar hand territory; 11. Radial hand territory; 12. Mesothenar territory; 13. Ulnar forearm territory; 14. Radial forearm territory; 15. Median forearm territory; 16. Connection between radial forearm territory and lateral upper arm territory ("long upper arm type"); 17. Medial upper arm territory; 18. Lateral upper arm territory; 19. Cephalic bundle.

drainage of lymphatic loads coming from the interphalangeal joints. From the dorsum of the hand, the lymph vessels pass the wrist to join the collectors of the forearm.

◆ **Collectors on the Forearm**

The 20 to 30 collectors in this area are subdivided into the radial, ulnar, and median territories. The *median forearm territory* represents a continuation of the mesothenar hand terri-

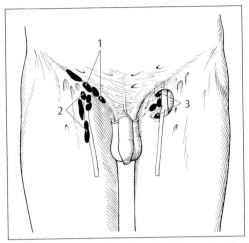

Figure 1–22 Inguinal lymph nodes. 1. Inguinal nodes, horizontal group (superficial); 2. Inguinal nodes, vertical group (superficial); 3. Deep inguinal nodes.

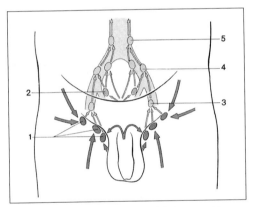

Figure 1–23 Inguinal nodes and drainage pathways. 1. Inguinal nodes (superficial); 2. Internal pelvic nodes; 3. Deep inguinal nodes; 4. Common pelvic nodes; 5. Lumbar nodes.

tory and is located on the anterior surface of the forearm. Collectors coming from the dorsum of the hand continue on the forearm with the *radial and ulnar forearm territories*, which accompany the cephalic and basilic veins, respectively. The collectors of both bundles conform around the forearm to converge together with the median territory in the antecubital area, where they decrease in number.

Antecubital lymph nodes, located adjacent to the basilic vein, may provide additional filter stations for the collectors of the ulnar territory. Antecubital lymph nodes vary in number.

Vessels belonging to the radial forearm territory occasionally ascend with the cephalic vein to the axillary or supraclavicular lymph node groups. Kubik describes this drainage pathway as the *long upper arm type* (present in 16% of the population), which may have an important function in the case of axillary lymph node dissection (e.g., individuals with long upper arm type may not develop secondary upper extremity lymphedema).

◆ Collectors on the Upper Arm

The collectors coming from the forearm continue to travel to the axillary lymph node group along the *medial upper arm territory*, which is located between the biceps and the triceps muscles on the medial upper arm. Collectors of this territory also drain the skin on the dorsomedial upper arm and shoulder.

The lateral upper arm territory is responsible for the drainage of the skin on the dorsolateral upper arm and shoulder. Its collectors drain partly into axillary and supraclavicular lymph nodes. The vessels passing to the supraclavicular nodes generally accompany the cephalic vein along the infraclavicular fossa. This pathway is also described as the *cephalic bundle*, which may contain a varying number of lymph nodes (deltoideopectoral nodes).

Deep Layer

Subfascial tissues (except metacarpophalangeal and interdigital joints) drain via the deep lymphatic system; its vessels accompany the deep blood vessels. In the forearm, they consist of four sets, corresponding with the radial, ulnar, volar, and dorsal interosseous arteries. On the upper arm, the collectors generally follow the brachial artery and transport the lymph fluid toward the axillary lymph nodes.

Lymphatic Drainage of the Lower Extremity

As with the arm, the lymph vessels on the lower extremity are divided into a superficial and deep layer with the exception of the toes. The fascia between the subcutis and the muscle layer is absent in toes; a distinction between the two layers is therefore not possible.

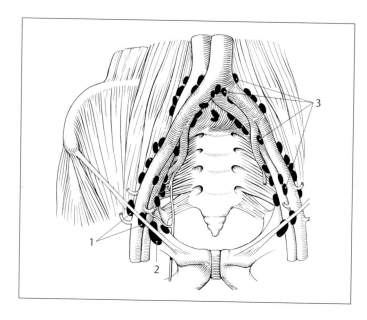

Both layers communicate via perforating precollectors. There are also connections between the superficial and deep layers of the inguinal lymph nodes (Figs. 1–7, 1–22, 1–23).

Superficial Layer

◆ **Superficial Inguinal Lymph Nodes (6–12)**

Location: grouped around the great saphenous vein and embedded in fatty tissue, these nodes are found in the upper part of the medial femoral triangle (outlined by the inguinal ligament, sartorius muscle, and adductors) and can be divided into two groups. The nodes belonging to the horizontal group are arranged as a chain situated immediately below the inguinal ligament. The nodes arranged around the saphenous perforation belong to the vertical group (Figs. 1–7, 1–22).

Tributaries: the horizontal group receives lymph fluid from the integument of the penis, scrotum, lower part of the vagina, perineum, anus, buttock, and anterior and posterior trunkal wall below the level of the umbilicus (lower quadrant). The vertical group is chiefly responsible for the superficial lymphatic vessels of the lower extremity; they also receive some of the vessels that drain the integument of the penis, scrotum, vagina, perineum, and buttock.

The efferent vessels perforate the fascia below the inguinal ligament, and most of the collectors follow the pelvic artery to connect with the pelvic lymph nodes (Figs. 1–7, 1–23, 1–24). From there the lymph fluid continues to pass through the lumbar lymph nodes (located along the vertebral levels L5–L1) and the lumbar trunks to reach the cisterna chyli and the thoracic duct (Figs. 1–7, 1–25).

◆ **Collectors on the Foot**

The meshes of the initial lymph vessel plexus, which pervades the skin everywhere, are finer on the sole of the foot and the flexor aspects of the toes. Collectors on the dorsum of the foot drain the majority of the sole, the toes, and the medial malleolus area and pass the ankle on the anterior and medial side to continue as part of the ventromedial territory on the lower leg. Collectors draining the lateral malleolus and the lateral and posterior border of the foot (including portions of the lateral sole) continue as collectors belonging to the dorsolateral territory on the leg in the proximal direction (Figs. 1–13, 1–26).

◆ **Collectors of the Lower Leg and Knee**

Two territories can be distinguished on the lower leg. The *ventromedial territory* drains the majority of the foot (continuation of the collectors coming from the dorsum of the foot and

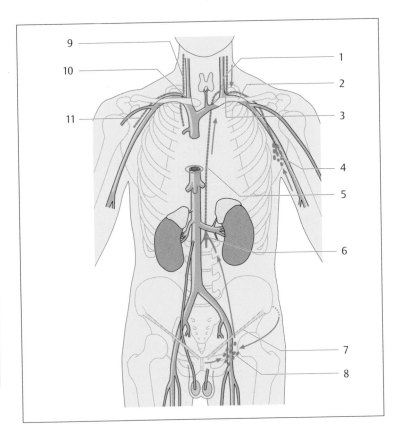

Figure 1–25 Lymphatic pathways. 1. Internal jugular vein; 2. Subclavian vein; 3. Left venous angle; 4. Axillary nodes; 5. Thoracic duct; 6. Cisterna chyli; 7. Inguinal ligament; 8. Inguinal nodes; 9. Jugular trunk; 10. Right venous angle; 11. Subclavian trunk.

the medial malleolus) as well as the skin of the lower leg, except an area of skin in the middle of the calf. Collectors of the ventromedial group are larger and more numerous than those belonging to the *dorsolateral territory*. Collectors of the dorsolateral group commence on the lateral and posterior border of the foot, drain the portion of skin located in the middle of the calf, and follow the small saphenous vein to the superficial popliteal lymph nodes. From the superficial popliteal lymph nodes, the lymph continues to the deep popliteal lymph nodes and from there, following subfascial collectors, to the deep inguinal lymph nodes (Figs. 1–7, 1–13, 1–27).

Collectors of the ventromedial territory run up the leg with the great saphenous vein and pass with it behind the medial condyle of the femur to the thigh (Figs. 1–13, 1–26, 1–28, 1–29). The vessels decrease in number below the medial knee to an average of 4 to 6 collectors (from 5 to 10 on the lower leg). Surgical interventions on the knee, especially incisions

on the medial aspect of the knee, may lead to more serious postoperative swelling involving tissues distal to this joint.

◆ Collectors on the Thigh

The vessels belonging to the ventromedial territory continue to follow the great saphenous vein to the superficial inguinal lymph nodes. The lateral thigh territory drains the skin of the lateral thigh and the lateral buttock. The medial thigh territory is responsible for the medial thigh, the medial buttock, and the perineum. A watershed running through the middle of the buttocks and the posterior thigh to the popliteal fossa separates both territories (gluteal watershed; Fig. 1–13).

Deep Layer

The deep lymphatic system in the lower extremities drains musculature, tendons, ligaments, and joint structures. The deep vessels

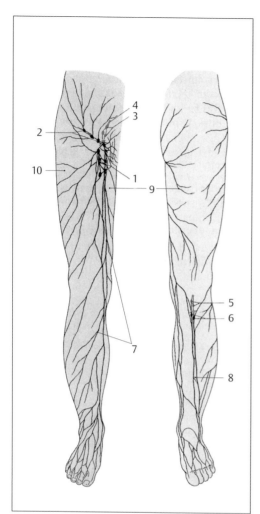

Figure 1–26 Drainage of the lower extremity. 1. Inguinal nodes (superficial), vertical group; 2. Inguinal nodes (superficial), horizontal group; 3. Deep inguinal nodes; 4. Deep collectors draining toward the pelvic nodes; 5. Deep popliteal nodes; 6. Superficial popliteal nodes; 7. Ventromedial territory on the thigh; 8. Dorsolateral territory on the thigh; 9. Medial thigh territory; 10. Lateral thigh territory.

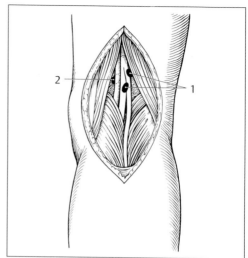

Figure 1–27 Popliteal nodes. 1. Superficial popliteal nodes; 2. Deep popliteal nodes.

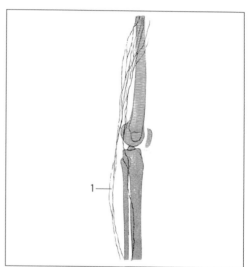

Figure 1–28 Ventromedial territory on the lower extremity. 1. Collectors of the ventromedial territory passing the knee behind the medial femur condyle.

below the knee consist of three sets, the anterior and posterior tibial and the peroneal, which accompany the corresponding blood vessels. All three transport the lymph to the deep popliteal lymph nodes.

The deep collectors on the thigh tend to follow the deep femoral artery and run toward the deep inguinal lymph nodes. Collectors in the gluteal area follow the gluteal artery and transport the lymph fluid to the pelvic lymph nodes.

◆ **Deep Popliteal Lymph Nodes (4–6)**

Location: embedded in the fat contained in the popliteal fossa (Figs. 1–7, 1–27)

Tributaries: portions of the skin drained by collectors belonging to the dorsolateral bundle

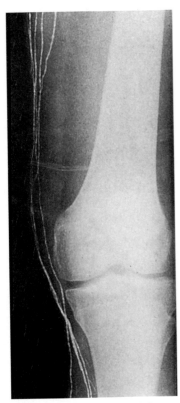

Figure 1–29 Radiograph of the ventromedial territory.

(superficial popliteal nodes drain into the deep popliteal lymph nodes); muscle and tendon tissue of the feet, lower legs, and distal part of posterior thigh; posterior portions of the ankle and knee joints

The efferent vessels of the deep popliteal lymph nodes pass through the adductor hiatus and follow the femoral artery to the deep inguinal lymph nodes.

◆ **Deep Inguinal Lymph Nodes (1–3)**

Location: below the fascia on the medial side of the femoral vein. If three nodes are present, the most inferior node is situated below the junction of the great saphenous and femoral veins, the middle in the femoral canal, and the superior node in the lateral part of the femoral ring. The upper lymph node is also known as the lymph node of Cloquet or Rosenmüller (Fig. 1–22, 1–24).

Tributaries: deep inguinal nodes receive the lymph transported by the deep lymph collectors accompanying the femoral artery, lymph fluid from the glans and corpus penis, and the outer layer of the clitoris. Lymph fluid previously filtered by the superficial inguinal lymph nodes also passes through the deep group.

Recommended Reading

1. Bates DO, Levick JR, Mortimer PS. Change in macromolecular composition of interstitial fluid from swollen arms after breast cancer treatment, and its implications. Clin Sci (Lond) 1993;85(6):737–746
2. Földi E, Földi M, Clodius L. The lymphedema chaos: a lancet. Ann Plast Surg 1988;22:505–515
3. Földi M, Földi E. Das Lymphoedem. Germany: Gustav Fischer Verlag; 1991
4. Földi M, Kubik S. Lehrbuch der Lymphologie. Germany: Gustav Fischer Verlag; 1999
5. Guyton AC. The lymphatic system, interstitial fluid dynamics, edema, and pulmonary fluid. In: Guyton AC. Textbook of Medical Physiology. 7th ed. Philadelphia: WB Saunders; 1986:361–373
6. Clodius L, Foeldi M. Therapy for lymphedema today. Inter Angio 1984;3
7. Olszewski W. Peripheral Lymph: Formation and Immune Function. Boca Raton, FL: CRC Press; 1985
8. Tortora GJ, Grabowski S. Principles of Anatomy and Physiology. 7th ed. New York: HarperCollins College; 1993
9. Weissleder H, Schuchardt C. Lymphedema, Diagnosis and Therapy. 3rd ed. Koln, Germany: Viavital-Verlag; 2001
10. Zöltzer H, Castenholz A. Die Zusammensetzung der Lymphe [in German]. Z Lymphologie 1985;9(1)

Chapter 1   Anatomy

2

Physiology

One of the main functions of the lymphatic system is to facilitate fluid movement from the tissues back to the blood circulation. A basic understanding of the complexities of fluid transfer between the blood capillaries, the tissues, and the lymph capillaries helps to understand the lymphatic system and its role in fluid homeostasis.

◆ Heart and Circulation

The cardiovascular system is an elaborate network designed to deliver oxygen and nutrients to body organs and to remove waste products of metabolism from the tissues. Its main components are the heart and a system of vessels that transport blood throughout the body. The part of the circulatory system that delivers blood to and from the lungs is called the pulmonary circulation, and the flow of blood throughout the rest of the body is administered by the systemic circulation (high-pressure system) (Fig. 2–1).

Blood that has been oxygenated in the lungs is pumped out of the left ventricle of the heart

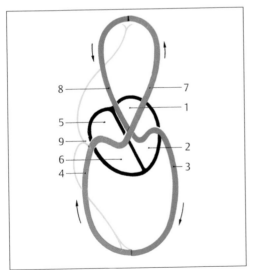

Figure 2–1 Pulmonary and systemic circulation. 1. Left atrium; 2. Left ventricle; 3. Aorta; 4. Inferior vena cava; 5. Right atrium; 6. Right ventricle; 7. Pulmonary artery; 8. Pulmonary vein; 9. Return of the lymphatic system to the low pressure system.

through the aorta, the largest artery in the body. The aorta arches upward from the left ventricle of the heart to the upper chest, then travels down toward the abdomen, forming the main trunk of the arterial circulation. It then branches off into numerous smaller arteries, which deliver oxygen-rich blood to the various body systems. These arteries further subdivide into smaller vessels, the precapillary arterioles. Precapillary arterioles in turn branch off into even smaller tubes, the blood capillaries, which are so thin that blood cells can only pass through them in single file. Blood capillaries consist of an arterial and a venous loop.

The walls of the larger arteries and arterioles are made up of an outer layer consisting of connective tissue (adventitia), smooth musculature in the middle layer (media), and an inner layer of endothelial cells (intima). The walls of the small capillaries do not contain any muscle fibers; they consist only of a single layer of endothelial cells (Fig. 2–2). This wall structure enables an exchange of certain substances between the blood capillaries and the surrounding tissues (wall permeability). The endothelial cells, which form the capillary wall, control its permeability. Across their walls exchanges occur between blood and tissue fluids, oxygen (O_2), carbon dioxide (CO_2), nutrients, water, inorganic ions, vitamins, hormones, immune substances, and metabolic waste. A large part of the waste products are extracted from the blood as it flows through the kidneys.

The average blood capillary is ~1 mm long, and the lumen diameter is ~8 μm. The flow velocity within a capillary amounts to ~2 cm per second, and the number or density of blood capillaries in a given tissue is proportional to its metabolic activity. Estimates indicate that if all capillaries of the body were placed end to end, they would reach 60,000 miles. If split in half, they would cover an area equal to one and a half football fields.

The blood leaving the blood capillaries through the postcapillary venules has a lower oxygen content. On its way back to the heart, the venous blood passes through progressively larger veins and connects with the right atrium via the superior and inferior vena cava. The pressure inside the thin-walled venous vessels is considerably lower than in the arterial sys-

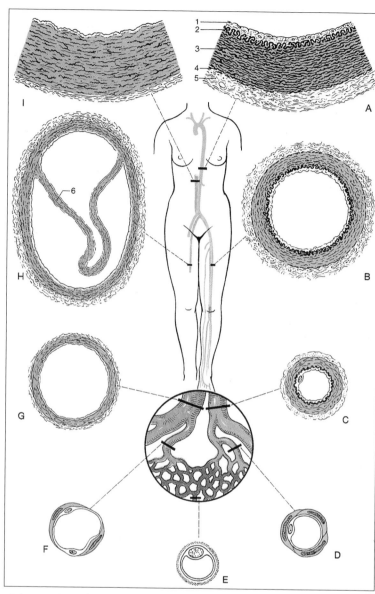

Figure 2–2 Layers in the walls of blood vessels in various parts of the systemic circulation. A. Aorta: 1. Intima; 2. Internal elastic membrane; 3. Media (with fenestrated elastic membranes) containing smooth musculature; 4. External elastic membranes; 5. Adventitia. B. Larger peripheral arteries. C. Smaller peripheral arteries. D. Precapillary arterioles (their media are formed by one or two circular layers of smooth musculature (precapillary sphincter). E. Blood capillaries (their walls do not contain smooth musculature). F. Postcapillary veins (their walls contain irregularly distributed muscle cells). G. Smaller peripheral veins (their walls consist of endothelium and a thin layer of spirally arranged smooth musculature, but most do not have a distinct three-layered structure). H. Larger peripheral veins (same wall structure as G; smaller and larger veins have numerous valves (semilunar pockets), which open in the direction of the heart. Valves are absent in the superior and inferior vena cava and the veins of the portal circulation, kidneys, and brain. 6. Cross section of a venous valve; I. Inferior vena cava (the wall has a well-developed intima; the longitudinal muscle strands in the media are arranged in small bundles).

tem (Fig. 2–3). A system of valves inside the larger veins prevents pooling of venous blood in the lower extremities. In fact, the pressure in the venous system is so low that a sufficient return of blood to the heart would not be possible without the help of the muscle and joint pumps, diaphragmatic breathing, and the suction effect of the heart during the relaxa-

tion phase, or diastole. Together with a functioning valvular system, these supporting mechanisms propel the venous blood back to the heart.

The blood leaves the right ventricle to reach the pulmonary circulation via the pulmonary artery, which carries blood with a low oxygen content to the lungs. There, it branches off into

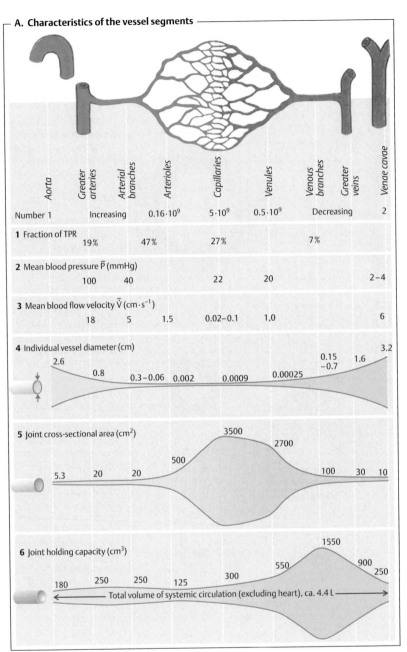

A. Characteristics of the vessel segments

	Aorta	Greater arteries	Arterial branches	Arterioles	Capillaries	Venules	Venous branches	Greater veins	Venae cavae
Number	1	Increasing		$0.16 \cdot 10^9$	$5 \cdot 10^9$	$0.5 \cdot 10^9$	Decreasing		2
1 Fraction of TPR		19%	47%		27%		7%		
2 Mean blood pressure $\bar{P}$ (mmHg)		100	40		22	20			2–4
3 Mean blood flow velocity $\bar{V}$ (cm·s⁻¹)		18	5	1.5	0.02–0.1	1,0			6

4 Individual vessel diameter (cm)

2.6 0.8 0.3–0.06 0.002 0.0009 0.00025 0.15–0.7 1.6 3.2

5 Joint cross-sectional area (cm²)

5.3 20 20 500 3500 2700 100 30 10

6 Joint holding capacity (cm³)

180 250 250 125 300 550 1550 900 250

← ——— Total volume of systemic circulation (excluding heart), ca. 4.4 L ——— →

Figure 2–3 Mean blood pressure values in different blood vessel segments and other characteristics. TPR, total peripheral flow resistance.

two arteries, one for each lung, to reach the thin-walled pulmonary capillaries, where CO_2 leaves and exits the body through the mouth and nose. Oxygen reenters the blood through the pulmonary capillaries, and the freshly oxygenated blood returns to the left atrium via the pulmonary vein. In pulmonary circulation, the roles of arteries and veins are opposite those in the systemic circulation (Fig. 2–1).

◆ Blood Pressure

Blood pressure is the force of blood pushing against the walls of blood vessels. It is measured in millimeters of mercury (mmHg) and reaches its highest value in the left ventricle and aorta during the systole, in which the blood is pumped from the heart into the systemic circulation. Its lowest value occurs during the diastole of the heart muscle.

> The blood pressure inside blood vessels is in inverse proportion to their distance from the heart; for example, it decreases as the distance increases and is lower in capillaries than in arteries.

Blood pressure varies with age, sex, and constitution of the individual. A rough rule of thumb for normal systolic pressure in adults is 100 plus the age of the individual. The diastolic pressure should be around two thirds of the value of the systolic pressure.

The mean blood pressure is a value half of the sum of systolic and diastolic values and should be around 100 mmHg for a normal individual in good health. Its value decreases continuously between the arterial and the venous end of the systemic circulation. In the veins near the heart, the pressure amounts to only 1.5 to 4 mmHg (Fig. 2–3). Sufficient venous return to the heart depends on supporting mechanisms described earlier.

The pulmonary circulation also belongs to the low-pressure system; its systolic value in the pulmonary artery amounts to ~25 mmHg.

Blood Capillary Pressure

The diameter of blood vessels in the arterial system decreases the farther they branch out; the resistance within these vessels is in inverse proportion to their diameter (i.e., the smaller the vessel, the greater the resistance). If the resistance within a vessel increases, the blood capillary pressure (BCP) will decrease (Fig. 2–3; see also Filtration and Reabsorption later in this chapter).

Because of the large diameter of the aorta and the larger arteries, the mean blood pressure in these vessels decreases only minimally. The resistance in the precapillary arterioles and the blood capillaries is notably higher (smaller diameter), causing a considerable decrease in pressure within these vessels. The mean pressure in the arterial end of the blood capillary amounts to ~29 mmHg (BCP_{art}), on the venous end to ~14 mmHg (BCP_{ven}).

Contraction or dilation of the ringlike smooth muscles in the media of precapillary arterioles (*precapillary sphincters*) also has an effect on blood capillary pressure. In the contraction phase of these sphincters, the lumen of the precapillary arterioles decreases, and the blood will be rerouted directly into postcapillary venules via arteriovenous anastomoses. Less blood reaches the blood capillaries, and the blood capillary pressure will decrease. If the sphincter dilates, more blood enters the blood capillaries, and the pressure inside the capillaries will subsequently increase (*vasodilation*).

The sympathetic branch of the autonomic nervous system controls the precapillary sphincter. It can regulate the flow of blood through the capillaries according to the metabolic needs of the tissue (e.g., hypoxia in the tissues supplied by the capillaries), external factors (temperature), or hormones.

The blood capillary pressure may also increase due to insufficient venous return (venous or cardiac insufficiencies, pregnancy). Venous stasis causes the thin-walled veins to dilate, resulting in venous pooling and a subsequent increase in venous pressure. The venous stasis will also affect the blood capillaries in that the blood volume inside the capillaries increases, thus leading to an increased blood capillary pressure (*passive vasodilation*). Variations in blood capillary pressure may have significant effects on lymphedema and swellings of other geneses due to increased filtration values (see also Combined Insufficiency later in this chapter).

◆ Capillary Exchange

The body can be viewed as being composed of two basic fluid volume compartments: intravascular and extravascular. The intravascular compartment is composed of cardiac chambers and blood vessels and contains blood; the

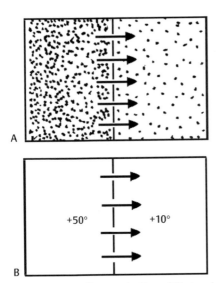

A

B

+50° +10°

Figure 2–4 Diffusion. A. Slow diffusion (a membrane separating the two media is slowing down the migration of molecules from a place of higher to a place of lower concentration). B. Temperature diffusion (temperature moves down the pressure gradient from high to low).

extravascular system represents everything outside of the intravascular compartment. The extravascular compartment is made up of many subcompartments, such as the interstitial, cellular, and lymphatic subcompartments, and a specialized system containing cerebrospinal fluid.

There is a constant exchange of fluids, gases, nutrients, and other substances between these compartments. The primary sites of this exchange are the blood capillaries within the blood capillary bed; the blood capillary bed consists of several capillaries supplied by the same precapillary arteriole. Some substances are transported across the endothelial membrane, but material (especially water) also leaves through pores in the capillary walls.

The clinical relevance of capillary exchange to lymphedema is discussed later in the section Filtration and Reabsorption.

Diffusion, osmosis, filtration, and reabsorption are the mechanisms involved in capillary exchange.

Diffusion

> Diffusion is the equilibrating movement of molecules and other particles in solution from an area of higher to an area of lower concentration (concentration gradient).

When areas of higher and lower concentrations are connected, more particles diffuse from the place of high concentration to the place of lower concentration than in the opposite direction (net diffusion). Substances undergoing net diffusion are said to move down their concentration gradient; for example, from higher to lower concentration. After a certain time these substances become evenly distributed: they reach *diffusional equilibrium*. In this state, there is no further net diffusion. The exchange of substances in diffusion is independent from energy (passive process) and influenced by the following factors:

Temperature: diffusion occurs more rapidly if temperature increases.

Concentration gradient: the larger the difference in concentration, the faster the diffusion.

Size of the molecules: smaller molecules (e.g., O_2) diffuse more rapidly than larger ones (e.g., protein).

Surface area: the larger the area, the faster the diffusion.

Diffusion distance: the shorter the distance, the more effective (and faster) the diffusion.

Diffusion can be differentiated between simple and slow. In simple diffusion, the migration of molecules from a place of higher to lower concentration (or temperature) occurs without any separation along the concentration gradient. In the body, this form of diffusion would occur within the interstitial spaces or the cells. In case of slow diffusion, a membrane separates the involved mediums (Fig. 2–4).

To better understand the movement of molecules through blood capillary walls or cell membranes, the following example is helpful. A container of water is separated by a membrane into two compartments. Sugar molecules are placed in one of the compartments but not in the other. The membrane is completely permeable for both the sugar and the water molecules. Although the sugar molecules will move in all directions, more of them will move (or diffuse) from the side of the container where they are in greater concentration to the other compartment of the container. At the same time, the water molecules will diffuse from the compartment where they are in greater concentration through the pores of the membrane to the side where they are in lesser concentration. Equilibrium (no more movement) will be reached with equal concentrations of sugar and water in both compartments (Fig. 2–5).

It is important to understand that diffusion is exclusively responsible for the exchange of O_2 and CO_2 in all the tissues in the body. The majority of the nutrients and other substances obtained by the body, as well as the removal of waste products, are supplied by diffusion as well. To ensure sufficient gas exchange and metabolism, a short diffusion distance is imperative. In healthy conditions, every tissue cell is usually within 2–3 cell diameters from the supplying blood capillary.

Clinical relevance: In cases of swelling, the distance between the blood capillaries and the cells supplied by these capillary increases. This increase in diffusion distance will result in a drastic decrease in the supply of the cells with oxygen and nutrients. Waste products and CO_2 will accumulate in the cells and interstitial tissues. This situation results in an environment extremely susceptible to infection, skin breakdown, cell damage, and delayed healing. It is imperative to initiate therapeutic decongestive measures in the very early stages of tissue swelling to avoid these complications or to promote healing in already damaged tissue.

Osmosis and Osmotic Pressure

Osmosis is the movement or diffusion of water molecules from a place of higher water concentration to a place of lower water concentration across a selectively permeable (or semipermeable) membrane, which is permeable only to water molecules but impermeable to other molecules.

Cell membranes in the body are generally permeable to water; water equilibrates throughout the body by osmosis.

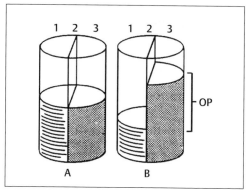

Figure 2–5 Osmosis. 1. A chamber containing water; 2. Membrane; 3. A chamber containing a solution of sugar and water. A. The membrane is permeable to water and sugar (slow diffusion). B. The selective membrane is impermeable to sugar but permeable to water. OP, Osmotic pressure (measured in mmHg). The increased water level in chamber 3 causes an elevation in hydrostatic pressure.

To better understand the process of water moving through cell membranes, the example of the water container will be used again. A container of water is separated by a membrane into two compartments. Sugar molecules are placed in one of the compartments but not in the other. The membrane is permeable only for the water molecules but impermeable for the sugar molecules. In the sugar solution, the concentration of water is lower; sugar molecules take up space that water molecules would otherwise occupy. The water molecules will diffuse from the side of the container where they are in larger concentration across the selective membrane to the other compartment of the container. The sugar molecules are unable to cross the membrane; osmosis occurs only toward one side of the container (toward the side with the sugar solution), leading to a rise of the water level on this side of the container. The hydrostatic pressure in this side of the container will increase, leading to a pressure difference between the two sides of the membrane. This is called the osmotic pressure (OP) and is measured in mmHg (Fig. 2–5).

To move the water back into the other side of the container (the compartment with the larger concentration of water molecules), a pressure equal to the osmotic pressure needs to be applied to the increased water level on one side of the container. This pressure is needed to overcome the hydrophilic effect of the sugar molecules.

The most abundant substance to diffuse through cell membranes is water. Enough water moves in each direction through the cell membranes per second to equal an amount ~100 times the volume of the cell itself.

Clinical relevance: Because the volume of water moving into and out of the cells is the same, the volume of the cells remains constant. However, under certain conditions a concentration difference for water may develop across a membrane. In the case of lymphedema and an impaired lymphatic system, the protein concentration within the interstitial tissue fluid will increase (high-protein edema) in that area. The hydrophilia of these proteins and the higher solute concentration in the interstitium will cause the water molecules to move toward the interstitial space, causing an increase in volume of the affected area. To overcome this osmotic pressure; that is, to force the water molecules back into the cells and blood capillaries, it is necessary to apply an appropriate pressure to the edematous area.

Colloid Osmosis and Colloid Osmotic Pressure

The concentration of proteins in the plasma amounts to ~75 g per liter of plasma. Proteins are the only dissolved substances in the plasma that do not diffuse readily through the blood capillary membranes. Those proteins leaving the blood capillaries into the interstitial fluid are soon removed from the interstitial spaces by the lymphatic system. Therefore, the concentration of the proteins in the plasma averages about three times more than the protein concentration in most interstitial fluids. Proteins in the plasma cause a higher colloid osmotic pressure (COP_{PL}; also known as oncotic pressure) than proteins in the interstitial fluid (interstitial fluid colloid osmotic pressure; COP_{IP}). Normal values for the COP_{PL} average ~25 mmHg.

Clinical relevance: The effects of increased protein concentration in lymphedema and the subsequent increase of the COP_{IP} of the interstitial fluid are already discussed in the section Osmosis and Osmotic Pressure. Patients and therapists should be cautious using external compression pumps in the treatment of lymphedema. These devices may temporarily re-

move water from the interstitial tissues, mechanically leaving the proteins behind. The result will be an increased COP_{IP} (i.e., the protein molecules will attract more water out of the blood capillaries). Diuretics may have the same effect (see Chapter 3, Therapeutic Approach to Lymphedema).

In case of a decrease in the amount of protein in the blood (hypoproteinemia), the oncotic pressure of the plasma proteins (COP_{PL}) will decrease. This will result in more water leaving the blood capillaries and accumulating in the tissues. The swelling resulting from hypoproteinemia affects the entire body surface (generalized edema) and should not be confused with lymphedema.

Filtration and Reabsorption

Another example for passive exchange of water across a membrane is filtration.

> This process depends on a pressure gradient between both sides of the membrane and always moves from the area of higher to the area of lower pressure.

As discussed earlier, the blood capillary membrane is permeable to water (solvent) containing micromolecules (solutes) but impermeable to larger molecules such as plasma proteins.

The pressure gradient is produced by the blood pressure; the pressure inside blood capillaries is greater than the pressure in the interstitial fluid. Another force affecting filtration is the colloid osmotic pressure of the plasma proteins.

Ernest Henry Starling (1866–1927) discovered that under normal conditions the average blood capillary pressure and the colloid osmotic pressure of the plasma proteins are approximately identical (Starling's equilibrium). But because the BCP in the arterial end of the capillary (29 mmHg) is higher than the COP (25 mmHg), water is filtered through the capillary membrane into the interstitium → filtration ($BCP_{art} > COP_{PL}$).

At the venous end of the capillary, the blood capillary pressure (14 mmHg) is lower than the colloid osmotic pressure of the plasma proteins (25 mmHg); water is reabsorbed back into the blood capillaries → reabsorption ($BCP_{ven} < COP_{PL}$) (Figs. 2–6, 2–7).

The water leaving the blood via filtration washes over the tissue cells carrying nutrients and other solutes with it. Fluid returning through reabsorption deposits waste products from the cells back into the venous system. This "balance" in filtration and reabsorption changes frequently by contraction or dilation of the precapillary sphincter (see Blood Capillary Pressure previously in this chapter). In the dilation phase of the sphincter, the blood capillary pressure may increase to a value allowing only filtration to occur. If the sphincter contracts, the blood capillary pressure may decrease so much that only reabsorption takes place over the entire length of the capillary (Fig. 2–8).

In the course of a day, about 20 L of fluid (representing 0.5 % of the plasma in the flowing blood) is filtered by the nonrenal blood capillaries into the interstitial space. About 80 to 90 % of this filtrate is reabsorbed back into the blood capillaries. The remaining fraction of about 10 to 20 % is also known as the net filtrate and accounts for the roughly 3 L that are returned to the blood circulation via the lymphatic system.

Additional factors affecting filtration and reabsorption are the interstitial fluid colloid osmotic pressure (COP$_{IP}$) and the interstitial fluid pressure (IP).

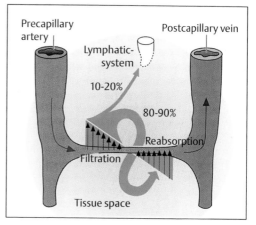

Figure 2–6 Filtration and reabsorption on the blood capillary level.

Interstitial fluid colloid osmotic pressure (COP$_{IP}$): Although the blood capillary membrane is usually impermeable toward the protein molecules, approximately half of the proteins circulating in the blood manage to leave the blood capillaries and the postcapillary venules in the course of a day. The permeability toward protein varies between the different tissues and depends on the individual microstructure. As outlined previously, the presence of proteins in the perivascular space results in colloid osmotic pressure in the interstitium (COP$_{IP}$), which aver-

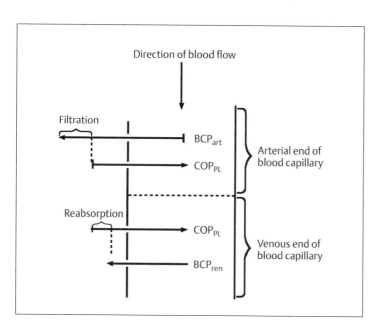

Figure 2–7 The effects of blood capillary pressure (BCP$_{art}$ and BCP$_{ven}$) and colloid osmotic pressure of the plasma proteins (COP$_{PL}$) on filtration and reabsorption.

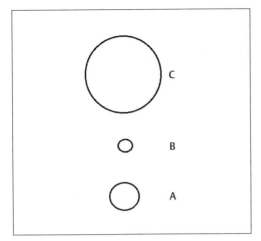

Figure 2–8 The effect of the precapillary sphincter musculature on blood capillary pressure and blood pressure in the precapillary arterioles. A. Lumen diameter of the precapillary arterioles in normal muscle tone. B. Contraction of the precapillary sphincter muscles causes a decrease in lumen diameter of the precapillary arterioles. Less blood reaches the blood capillaries, causing a decrease in blood capillary pressure. The blood pressure proximal to the precapillary arterioles increases. C. Dilation of the precapillary sphincter muscles causes an increase in the lumen diameter of the precapillary arterioles. More blood reaches the blood capillaries, causing an increase in blood capillary pressure. The blood pressure proximal to the precapillary arterioles decreases.

ages ~8 mmHg. COP_{IP} will cause the water molecules to move toward the interstitial space and thus "works against" the effort of the proteins in the blood to reabsorb the fluid.

Interstitial fluid pressure (IP): This is the pressure located in the interstitial fluid. For reasons not further elaborated in this book, it is extremely difficult to measure the value of this pressure. Some authors report negative (subatmospheric) values, others positive values. If the value is positive, it represents a force working against filtration and supporting reabsorption; if it is negative, it supports filtration and works against reabsorption.

Net Filtration Pressure

To determine this value at the arterial end of the blood capillary, it is necessary to subtract all the inward forces from the outward forces on the capillary.

Outward forces: BCP_{art}, COP_{IP}, IP (if negative)

Inward forces: COP_{PL}, IP (if positive)

> Under normal conditions, the outward forces are greater than the inward forces on the arterial end of the capillary.

Net Reabsorption Pressure

To determine the net reabsorption value on the venous end of the blood capillary, the outward forces have to be subtracted from the inward forces.

Inward forces: COP_{PL}, IP (if positive)

Outward forces: BCP_{ven}, COP_{IP}, IP (if negative)

> Under normal conditions, inward forces outweigh outward forces on the venous end of the blood capillaries.

Clinical relevance: Almost all therapeutic measures and activities (as well as pathologies) will have an effect on net filtration and net reabsorption. Knowing about the relationship and interactions between filtration and reabsorption, it is easy to understand why some therapeutic measures or activities help and support the lymphatic system, whereas others work against it.

Increased net filtration: An increase in blood capillary pressure results in more water leaving the blood capillaries. BCP increases if the blood volume entering the capillary increases (vasodilation). Possible causes are massage, changes in temperature (ice, heat, sauna, sunburn), passive vasodilation (insufficient venous return), strenuous exercise, infection, and other factors (Fig. 2–9).

More water leaving the blood capillaries results in an increase in lymphatic load of water. In most cases this will not present a problem for healthy individuals with a functioning lymphatic system. The lymphatic system is capable of coping with an increase of lymphatic load by activating its safety factor (see Safety Factor of the Lymphatic System later in this chapter).

However, if the lymphatic system is impaired or already overloaded, such as in edema and lymphedema, the lymphatic system in many cases is unable to respond to a local increase in

A. Exchange of fluids via capillaries and venules

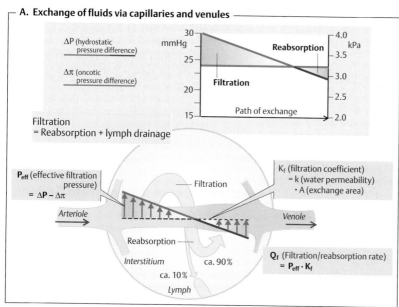

ΔP (hydrostatic pressure difference)

$\Delta\pi$ (oncotic pressure difference)

Reabsorption

Filtration

Path of exchange

mmHg / kPa scale: 30 / 4.0, 25 / 3.5, 20 / 3.0 / 2.5, 15 / 2.0

Filtration
= Reabsorption + lymph drainage

P_{eff} (effective filtration pressure)
$= \Delta P - \Delta\pi$

Arteriole

Filtration

Venole

Reabsorption

Interstitium

ca. 90%

ca. 10%

Lymph

K_f (filtration coefficient)
$= k$ (water permeability)
$\cdot A$ (exchange area)

Q_f (Filtration/reabsorption rate)
$= P_{eff} \cdot K_f$

B. Causes of edema

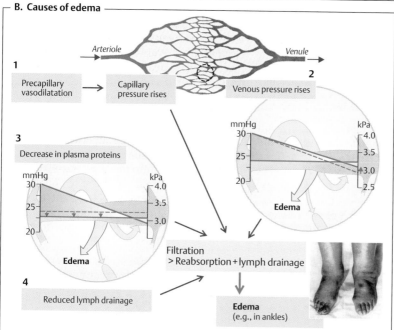

Arteriole

Venule

1

Precapillary vasodilatation → Capillary pressure rises

2

Venous pressure rises

3

Decrease in plasma proteins

Edema

4

Reduced lymph drainage

Filtration
> Reabsorption + lymph drainage

Edema

Edema
(e.g., in ankles)

mmHg / kPa scales shown in graphs: 30 / 4.0, 25 / 3.5, 20 / 3.0, 2.5

Figure 2–9
Causes of edema. 1. Vasodilation (heat, massage, infection, strenuous exercise); 2. Passive vasodilation due to insufficient venous return (venous or cardiac insufficiency, pregnancy); 3. Hypoproteinemia (malnutrition, kidney and liver diseases); 4. Reduced transport capacity of the lymphatic system.

net filtrate. To avoid additional problems and setbacks in treatment progress, it is necessary to avoid causes responsible for a significant increase in net filtration (heat, infection, strenuous exercises, impaired venous return).

Increased net reabsorption: Supporting the reabsorption of water from the interstitial areas back into the blood capillaries is a therapeutic goal in the management of edema and lymphedema. Increasing the tissue pressure by the skillful application of compression, either with special bandage materials or compression garments, will help to achieve that goal (see Chapter 4, Compression Therapy). Simultaneous to increasing the net reabsorption, the net filtration will be decreased.

◆ Physiology of the Lymphatic System

Now that the different factors affecting the movement of fluid through the capillary membranes have been covered, it becomes necessary to discuss the physiological capabilities of the lymphatic system to understand one of its most vital functions: the removal of proteins and other substances, along with active edema protection by the removal of interstitial fluid.

Lymph Time Volume and Transport Capacity of the Lymphatic System

The lymph time volume (LTV) is the amount of lymph fluid the lymphatic system is able to transport in a unit of time. LTV is lower at rest and higher during activity.

> The transport capacity (TC) of the lymph vascular system represents the amount of lymph fluid transported by the lymphatic system utilizing its maximum amplitude and frequency. It is equal to the maximum lymph time volume (TC = LTV_{max}).

Under physiological conditions, the lymph time volume at rest is equal to ~10% of the transport capacity of the lymphatic system. The difference between LTV and TC represents the *functional reserve* (FR) of the lymphatic system (Fig. 2–10).

To clarify the relationship between normal lymph time volume, the transport capacity,

and the functional reserve of the lymphatic system, the example of the thoracic duct will be used. As discussed in Chapter 1, the normal volume of lymph fluid returned to the blood circulation by the thoracic duct equals 2 to 3 L in 24 hours. In certain pathologies, volumes of more than 20 L of lymph fluid per day were measured. The functional reserve enables the lymphatic system to respond to a volume increase in lymph fluid and proteins in the tissue with an increase in LTV.

Safety Factor of the Lymphatic System

The body's ability to respond to an increase in the lymphatic load of water (increase in net filtrate) and protein consists of active and passive edema protective measures.

Passive edema protection: An increase in the volume of water leaving the blood capillaries results in an elevated volume of fluid accumulating in the interstitial tissue; the interstitial fluid pressure will subsequently increase. Referring to the earlier discussions in the sections Net Filtration Pressure and Net Reabsorption Pressure, it is clear that an increase in IP will decrease net filtration and increase net reabsorption pressures, thus enhancing edema protection. The additional water in the interstitium will lower the concentration gradient of the interstitial proteins, thus lowering COP_{IP}. These passive measures allow more fluid to be reabsorbed back into the blood capillaries.

Active edema protection: The lymphatic system activates its safety factor; that is, it responds to an increase in lymphatic load of water and protein with an increase in lymph

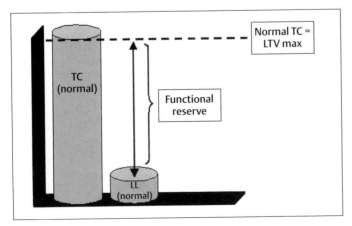

Figure 2–10 Functional reserve of a sufficient lymphatic system. FR, functional reserve of the lymphatic system; LL, lymphatic loads or lymph volume; LTV, lymph time volume (TC = LTVmax); TC, transport capacity of the lymphatic system.

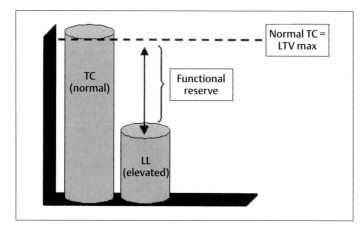

Figure 2–11 Lymphatic safety factor. The sufficient lymphatic system reacts to an increase of lymph volume with an increase in lymph angiomotoricity. FR, functional reserve of the lymphatic system; LL, lymphatic loads or lymph volume; LTV, lymph time volume (TC = LTVmax); TC, transport capacity of the lymphatic system.

formation on the lymph capillary level, as well as an elevated contraction frequency in lymph collectors and trunks (increase in LTV) (Fig. 2–11).

The effects of fluid accumulation in the interstitial tissues on lymph capillaries and anchoring filaments are discussed in Chapter 1, Lymph Capillaries. The increased intralymphatic pressure in collectors and trunks stimulates the smooth musculature inside the wall of the lymph angions, which leads to an increase in contraction frequency and amplitude in these vessels.

An increase in the amount of protein in the tissue (inflammation) will also activate the safety factor. Protein accumulation causes COP_{IP} to increase, which in turn results in more water leaving the capillaries. The resulting elevated water load has the same effect on the lymphatic system as previously outlined.

> The lymphatic system is said to be sufficient if the transport capacity is greater than the lymphatic load of water and protein.

◆ Insufficiencies of the Lymphatic System

Insufficiency occurs if the transport capacity of the lymphatic system is smaller than the lymphatic load (TC < LL); lymphatic insufficiency will induce edema (local or generalized) in the interstitial area.

There are three forms of insufficiencies, which can result in either edema or lymphedema: dynamic, mechanical, or combined insufficiency.

Dynamic Insufficiency

Dynamic is the most common insufficiency and is also known as *high-volume insufficiency*. In this case, the lymphatic load (of water or of protein and water) exceeds the transport capacity of the anatomically and functionally intact lymphatic system (LL > TC); as discussed earlier, the limit of the functional reserve of the lymphatic system is its transport capacity (Fig. 2–12).

> Dynamic insufficiency occurs if active and passive edema protective measures are exhausted, and results in edema.

> Edema is a swelling caused by the accumulation of abnormally large amounts of fluid in the intercellular tissue spaces of the body, which is visible and/or palpable (pitting). It is a symptom rather than a disease or disorder and may be caused by cardiac insufficiency, immobility, chronic venous insufficiency (stage I and II), hypoproteinemia, pregnancy, and other factors.

Clinical relevance: If dynamic insufficiency is present over long periods of time (e.g., months; the duration varies depending on the condition and severity), secondary damage to the lymphatic system is imminent. The intra-

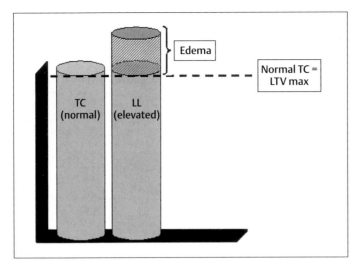

Figure 2-12 Dynamic insufficiency. The lymph volume exceeds the transport capacity of the healthy lymphatic system, resulting in the onset of edema. FR, functional reserve of the lymphatic system; LL, lymphatic loads or lymph volume; LTV, lymph time volume (TC = LTVmax); TC, transport capacity of the lymphatic system.

lymphatic pressure increases in lymph collectors working at their transport capacity over extended time periods, resulting in possible damage to the collector walls and their valvular system. Secondary damage to the lymph collectors could cause a reduction in their transport capacity, which would exacerbate the situation.

To avoid secondary damage to the lymphatic system and the tissues, it is imperative to reduce the lymphatic load of water (or protein and water in the case of inflammation) as soon as possible. In localized edema, this is usually achieved by elevation, compression, and exercises. Manual lymph drainage (MLD) is not the therapy of choice in cases of dynamic insufficiency. MLD increases a reduced transport capacity of the lymphatic system; it is not possible to elevate the normal transport capacity of an overloaded but otherwise healthy lymphatic system by use of manual lymph drainage.

Compression therapy and MLD are strictly contraindicated in edema caused by cardiac insufficiency (*hemodynamic insufficiency*) due to the elevated fluid volumes returning to the heart, which may cause cardiac overload or additional damage.

Mechanical Insufficiency

Typical for mechanical insufficiency, also known as *low-volume insufficiency*, is a reduction in the transport capacity of the lymphatic system due to functional or organic causes (Fig. 2-13).

> The impairment is so severe that the lymphatic system is unable to manage a normal amount of lymphatic load (TC < LL [normal]) or to respond to an increase in the lymphatic load of water and protein.

Surgery, radiation, trauma, or inflammation (organic causes) involving the lymphatic system can result in mechanical insufficiency. Functional causes may involve paralysis of the lymph vessels as a response to certain drugs or toxins (filariasis), as well as valvular insufficiency as a result of lymph vessel dilation. The walls of the lymph angions may become fibrotic due to high intralymphatic pressure and subsequent seepage of proteins into the wall structure (mural insufficiency).

> The inability of the lymphatic system to perform one of its basic functions; for example, the removal of water and protein from the tissues, will result in high-protein edema or lymphedema.

Clinical relevance: Lymphedema, if left untreated, will lead to serious consequences. The stagnation of water, protein, and other waste products in the interstitium may cause tissue damage. The protein-rich swelling elongates the diffusion distance and thus reduces the ability of the body's defense mechanisms as a

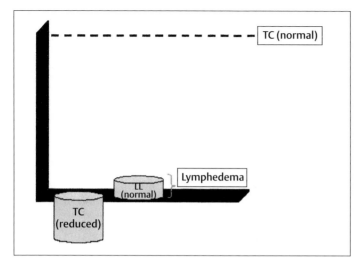

Figure 2–13 Mechanical insufficiency. The transport capacity falls below the normal lymph volume. FR, functional reserve of the lymphatic system; LL, lymphatic loads or lymph volume; LTV, lymph time volume (TC = LTVmax); TC, transport capacity of the lymphatic system.

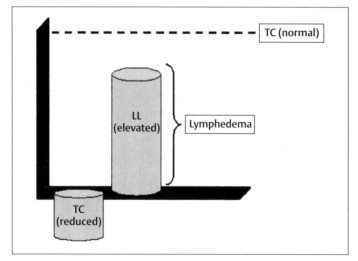

Figure 2–14 Combined mechanical/dynamic insufficiency. FR, functional reserve of the lymphatic system; LL, lymphatic loads or lymph volume; LTV, lymph time volume (TC = LTVmax); TC, transport capacity of the lymphatic system.

result of the impaired circulation of macrophages and lymphocytes. This leads to a high susceptibility to infections (cellulitis).

To reduce lymphedema and to avoid further damage, it is imperative to treat this condition by means of complete decongestive therapy (CDT; see Chapter 4) and to avoid conditions that may lead to excessive vasodilation (increased net filtrate) and infections. CDT has little or no side effects and shows excellent long-term results.

Combined Insufficiency

In combined insufficiency, the transport capacity of the lymphatic system is reduced, and the volume of the lymphatic loads is simultaneously elevated (Fig. 2–14).

The maximum degree of this insufficiency is reached if the transport capacity is reduced below the level of normal lymphatic loads (mechanical insufficiency), and the volume of lymphatic loads is greater than the transport capacity of a healthy lymphatic system (dynamic insufficiency). The combination of these insufficiencies may lead to severe tissue damage (necrosis) and chronic inflammation in the affected areas.

The presence of either dynamic or mechanical insufficiency may lead to combined insufficiency. As discussed earlier in this chapter, if dynamic insufficiency presents over long periods of time the walls and valves of lymph collectors may experience damage. The resulting reduction of its transport capacity will lead to combined insufficiency.

If mechanical insufficiency is present and the lymphatic load of water or protein and water increases, combined insufficiency will be the result.

Clinical relevance: To avoid further complications in the presence of dynamic insufficiency, the primary goal is to reduce the lymphatic loads. The clinical goal in lymphedema (mechanical insufficiency) is to reduce the interstitial swelling as soon as possible. It is also important to understand that infection, trauma, and certain forms of exercises result in an increase in lymphatic loads, which may lead to combined insufficiency with further complica-

tions. To avoid this situation and to further compliance, it is necessary to provide patients suffering from lymphedema with as much information as possible (see Chapter 5, Precautions).

The pathophysiology of lymphedema is discussed in the following chapter. Chapters 4 and 5 cover the various intervention techniques for this condition.

Recommended Reading

1. Despopoulos A, Silbernagl S. Color Atlas of Physiology. 4th ed. New York: Thieme Medical Publishers; 1991
2. Földi M, Kubik S. Lehrbuch der Lymphologie. Germany: Gustav Fischer Verlag; 1999
3. Guyton AC, Hall JE. Textbook of Medical Physiology. 9th ed. Philadelphia: WB Saunders; 1996.
4. Kugler C, Strunk M, Rudofsky G. Venous pressure dynamics of the healthy human leg: role of muscle activity, joint mobility and anthropometric factors. J Vasc Res 2001;38:20–29
5. Kuhnke E. Die Physiologischen Grundlagen der Manuellen Lymphdrainage. Physiotherapie 1975;12
6. Weissleder H, Schuchardt C. Erkrankungen des Lymphgefaessystems. Viavital Verlag Koeln; 2000

3
Pathology

◆ Lymphedema

Definition

Lymphedema is a very common and serious condition, affecting at least 3 million Americans. It occurs if the transport capacity (TC) of the lymphatic system has fallen below the normal amount of lymphatic load (LL; see Chapter 2, Mechanical Insufficiency), resulting in the abnormal accumulation of water and proteins principally in the subcutaneous tissues.

Lymphedema may be present in the extremities, trunk, abdomen, head and neck, external genitalia, and inner organs; its onset is gradual in some patients and sudden in others. Most patients in the Western Hemisphere develop lymphedema after surgery and/or radiation therapy for various cancers (breast, uterus, prostate, bladder, lymphoma, melanoma), in which case it is referred to as secondary lymphedema. Other patients develop it without obvious cause at different stages in life (primary lymphedema), and still others develop it after trauma or deep vein thrombosis. In third world countries, parasites (filariasis) account for millions of cases.

Lymphedema is serious because of its long-term physical and psychosocial consequences for patients; it continues to progress if left untreated. If lymphedema combines with other pathologies (cardiac and venous insufficiencies, chronic arthritic conditions, etc.), the pathophysiological effects are further exacerbated due to the additional stress placed on the already compromised lymphatic system (see Chapter 2, Combined Insufficiency). Its cosmetic deformities are difficult to hide, and complications do occur frequently (fibrosis, cellulitis, lymphangitis, lymphorrhea, etc.). Lymphedema is also serious because of the pervasive lack of medical expertise in the diagnosis and treatment of this condition and the tendency of clinicians to trivialize lymphedema in patients who have been treated for cancer.

Incidence of Lymphedema

No specific studies on the incidence of lymphedema have been performed to date, and estimated rates reported in the literature vary widely. Worldwide, 140 million to 250 million cases of lymphedema are estimated to exist, with filariasis, a parasitic infestation (see Secondary Lymphedema later in this chapter), being the most common cause.

In the United States, the highest incidence of lymphedema is observed following breast cancer surgery, particularly among those who undergo radiation therapy following axillary lymph node dissection.

Other than skin cancer, breast cancer is the most common type of cancer among women in the United States. All women are at risk for developing breast cancer. A woman's chance of developing breast cancer increases with age. The majority of breast cancer cases occur in women over 50 years of age. Although breast cancer is less common at a young age, younger women tend to have more aggressive types of breast cancer than older women, which may explain why survival rates are lower among younger women. Incidence also varies within ethnic groups and geographical location within the United States (Table 3–1).

Generally, it can be said that 1 out of 8 women in the United States will develop breast cancer during the course of their lives. (More information can be found on the National Institute for Cancer Web site at http://cancer.gov/cancerinformation.)

Other cancer survivors at risk for lymphedema include those who have undergone surgery and/or radiation treatment for malignant melanoma of the upper or lower extremities; prostate cancer; gynecologic cancers; ovarian, testicular, and prostate cancers; and colorectal, pancreatic, or liver cancers. Some studies report an incidence of lower extremity lymphedema (and/or genital lymphedema) after radical lymph node dissection in prostate cancer to be more than 70%.

Table 3–1 Incidence of Breast Cancer by Age

By age 30	1 out of 2212
By age 40	1 out of 235
By age 50	1 out of 54
By age 60	1 out of 23
By age 70	1 out of 14
By age 80	1 out of 10
Ever	1 out of 8

Source: National Cancer Institute, 1999

It is generally thought that the more lymph nodes are removed during any surgical procedure, the higher the incidence of lymphedema. The true numbers of patients suffering from any form of lymphedema are unknown.

Most statistics are available on the incidence of upper extremity lymphedema following breast cancer surgery in women. Studies show incidences varying from 6 to 70% of breast cancer patients (a report in the April 1984 issue of *Breast Cancer Digest* found that ~50 to 70% of patients who have had axillary node surgery will develop lymphedema). In general, studies with longer follow-up show higher incidence and more severe swelling. Some authors feel that with the more conservative surgical procedure (modified radical mastectomy), the incidence has decreased. Surgeons hope that the sentinel node procedure (see discussion in Secondary Lymphedema later in this chapter) will reduce lymphedema because it removes fewer nodes. Presently, there is not enough follow-up information available to state this with certainty.

Based on the numbers above and other statistics, it is estimated that 2 million to 3 million secondary and 1 million to 2 million primary lymphedema cases are currently in existence in the United States.

> Lymphedema may develop anytime during the course of a lifetime in primary cases. Secondary cases may occur immediately postoperative, within a few months, a couple of years, or twenty years or more after surgery.

Etiology of Lymphedema

Lymphedema can be classified as primary or secondary, based on underlying etiology. However, this classification usually has little significance in determining the method of treatment (Table 3–2).

Primary Lymphedema

> Primary lymphedema represents a developmental abnormality (dysplasia) of the lymphatic system, which is either congenital or hereditary. It can present as a variety of abnormalities.

◆ **Hypolasia.** This most common form of dysplasia refers to the incomplete development of lymph vessels; that is, the number of lymph collectors is reduced, and the diameter of existing lymph vessels is smaller than normal.

◆ **Hyperplasia.** The diameter of lymph collectors is larger than normal in this dysplasia (*lymphangiectasia* or *megalymphatics*). The dilation of the lymph collectors results in a malfunction of the valvular system within the collectors, which often leads to lymphatic reflux.

◆ **Aplasia.** The absence of single lymph collectors, capillaries, or lymph nodes associated with this abnormality may be a cause for the development of primary lymphedema.

Table 3–2 Etiology of Lymphedema

Primary Lymphedema	Secondary Lymphedema
◆ Aplasia	◆ Dissection of lymph nodes
◆ Hypoplasia	◆ Radiation
◆ Hyperplasia (lymphangiectasia/megalymphatics)	◆ Trauma
	◆ Surgery
◆ Fibrosis of lymph nodes	◆ Infection
◆ Agenesis of lymph nodes	◆ Malignancies
	◆ Chronic venous insufficiencies
◆ Congenital	◆ Immobility
◆ <35 years of age: lymphedema praecox	◆ Self-induced
◆ >35 years of age: lymphedema tarda	

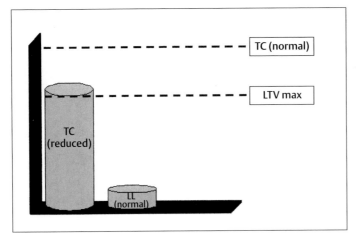

Figure 3–1 Reduced transport capacity in the subclinical stage of lymphedema. LL, lymphatic loads or lymph volume; LTV, lymph time volume (TC = LTV$_{max}$); TC, transport capacity of the lymphatic system.

Fibrosis of the inguinal lymph nodes (Kinmonth syndrome) presents an additional cause for the onset of primary lymphedema. The fibrotic changes primarily affect the capsular and trabecular area of the involved lymph nodes. This may affect lymph transport in the afferent lymph collectors.

With the understanding of basic lymphatic system physiology, it becomes evident that the transport capacity of the lymphatic system in all the abnormalities listed above is reduced (Fig. 3–1). As discussed in Chapter 2, lymphedema occurs if the transport capacity of the lymphatic system falls below the normal amount of lymphatic loads.

Although the developmental abnormalities are present at birth, lymphedema may develop at some point later in life. It may not develop at all as long as the (reduced) transport capacity of the lymphatic system is sufficient enough to manage the lymphatic loads. Primary lymphedema is often classified by the age of the patient at the onset of swelling.

Congenital lymphedema is clinically evident at birth or within the first 2 years of life. A subgroup of patients with congenital lymphedema has a familial pattern of inheritance, which is termed Milroy's disease. If primary lymphedema presents after birth but before the age of 35, it is called *lymphedema praecox*, which is the most common form of primary lymphedema and most often arises during puberty or pregnancy. *Lymphedema tarda* is relatively rare and develops after the age of 35.

Primary lymphedema almost exclusively affects the lower extremity (unilateral and bilateral) and involves mostly females. The swelling usually starts at the foot and ankle and gradually involves the remainder of the extremity. It may occur without any known impetus or may develop after minor trauma (insect bites, injections, sprains, strains, burns, cuts), infections, or immobility. These triggering factors produce additional stress to the already impaired lymphatic system, resulting in mechanical insufficiency (Fig. 3–2).

Secondary Lymphedema

The mechanical insufficiency present in secondary lymphedema is caused by a known insult to the lymphatic system.

> Most common causes for secondary lymphedema include surgery and radiation, trauma, infection, malignant tumors, immobility, and chronic venous insufficiencies.

Lymphedema may also be self-induced.

Surgery and radiation: As outlined earlier, this is by far the most common cause for secondary lymphedema in the United States. Surgical procedures in cancer therapy commonly include the removal (dissection) of lymph nodes. The goal of these procedures is to eliminate the cancer cells and to save the patient's life.

A side effect in lymph node dissection is the disruption in the lymph transport. If the remaining lymphatics are unable to manage the lymphatic load, secondary lymphedema will develop.

In the early years of breast cancer surgery, *radical mastectomy* was the only option available for patients. Radical mastectomy includes the removal of the entire mammary gland, the axillary lymph nodes, and the pectoralis muscles under the breast. Although common in the past, radical mastectomy is now rarely performed and is recommended only if the cancer cells have spread to the muscles under the mammary gland. *Modified radical mastectomy* is now more commonly performed. This procedure includes the removal of the breast and part of the axillary lymph nodes. In certain forms of breast cancer, a *simple* or *total mastectomy* is performed, in which only the mammary gland, but not the axillary lymph nodes, is removed.

Today, many women with breast cancer are given the choice between mastectomy and *lumpectomy*. In lumpectomy, also referred to as breast-conserving surgery, only the part of the mammary gland containing the malignant tumor and some of the normal surrounding tissue are removed. Most women after breast surgery, especially after lumpectomy, receive radiation treatments (Fig. 3–3).

Sentinel lymph node biopsy, a relatively new technique, was developed to determine if cancer cells have spread to the axillary nodes and trunks, without having to perform a traditional axillary lymph node dissection during which, on average, ~10 to 15 axillary lymph nodes are removed. A sentinel lymph node

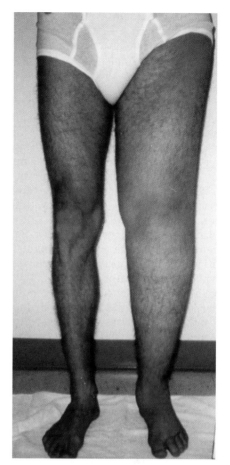

Figure 3–2 Primary lymphedema of the left lower extremity.

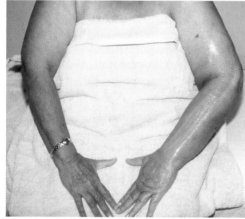

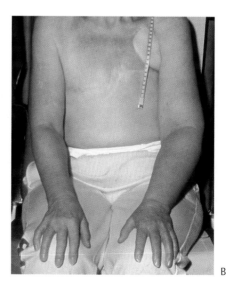

A

Figure 3–3 A. Secondary lymphedema of the left upper extremity. B. Secondary lymphedema of the left upper extremity following bilateral mastectomy.

B

biopsy requires the removal of only those lymph nodes to which the mammary gland drains first (sentinel nodes) before reaching the rest of the axillary lymph nodes. A pathologist then closely reviews these one to three lymph nodes. If they do not contain malignant cells, the chance that the remaining axillary nodes are cancer free is ~95%, and removal of additional axillary nodes may be avoided.

Radiation (or radiotherapy) is the treatment of cancer and other diseases with ionizing radiation. The goal of this therapy is to destroy cancer cells that may linger after surgery. It uses either precisely aimed, high-energy, external beam radiation or radioactive seeds that are implanted in the tumor area. Malignant cells often grow at a faster rate than normal cells; this makes many cancers very sensitive; that is, vulnerable to radiation.

Although radiation damages both cancer cells and normal cells, the normal cells are able to repair themselves and continue to function properly. Radiation is usually administered 5 days a week for several weeks and may also contribute to the onset of lymphedema. Rays can cause fibrosis in the tissues, leading to an impaired lymph transport, and hinder the regeneration of lymph vessels. Radiation may also affect nervous tissue, which can result in numerous problems affecting either the lymphedema itself or the patient's ability and compliance during the treatment of the lymphedema (radiation plexopathy; see Complications in Lymphedema later in this chapter).

Trauma: Traumatic insults involving the lymphatic system may cause a significant reduction in lymph flow, resulting in secondary lymphedema (burns, larger skin abrasions). Scar tissue hinders regeneration (lympholymphatic anastomosis) of lymph collectors, further exacerbating the problem. Post-traumatic secondary lymphedema develops from a mechanical insufficiency of the lymphatic system as a result of tissue lesions and should not be confused with post-traumatic edema. Post-traumatic edema is a local result due to trauma, which usually recedes after a few days (see Lipedema later in this chapter).

Infection: Recurrent acute or chronic inflammatory processes affecting the lymphatic system may result in mechanical insufficiency. If inflammation involves lymph nodes (lymph-adenitis) or collectors (lymphangitis), the walls tend to become fibrotic and the lymph fluid coagulates and obliterates the lymphatics, thus creating blockage to the lymph flow. In addition to the existing mechanical insufficiency, there is an increase in the volume of lymphatic load, resulting in combined insufficiency.

Lymph node and lymph vessel infections can be caused by bacteria (especially *Streptococcus*) and fungal infections. The inflammatory process affecting intra and periarticular tissues in rheumatoid arthritis may spread to the lymphatics, presenting another cause for mechanical insufficiency (see Traumatic Edema later in this chapter).

The most common cause for inflammation of the lymphatic system and lymphedema in general is filariasis (Fig. 3–4A).

> Lymphatic filariasis is endemic in more than 80 countries in the tropics and subtropics and is caused by threadlike, parasitic filarial worms, *Wuchereria bancrofti*, that live almost exclusively in humans.

Lymphatic filariasis is transmitted when an infected mosquito bites a person, then goes on to bite others, thus infecting them with the parasites. The worms live for 4 to 6 years lodged in the lymphatic system, where they reproduce. The toxicity of the waste products produced by these worms results in inflammation and obliteration of the lymphatic system, leading to swelling (often extreme) of the lower extremities and genitalia (Fig. 3–4B).

Lymphatic filariasis has been identified by the World Health Organization as a leading cause of permanent and long-term disability in the world. It is estimated that over 120 million people have some form of the disease, with over 40 million people having recurrent infections and abnormalities. Lymphatic filariasis is very rare in the United States, but it may be contracted by visitors to the endemic areas.

The goal of the Global Alliance to Eliminate Lymphostatic Filariasis is to stop the spread of filarial infection, thus interrupting transmission. This is done through the distribution of free medication in the endemic areas. Lymphedema caused by filariasis can be treated successfully with complete decongestive therapy.

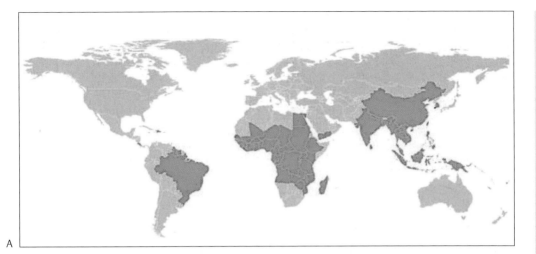

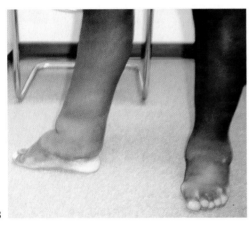

Figure 3–4 A. Lymphatic filariasis endemic countries (Used with permission from the World Health Organization). B. Lymphatic filariasis on both lower extremities.

Malignant tumors: Malignant tumors may mechanically block the lymph flow by pressing against lymphatic structures from the outside (see Complications in Lymphedema later in this chapter). Malignant cells may also infiltrate the lymphatic system and proliferate in either lymph vessels (malignant lymphangiosis) or lymph nodes, thus blocking the flow of lymph (Fig. 3–5). Modified CDT protocols may be applied to address the symptoms associated with malignancies (Fig. 3–6).

Chronic venous insufficiencies: Insufficient venous return results in an increase in venous blood pressure. The subsequent elevation in blood capillary pressure causes an increase in net filtrate (see Chronic Venous and Lymphovenous Insufficiency later in this chapter). In its primary function to actively prevent edema, the lymphatic system tries to compensate for the higher volume of the lymphatic

load of water by the activation of its safety factor (see Chapter 2, Safety Factor of the Lymphatic System). Without initiation of adequate therapy for the venous problem, the lymphatic system may develop a mechanical insufficiency (combined insufficiency) over time, due to the constant strain (Fig. 3–7).

Immobility: If left without proper care, immobility caused by injuries to the spinal cord, stroke, or cerebral hemorrhage may eventually result in similar problems as discussed earlier (e.g., insufficient venous return with subsequent lymphatic overload).

Self-induced lymphedema: By use of a tourniquet (bandages, rubber band), some individuals produce a combination of venous and lymphatic obstruction on an extremity to produce the signs and symptoms of lymphedema. The ligature mark is usually easily identifiable just proximal to the swelling. This

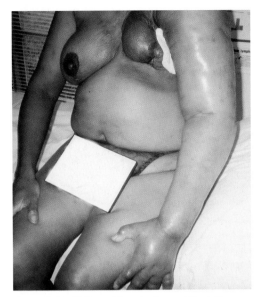

Figure 3–5 Malignant lymphedema of the left upper extremity.

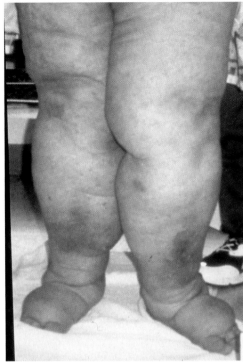

Figure 3–7 Lymphedema in combination with venous insufficiency (stage 2) on both lower extremities.

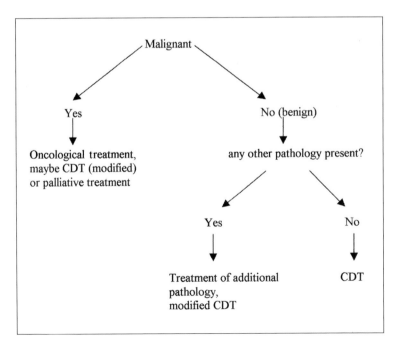

Figure 3–6 Therapeutic approach in malignant lymphedema.

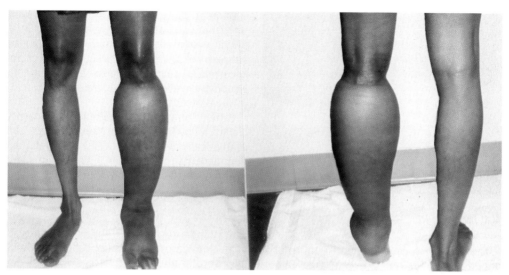

Figure 3–8 Self-induced lymphedema of the left lower extremity (note the ligature mark on the left knee).

condition is extremely rare. If a therapist suspects self-induced lymphedema (also known as artificial lymphedema), it is recommended that he or she contact the referring physician following the evaluation (Fig. 3–8).

If lymphedema is present, the lymphatic system is mechanically insufficient; that is, the transport capacity has fallen below the normal amount of lymphatic load.

Stages of Lymphedema

Currently, there is no cure or permanent remedy for lymphedema. The transport capacity in the damaged lymph vessels cannot be restored to its original level (see Chapter 2, Fig. 2–13).

Although the swelling may recede somewhat during the night in some early-stage cases, lymphedema is a progressive condition. Regardless of genesis, lymphedema, in most cases, will gradually progress through its stages, if left untreated (Table 3–3).

Table 3–3 Stages of Lymphedema with Typical Symptoms

Stages of Lymphedema	Characteristics
◆ Latency stage ◆ Lymphangiopathy (also Stage 0/Prestage/Subclinical stage)	◆ No swelling ◆ Reduced transport capacity (TC) ◆ "Normal" tissue consistency
Stage 1 (reversible stage)	◆ Edema is soft (pitting) ◆ No secondary tissue changes ◆ Elevation reduces swelling
Stage 2 (spontaneously irreversible stage)	◆ Lymphostatic fibrosis ◆ Hardening of the tissue (no pitting) ◆ Stemmer sign positive ◆ Frequent infections
Stage 3 (lymphostatic elephantiasis)	◆ Extreme increase in volume and tissue texture with typical skin changes (papillomas, deep skinfolds, etc.) ◆ Stemmer sign positive

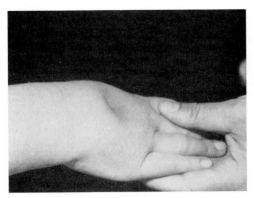

Figure 3–9 Pitting lymphedema (stage 1) on the right hand.

There is no specific period of time for a patient to remain in a particular stage. For example, a patient will not be in stage 1 for 4 months and then progress to stage 2 for 6 months before moving to stage 3.

Stage 0

This stage is also known as the subclinical stage, or prestage, of lymphedema. In this stage, the transport capacity of the lymphatic system is subnormal, yet remains sufficient to manage the (normal) lymphatic load (Fig. 3–1). This situation results in a limited functional reserve (FR) of the lymphatic system (see Chapter 2, Lymph Time Volume and Transport Capacity of the Lymphatic System).

Patients who underwent surgery (or had trauma) involving the lymphatic system and do not experience the onset of lymphedema are said to be in a *latency stage*, which is a subcategory of stage 0. For example, those women who had surgery for breast cancer (with or without lymph node dissection and radiation) and do not present with postmastectomy/lumpectomy lymphedema are considered to be in a latency stage. Again, in these cases, the TC is subnormal but still sufficient to drain the normal LL.

A condition known as *lymphangiopathy* presents if the TC is reduced by congenital malformations (dysplasia) of the lymphatic system. As long as the subnormal TC can manage the LL, lymphedema is not clinically present.

Patients in a prestage are "at risk" to develop lymphedema. The reduction in functional reserve results in a fragile balance between the

subnormal TC and the LL. The onset of lymphedema correlates to the ability of the lymphatic system to compensate for any added stress to the system or the frequency of certain occurrences that may cause an increase in lymphatic load of water (or water and protein) in the limb at risk.

Patient information and education, especially following surgical procedures, can dramatically reduce the risk of developing lymphedema (see Chapter 5, Precautions and Lymphedema and Air Travel).

Stage 1

This stage, also known as the *reversible stage*, is characterized by soft tissue pliability without any fibrotic alterations. Pitting is easily induced, and the swelling retains the indentation produced by the (thumb) pressure for some time (Fig. 3–9). In early stage 1, it is possible for the swelling to recede overnight.

With proper management in this early stage, it is possible for the patient to expect reduction of the extremity to a normal size (compared with the uninvolved limb). Without proper care, progression into stage 2 in the vast majority of the cases is inevitable.

It is difficult to distinguish stage 1 lymphedema from edemas of other geneses. The clinician needs to rely on the patient's history and whether the swelling resolves with conventional management (compression, elevation) or not (refer to Diagnosis and Evaluation of Lymphedema later in this chapter).

Stage 2

Stage 2, also known as *spontaneously irreversible lymphedema*, is primarily identified by tissue proliferation and subsequent fibrosis (lymphostatic fibrosis). Over time the tissue becomes more indurated, and pitting is difficult to induce. In stage 2, the Stemmer sign is positive (Fig. 3–10). A Stemmer sign is positive if the skin from the dorsum of the fingers and toes cannot be lifted, or lifted only with difficulty (compared with the uninvolved side). A positive Stemmer sign is considered accurate to diagnose lymphedema of the extremities; the absence of a Stemmer sign, however, does not exclude the presence of lymphedema (false-negative Stemmer sign).

In many cases, the volume of the swelling increases, which exacerbates the already compromised local immune defense (increased diffusion distance). Because of this, infections (cellulitis) in this stage are common.

Volume reduction can be expected if proper treatment is initiated in this stage of lymphedema. In most cases, the indurated tissue will not completely recede in the intensive phase of Complete Decongestive Therapy (see Chapter 4). Reduction of fibrotic tissue is achieved mainly in the second phase of CDT with compression and good patient compliance (Fig. 3–11).

Lymphedema often stabilizes in stage 2. In those patients suffering from recurrent infections, the lymphedema may develop into stage 3, lymphostatic elephantiasis.

Stage 3 (Lymphostatic Elephantiasis)

Typical for this stage are an increase in volume of the lymphostatic edema and further progression of the tissue changes. Lymphostatic fibrosis increases in firmness, and other skin alterations, such as papillomas, cysts, and fistu-

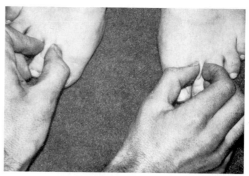

Figure 3–10   Positive Stemmer sign on the second toe of the right foot in lower extremity lymphedema.

las, hyperkeratosis, mycotic infections of the nails and skin, and ulcerations, develop frequently. Pitting may or may not be present. The natural skinfolds, especially on the dorsum of the wrist and ankle, deepen, and the Stemmer sign becomes more prominent. In many cases, cellulitis is recurrent (Fig. 3–12).

If lymphedema management starts in this stage, reduction can still be expected. To achieve good results, it is necessary to extend the duration of the intensive phase of complete

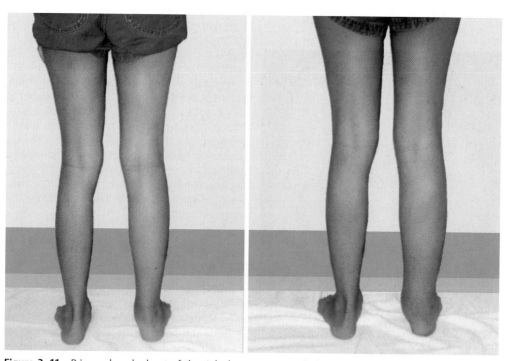

Figure 3–11   Primary lymphedema of the right lower extremity before (right) and after (left) complete decongestive therapy.

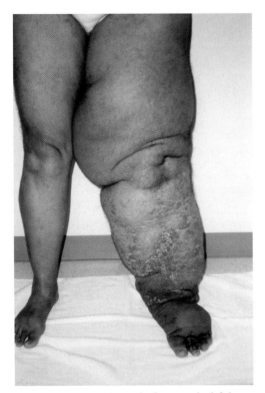

Figure 3–12   Stage 3 Lymphedema on the left lower extremity.

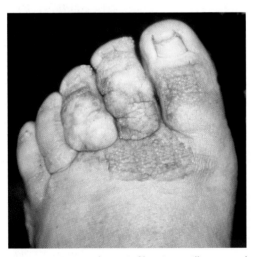

Figure 3–13   Lymphostatic fibrosis, papillomas, and fungal infections of the left foot.

decongestive therapy (CDT). In many cases, the intensive phase has to be repeated several times. Even extreme cases of lymphostatic elephantiasis can be reduced to a normal or near normal size with proper care and patient compliance (see Therapeutic Approach to Lymphedema later in this chapter).

> Tissue changes or the progression of fibrosis remains the clinical trait to distinguish between the stages of lymphedema.

Tissue changes commonly seen in the progression of lymphedema are proliferation of connective tissue cells, production of collagen fibers, and an increase in fatty deposits and fibrotic changes (lymphostatic fibrosis). The fibrotic tissue tends to become sclerotic over time, increasing in firmness. Lymphostatic fibrosis is initially noticed at the distal end of the extremities, fingers, and toes (Fig. 3–13).

Pitting is generally more pronounced in the early stages of lymphedema and occurs if pressure is applied with the examiner's thumb on the edematous tissue. Pitting is usually tested on the distal extremity (preferably over bony prominences) and occurs because of the displacement of fluid in the tissue caused by pressure with the flat thumb. The pitting response (indentation produced by pressure) can remain on the tested area for some time if there are minimal fibrotic skin changes present.

Angiosarcoma (Stewart-Treves syndrome; see also Complications in Lymphedema later in this chapter) may develop in long-lasting lymphedema, particularly in patients with stage 3 lymphedema. This type of angiosarcoma may develop in primary or secondary lymphedema and is characterized by extensive malignancy; it is highly lethal. Reliable data on the incidence of angiosarcoma in lymphedema are not available at this time.

Grading of Lymphedema Based on Severity

Extremity volume is not considered within the different stages of lymphedema. The severity of unilateral lymphedema in relation to volume can be assessed within each stage as minimal (less than 20% increase), moderate (20–40% increase), or severe (more than 40%) increase in limb volume (Table 3–4).

Table 3–4 Grading of Lymphedema Based on Severity

Severity of Lymphedema	Volume Increase
Minimal	<20%
Moderate	20–40%
Severe	>40%

Precipitating Factors for Lymphedema

For a patient "at risk," the possible development of lymphedema depends on many factors (see Avoidance Mechanisms later in this chapter). Some patients are able to effectively compensate for a decrease in transport capacity and functional reserve by the regeneration of lymph vessels, utilizing alternative collateral circulation routes and lymphovenous anastomoses and increasing the lymph time volume of remaining collectors. These patients may not exhibit signs or symptoms of lymphedema as long as the lymphatic system has found a way to compensate.

As discussed earlier, lymphedema may develop anytime during the course of a lifetime in primary cases. In secondary cases, the swelling may occur immediately postoperative, within a few months or a couple of years, or twenty years or more after surgery.

Based on the pathology and pathophysiology, as well as patient reports, certain triggers that cause the onset of lymphedema can be identified (for a more detailed review of precipitating factors and prevention of lymphedema, refer to Chapter 5, Precautions).

Increase in blood capillary pressure: Active hyperemia (vasodilation) that results from a local or systemic application causes an increase in blood flow, which ultimately will increase the lymphatic load of water and stress a compromised lymphatic system (see Chapter 2, Fig. 2–9). Examples of active hyperemia include local hot pack, other thermal modalities (diathermy, electrical stimulation, ultrasound), massage, vigorous exercise, and infection of the limb "at risk." Hot tubs and saunas, hot weather and high humidity, as well as injuries, are additional triggering factors.

Passive vasodilation as a result of the obstruction of the venous return will also result in increased net filtrate and place additional stress on the compromised lymphatic system. Examples include chronic venous insufficiencies, cardiac insufficiencies, and immobility, as well as the examples listed under the next category.

Fluctuation in weight gain and fluid volumes: Pregnancy and obesity, excessive weight gains during the menstrual cycle (cyclic idiopathic edema), and certain medications are known to trigger the onset of lymphedema by causing additional stress (lymphatic load) on the compromised lymphatic system.

Injury: Even in subclinical stages of lymphedema, the immune response is reduced as a result of edematous saturation of the tissues on a microscopic level. Any insult to the integrity of the skin may cause infection, thus triggering the onset of lymphedema. Examples include insect bites, pet scratches, injections, intravenous cannulation, blood pressure measurements on the involved extremity, cuts, and abrasions.

Changes in pressure: The change in cabin pressure during an airline flight, coupled with inactivity, may trigger the onset of lymphedema. The reduced cabin pressure may allow more fluid into the tissue spaces. Additional inactivity allows for venous pooling, which will eventually cause an increased pressure at the blood capillary level, thereby increasing filtration and the lymphatic loads (see Chapter 5, Lymphedema and Air Travel).

Avoidance Mechanisms

In an effort to maintain fluid homeostasis, the body has the ability to respond to lymphostasis, which may prevent the manifestation of lymphedema. The following discussion will focus on the body's compensatory mechanisms.

Safety Factor

Lymph collectors not affected by either blockage (surgery, radiation, trauma) or malformation will increase their contraction frequency and amplitude (lymphangiomotoricity) in an effort to compensate for those collectors affected by mechanical insufficiency. These compensating collectors are located in the same tributary area. The mechanisms involving the

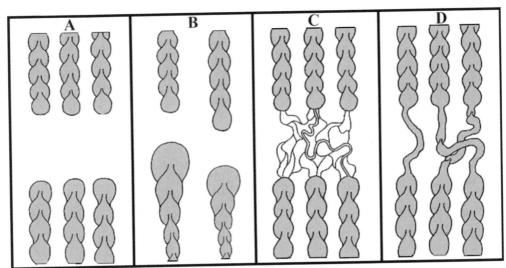

Figure 3–14 Reconnection of lymph collectors following blunt trauma.
A. Severed lymph collectors. B. Intralymphatic pressure in the distal lymph collector stump increases. C. Newly formed lymph vessels connecting the distal and proximal lymph vessel stumps. D. Lympho-lymphatic regeneration.

lymphatic safety factor are described in Chapter 2, Safety Factor of the Lymphatic System.

Collateral Circulation

Lymph collectors circumnavigating blocked areas may be able to avoid the onset of lymphedema by redirecting lymph fluid into areas with sufficient lymph drainage. Lymph collectors of the lateral upper arm, for example, may drain into the supraclavicular lymph nodes. This may be significant in case of axillary lymph node dissection because part of the lymph fluid may be rerouted around the axillary area into the supraclavicular nodes. The chance to avoid the manifestation of lymphedema, in this case, of the arm, is even greater if the individual's collectors of the lateral upper arm communicate with those located in the radial forearm territory (long upper arm type; see Chapter 1, Superficial Layer). If this connection exists, lymph fluid from the forearm and upper arm would be able to bypass the blocked axillary area into the supraclavicular nodes.

Interterritorial anastomoses present another possible bypass for lymph fluid. If the normal flow of lymph within a truncal territory is interrupted by lymph node dissection, the interterritorial anastomoses may prevent the onset of swelling in those quadrants that would normally drain into the dissected lymph node groups. The higher the number of anastomoses, as described in Chapter 1, Interterritorial Anastomoses, the better the chance to avoid lymphedema.

Lympho-Lymphatic Anastomosis

Severed lymph collectors tend to reconnect after a relatively short time (2–3 weeks). Newly formed lymph vessels reconnect the distal with the proximal lymph vessels stump (Fig. 3–14). Scar tissue may prevent lympholymphatic anastomoses. Lymph collectors separated due to blunt trauma (no skin breakage) will regenerate more effectively than collectors disconnected by incisional trauma.

Lympho-Venous Anastomosis

The distal end of a severed lymph collector may connect with an adjacent vein, creating a natural shunt. Lymph fluid then directly voids into venous blood.

Lymph Vessels in the Adventitia of Blood Vessels

Larger blood vessels have their own nutrient blood vessels (vasa vasorum vessels), which supply the wall of the larger arteries and veins with oxygen and nutrients.

There are also lymph vessels in the adventitia of larger blood vessels (lymph vasa vasorum). With lymphedema present, lymphatic loads may reach these lymph vasa vasorum vessels via tissue channels. Lymph vessels in the adventitia of blood vessels have the ability to increase their activity, thus providing an additional drainage pathway for stagnant lymph fluid.

Macrophages

If protein-rich fluid accumulates in the tissues, monocytes leave the blood capillaries in large numbers. Once in the tissues, they are macrophages (phagocytes) and will digest accumulated protein molecules. The subsequent decrease in tissue protein concentration will result in an increased reabsorption and a decrease in net filtrate, which will help to reduce the lymphatic loads. The digested protein molecules are broken down into amino acids, which do not present a lymphatic load, and are removed by the blood circulatory system.

Complications in Lymphedema

Lymphedema is often combined with other pathologies and conditions, which either aggravate the existing symptoms or present additional complicating factors in the treatment of lymphedema.

The following is a list of the most common complications.

Reflux: Retrograde flow of lymph fluid caused by valvular insufficiency of lymph collectors. Valvular insufficiencies are the result of hyperplasia, dilation of collectors due to constant strain or blockage of lymph flow, or organic changes in the walls of lymph collectors (mural insufficiency; see Chapter 2, Mechanical Insufficiency).

If valvular insufficiency is present, lymph fluid is propelled not only to proximal but also to distal (retrograde flow) during the contraction of lymph angions. Reflux presents as blis-

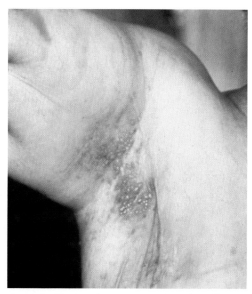

Figure 3–15   Lymphatic cysts in the right axilla.

terlike formations (*lymphatic cysts*) on the surface of the skin, commonly in the axillary (Fig. 3–15), cubital, genital (see Chapter 5, Fig. 5–23), and popliteal areas. Lymphatic cysts contain lymph fluid, which may be clear or chylous. If chylous, the reflux originates from the intestinal lymph system.

Clinical relevance: Lymphatic cysts may easily break open, presenting an entryway for pathogens, which can cause infection. Burst cysts associated with leaking of lymph fluid (lymphorrhea) are termed *lymphatic fistulas.*

To avoid damage to cysts and to prevent infection, it is recommended to cover the cyst with sterile gauze during treatment (local antibiotics should be applied around the fistulas), and not manually work on or around the cysts and fistulas. Cysts should be padded with soft foam material (donut or U-shaped padding) to avoid direct contact with the bandage materials while the patient wears the bandages.

Radiation fibrosis: Reaction of the skin to irradiation, leaving visible and/or palpable changes in the skin and subcutaneous tissue. The skin in radiation fibrosis appears reddish brown (Fig. 3–16), and superficial blood vessels may be dilated in the irradiated area (telangiectasia) (Fig. 3–17). The newly formed scar tissue may be soft or hard, and the skin may be adhered to the underlying fascia.

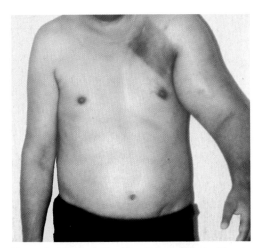

Figure 3–16 Radiation fibrosis in a patient with secondary lymphedema on the left upper extremity.

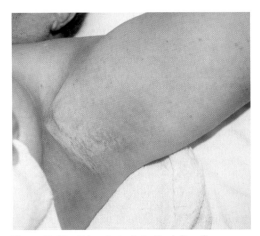

Figure 3–17 Telangiectasia in the left axilla.

Clinical relevance: The tissue changes in radiation fibrosis tend to get worse over time, possibly resulting in compression of venous blood vessels and subsequent dilation of superficial veins.

Radiation fibrosis may cause pain, limitations in range of motion if near a joint, paresthesia, pareses, and paralysis, which can occur even years after the radiation therapy was administered.

The skin in radiation fibrosis may also be more fragile. To avoid mechanical damage to the ir-

radiated skin, CDT presents a local contraindication in radiation fibrosis if there is adhesion to the fascia or if the radiated area is painful. Movements designed to mildly stretch the affected skin area should be incorporated into the exercise program. CDT techniques may be applied with lighter pressures if skin discoloration or telangiectasia and/or dilated superficial veins are present and the skin is pliable.

Infection: Bacterial (especially *Streptococcus*) and fungal infections are common in patients with lymphedema (especially stages 2 and 3). Clinical symptoms of cellulitis are fever and tenderness; the skin is red with indistinct margins (Fig. 3–18).

Fungal infections may involve the skin and/or nails and most often affect the lower extremities (Fig. 3–19). Nails generally take on yellow color, split, flake, and grow too thick. Symptoms in fungal infections of the skin include itching, crusting, scaling, and maceration between the toes. The skin may be moist or dry and may show a grayish white film. A sweet odor is often associated with fungal infections.

Clinical relevance: Episodes of cellulitis (or erysipelas) usually require a course of systemic antibiotics. CDT is generally contraindicated until the infection has cleared. Therapy for the fungal infection with local or systemic antifungal medication precedes lymphedema treatment.

Hyperkeratosis: Hypertrophy of the corneous layer of the skin. This condition is often associated with lymphedema, especially on the lower extremity. Wartlike papillomas are generally observed on the feet and toes. Skinfolds may be deepened.

Clinical relevance: Good skin hygiene is necessary to avoid possible infections in the moist skinfolds. Hyperkeratosis may be treated with over-the-counter medication or, in extreme cases, may be surgically removed (after decongestion), especially if papillomas interfere with the donning of compression garments. Because papillomas are elevated nodules, care must be taken to not tear the papillomas while donning the garments.

Scars: Scars located perpendicular to lymph collectors may present a blockage to lymph drainage, especially if the scar tissue adheres to the underlying tissues and/or exceeds 3 mm in width.

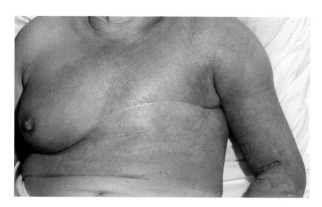

Figure 3-18 Cellulitis in a patient with secondary lymphedema of the left upper extremity.

Clinical relevance: The treatment of fresh scars is covered later in this chapter under Traumatic Edema. Older scars causing discomfort, blocking lymph flow, or hindering exercise protocols may be treated with techniques and materials designed to soften the indurated tissue (foam, manual techniques, nonthermal ultrasound).

Malignancies: Blockage of the lymphatic return may be caused by malignant tumors, in which case the swelling would be categorized as malignant lymphedema. As described earlier in this chapter, a rare form of malignancy may develop as a result of long-standing lymphedema (angiosarcoma or Stewart-Treves syndrome). Malignant cells may also infiltrate the lymphatic system, causing blockage to the lymph flow (malignant lymphangiosis) (Fig. 3–20).

Signs and symptoms of malignancies include sudden onset and fast progression of the swelling, pain (especially in the swollen extremity), paresthesia, paresis and paralysis, enlarged lymph nodes, ulcerations on the skin, varicose veins on the thorax, and elevated shoulder due to pain on the involved side in upper extremity involvement (Fig. 3–21).

Changes in the color and integrity of the skin may also indicate malignancies: cellulitis-like redness is often associated with malignant lymphangiosis (Fig. 3–20) (the redness does not appear suddenly as in cellulitis but develops slowly over the course of weeks and months). Hematoma-like discolorations on the skin may indicate the presence of angiosarcoma.

Clinical relevance: If any of the above symptoms are present, if lymphedema is therapy-resistant, or if there is a sudden relapse in swelling in previously treated lymphedema, a physician must be consulted immediately. Modified CDT protocols may be applied to reduce and alleviate the symptoms associated with malignancies (palliative care).

Paresis and paralysis: Partial or complete loss of motor function may be caused by injuries to peripheral nerves, the spinal cord, stroke or

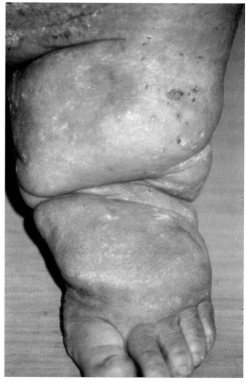

Figure 3-19 Fungal infections and lymphorrhea on lymphedema of the left lower extremity.

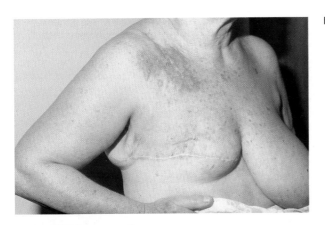

Figure 3–20 Malignant lymphangiosis.

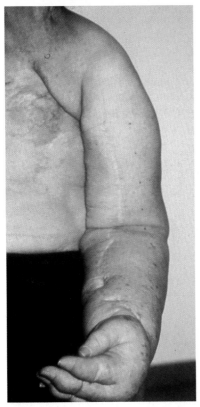

Figure 3–21 Malignant lymphedema of the left upper extremity.

cerebral hemorrhage, infiltration of nervous tissue by malignant tumors, or radiation (radiation plexopathy).

Clinical relevance: Immobility is detrimental to the lymphatic return. Modifications to the exercise program are necessary to address im-

paired motor function. Patients may need assistive devices to enhance mobility.

Genital swelling: Frequently present in combination with lower extremity lymphedema. In 40 to 60 % of the male lymphedema population, the external genitalia (scrotum and/or penis) may also present with significant swelling, in addition to the lower extremity involvement. Females are affected less frequently.

Clinical relevance: These patients should be thoroughly instructed in self-management issues (e.g., hygiene, the application of bandages or pads to the swollen area, appropriate clothing, etc.). It is important that compression garments incorporate the genital swelling (pantyhose, compressive body parts; refer to appropriate sections in Chapters 4 and 5).

Other pathologies combined with lymphedema: Lymphedema is often combined with other conditions and pathologies that may worsen the symptoms associated with lymphedema or complicate the treatment protocol with additional obstacles.

Clinical relevance: It is necessary to incorporate modifications in the treatment protocol for lymphedema to appropriately address signs and symptoms associated with any additional pathologies.

Examples

◆ **Lymphedema and cardiac insufficiency.** Abdominal techniques are contraindicated; the affected extremity (especially in leg lymphedema) should be treated only in sections to avoid too much venous blood and lymph fluid returning to the heart during the

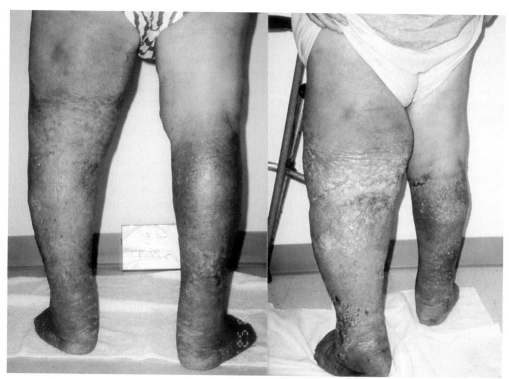

Figure 3–22 Lymphedema in combination with venous insufficiency (stage 3), ulcerations, and lymphorrhea on both lower extremities before (right) and after (left) complete decongestive therapy.

treatment. Lighter compression is necessary for the same reason.

◆ **Lymphedema and obesity.** Obesity contributes to the onset of lymphedema and, depending on the degree of obesity, may seriously hamper treatment progress and worsen already existing symptoms. It is often difficult to apply bandages and to prevent the materials from sliding. Compression garments may have to be custom ordered, creating a financial burden to the patient. Exercise protocols have to be modified accordingly. Patients should be advised to achieve and maintain normal weight to reduce the risk factors associated with obesity and to improve compliance.

◆ **Lymphedema and orthopedic problems.** Symptoms associated with lymphedema and orthopedic pathologies will magnify each other and may even exacerbate the current presentation of either or both pathologies. Relevant combinations are "frozen" shoulder and upper extremity lymphedema or hip/knee problems associated with lymphedema of the leg. To interrupt the vicious cycle, it is necessary to address all involved pathologies. It is often advised to prioritize treatment according to the more limiting factors found during the assessment.

◆ **Lymphedema and venous insufficiencies.** Venous insufficiencies contribute to the onset of lymphedema and worsen symptoms of existing lower extremity lymphedema (see Chronic Venous and Lymphovenous Insufficiency later in this chapter). The additional presence of venous ulcerations necessitates proper wound care (Fig. 3–22; see also Wounds and Skin Lesions later in this chapter). It is recommended that the lymphedema therapist incorporate the materials prescribed by the physician into the compression bandage.

Although venous insufficiencies will benefit from CDT for lower extremity lymphedema, it is imperative to observe possible complications associated with venous insufficiencies (thrombophlebitis). These complications may present a contraindication for the treatment of lymphedema.

◆ **Lymphedema and diabetes.** Diabetes is often associated with dry skin, frequent infections, neuropathy, slow-healing wounds, and high blood pressure. To address these problems, the treatment protocol for lymphedema may be modified accordingly, with more emphasis on skin hygiene. If ulcerations are present, the incorporation of wound care into the protocol becomes necessary. As with venous ulcers, it is recommended that the lymphedema therapist use and incorporate the materials prescribed by the physician into the compression bandage.

Diagnosis and Evaluation of Lymphedema (by Michael King, M.D.)

A complete history and physical examination during the initial evaluation of a patient with lymphedema are most important. These should involve a physician or, in many cases, multiple physicians working together. Cooperation should continue throughout all levels of treatment. Initial medical evaluation is essential, but so is continued follow-up throughout the patient's course of therapy. Unfortunately, the teaching of lymphedema in medical schools is inadequate in the United States at the present time. The result is often an inability to adequately evaluate and treat patients with lymphedema. A physician is able to evaluate historical information and, based on this, perform a physical examination, looking for specific physical findings, which might otherwise be overlooked. Appropriate diagnostic studies can then be ordered and interpreted, and the patient's entire medical condition can be understood. At this level, a physician is most qualified to plan and coordinate medical treatment. It is only after that initial evaluation that a patient can be cleared for lymphedema therapy. Therapists should not treat a patient without a physician's knowledge and backup. Communication between the therapist and the physician is essential. This is required to exchange medical information and explain to the therapist possible complications of therapy, what to look for, and when not to continue treatment without further medical consultation. This is especially true when manual lymphatic drainage on the neck or abdominal area is required. Potential problems, such as carotid sinus hypersensitivity, aortic aneurysm, and others, may necessitate modifications to the treatment protocol that need to be discussed with the referring physician.

Physical examination may reveal a swollen limb; however, it must be understood that lymphatic congestion involves not only the extremity but, in many cases, also parts of the torso, and goes far beyond what is clinically evident. To properly treat lymphedema, this must be recognized. Treatment of what appears to be a local symptom probably will not solve the ultimate problem. This is why pumps or simple elevation is generally inadequate in the treatment of a lymphatic congestion. Congestion of the lymph system exists more extensively than may be clinically apparent. The physician must understand this to prescribe appropriate treatment; he or she must also realize that lymphedema is a chronic condition.

It is important for physicians to understand that lymphedema is a disease. Most other kinds of edema are symptoms of other problems that need to be evaluated and understood.

Understanding the pathophysiology of edema dictates its proper therapy. Most patients and physicians look upon swelling as "fluid retention," and a diuretic is often given. Fluid retention states, which might include endocrine, cardiac, renal, hepatic, and other medical conditions resulting in the body retaining fluid, might be usefully treated with diuretics.

Drainage problems, that is, the mechanical inability to get rid of "normal" fluid, should not be treated with diuretics, which in some cases can be harmful. Many problems are mixed and involve multiple treatments, some of which are contradictory. A physician may be required to assess the medical situation and seek appropriate help to advise therapists on how to proceed. Also, a physician must understand that some forms of an inherited lymphedema may not appear until adolescence or in people over 30 years of age.

Basic clinical hints for evaluation

◆ **Upper Extremities**

◆ Diagnosis is usually clear, especially with history of breast, axillary, or chest surgery.

◆ Physicians should be aware of infectious disease past or present, or other pulmonary diseases. Computed tomography (CT) scans, chest x-rays, and other appropriate tests may be required. Men get breast cancer also.

◆ Some treatment is palliative. Be sure the patient and other physicians are aware of the patient's medical condition and what the therapeutic and prognostic expectations are.

◆ **Lower Extremities**

◆ Symmetrical swelling is generally a sign or symptom of other problems: think of systemic disease, and arrive at a differential diagnosis. Aside from cardiac, pulmonary, liver, and kidney disease, less common diagnoses, such as constrictive pericarditis, abdominal aortic aneurysm, and occult lymphoma should be taken into consideration.

◆ An infectious disease may play a role.

◆ Gastrointestinal, gynecological, urological, and, of course, chronic venous disease with deep venous thrombosis (DVT) must be ruled out.

Many of the above problems can lead to protein-loosing states, especially where the kidney, liver, or gastrointestinal system is involved. Hypoproteinemia will lead to edema— this is not lymphedema. In any case, edema of the lower extremities should not be taken lightly, and a physician must evaluate the etiology before referring a patient for "edema therapy." The therapist is depending on his or her diagnosis and direction. Compression bandaging, stockings, and manual lymph drainage (MLD) may seem standard treatment, but they vary from person to person according to the individual's medical needs. If a physician is unsure, it is in his or her best interest to refer a patient to a clinical lymphologist who deals with these problems on a daily basis.

A common question asked is, Will the current treatment of lymphedema spread cancer cells? There is no proof that it does, but this is an understandable concern. Physicians should remember that lymphedema itself can lead to immediate life-threatening problems, and in correctly chosen cases, appropriate lymphedema therapy can prevent additional problems. Patients with malignant lymphedema already have metastatic disease; to them, the treatment is palliative, that is, to relieve symptoms and reduce complications. The spread of malignant cells in this case is irrelevant. It is also irrelevant to those who have been cured and to whom lymphedema itself is a problem.

Physicians must be involved and understand the problems people with lymphedema are dealing with. It affects the patients both medically and socially.

Evaluation of Lymphedema (by Kim Leaird, P.T.)

Before evaluation, it is imperative that the patient has been cleared by a physician as an appropriate candidate for complete decongestive therapy. The referring practitioner should be aware of the possible multisystem involvement that can accompany lymphedema and the possible effects CDT can have on other body systems (e.g., cardiovascular).

A thorough evaluation will enable the therapist to set appropriate patient goals, use appropriate modalities, assess the progress of treatment, and plan for discharge of the lymphedema patient. The certified lymphedema therapist will also be a valued resource of information for the patient.

The evaluation process is an investigation into the patient's past and recent history that "paints a picture" to reflect the patient's current state. Patient history should reflect the following information:

◆ Past and current information regarding surgical history. The patient may be able to specifically identify a surgical event that precipitated swelling.

◆ Inclusion of coexisting health factors: diabetes, history or family history of cancer, vascular problems, thyroid problems, high blood pressure, pulmonary or asthma conditions, kidney dysfunctions, heart disease, or pregnancy

◆ If a surgical procedure was performed to remove a cancerous lesion or to remove involved lymph nodes, the patient may be able to convey the number of nodes removed, how many were positive, and if and when any other treatments for the cancer were administered (e.g., chemotherapy, radiotherapy).

◆ Has the patient experienced recent infections or had a chronic history of infections? Acute cellulitis is an absolute contraindication for CDT. Frequent and recurrent infections can cause the patient to progress through the stages of lymphedema more rapidly.

◆ How long has the swelling/lymphedema been present? Benign lymphedema will progress slowly, whereas a rapid progression of swelling could indicate a malignancy.

◆ Has the patient had previous intervention for lymphedema? Some patients may have used other methods of treatment for managing lymphedema, such as pumps, compression sleeves, or oral medications.

◆ Review of medications: Include a list of current medications the patient is taking and any specific allergies.

◆ Social history: involvement in sports or other recreational activities

◆ Support system: It is important to have some idea if the patient has a support system at home or from neighbors, other relatives, and so on, to plan appropriately for discharge.

◆ Work status: Provisions may be required for occupations involving long periods of standing, sitting, or highly repetitive activities. Given the specifics of the job, the patient's previous work environment may not be an optimal situation to return to with the lymphedematous limb. These work environments may provide a challenge for bandaging during phase 1 of treatment and govern the decision-making process when considering the appropriate compression class for garments.

◆ Review of current and available laboratory tests, diagnostic testing, and so on. Certain diagnostic testing for lymphedema, such as direct and indirect oily lymphography, may exacerbate symptoms.

◆ Does the patient currently wear a compression garment?

◆ Has the patient ever leaked lymph fluid?

◆ Has the patient ever had open sores on the affected limb? Did the sores heal? If so, how long did it take for the wounds to heal?

◆ Are there any changes in skin color? With long-standing lymphedema, skin changes can occur. The skin can develop a reddish tone, *lymphedema rubra*, or a brownish color, *lymphedema nigra*.

◆ Has the patient ever traveled outside the United States? Patients who travel abroad may develop a filarial infection from the bite of an infected mosquito. Filariasis is the leading cause of lymphedema worldwide.

◆ Does the patient exercise regularly? A regular exercise routine will increase the patient's tolerance to activity and help the clinician gauge the appropriate level of decongestive exercises to prescribe for the patient.

◆ How would the patient describe his or her daily activity: light, moderate, or heavy? Patients accustomed to a moderate or heavy schedule of activities may require additional encouragement to avoid activities that could exacerbate their symptoms during the initial phases of treatment.

◆ Does the swelling/lymphedema limit the patient in any way? A heavy arm may discourage the patient from moving the extremity, which could lead to adhesive capsulitis. Repetitive lifting of a heavy arm can lead to shoulder impingement, and repetitive lifting of a heavy leg could lead to back or hip involvement.

◆ Does the patient wear tight jewelry or clothing on the involved limb? Garments and jewelry that are too tight may restrict lymph flow and exacerbate symptoms.

Inspection of the involved area should note any skin or nail changes, wounds, or the presence of infections or fungal growth. Measurement of the ulcer or wound areas should be documented with other objective measurements, such as photographic imaging and planimetric measurements.

Palpation should note the temperature of the involved area. The grades for edema and pitting will help determine the stage of lymphedema. Test the presence of a Stemmer sign at the dorsum of the fingers and toes. Fibrotic areas of skin will be less pliable and mobile. The skin may also be thin and fragile or thick and "woody."

The physician must determine how the swelling presents. Lymphedema presents in an asymmetrical fashion, either one extremity is involved or, if both extremities are involved, one will be larger. If bilateral, symmetrical swelling is present, a process to differentiate other diagnoses (e.g., cardiac involvement) should be considered. If an involved limb presents with more swelling at the proximal portion, this could indicate a malignancy or the initial stage of secondary benign lymphedema.

The presence of lymphatic cysts and/or fistulas should be noted. These areas should be cleaned and padded generously to protect the cysts against compression. If fistulas are present, a local antibiotic should be applied, and the area should be covered with gauze to absorb any drainage and to protect the bandages from staining. With MLD techniques, place gauze over the area as a visual reminder to avoid pressure and strokes over the cysts and fistulas.

Document the presence of scars and papillomas. Scars can provide a challenge if they are oriented perpendicular to lymph collectors. As a general rule, lympholymphatic regeneration may be inhibited by scars that are wider than 3 mm, immobile, and bound to the fascia beneath. Papillomas are benign skin tumors, similar to large skin tags. These areas are not problematic with bandages, but they may need to be removed for the patient to don garments safely without avulsing the papillomas. Collateral veins may be present that indicate incompetent veins from clotting or valvular failure.

Objective information should include range of motion and strength measurements to determine functional limitations and to gauge progress. Measurements to document girth size of the involved extremity or extremities are also imperative. Girth or circumferential measurements should be from a standard point of reference on the extremity that is replicable each time the patient is measured.

The assessment should create a summative statement to include functional deficits and physical limitations and to identify the need for skilled intervention by a trained therapist. Frequently, lymphedema will accompany strength deficits, restrictions in range of motion, difficulties with activities of daily living, and balance deficits, depending on the age of the patient and the degree of involvement.

The initial evaluation session will involve not only the physical exam but also extensive education regarding the course of treatment and the requirements for successful completion of CDT. The therapist should inform the patient of the basic requirements: a daily treatment regime, the need for appropriate, accommodating clothing (larger shirts, pants, and shoes), and consistency and compliance from the patient. The bandages will be bulky and warm, and may not easily fit comfortably under normal clothing. Larger clothing may be needed so the patient can continue with daily activities of work, shopping, exercise, and so on. Patients should understand the requirements and necessity of compression.

The first day the patient is seen in the clinic should be for evaluation only. The evaluation process, discussions of requirements, and determination of the appropriate bandaging materials, as well as answering patient questions, will incorporate the appointed time. The first hands-on day for MLD should be separate from the evaluation. For example, if the evaluation is held on Tuesday of one week, the first day of CDT should be the following Monday. It is recommended the patient be seen for at least 4 or 5 days the first week of CDT. It is imperative patients understand and be comfortable with handling the bandages by the end of the first week of treatment. Initially, most patients will be intimidated by the reality that they must manipulate and don the bandages themselves, or with the help of a family member over the weekends. This will be one of the first major obstacles the therapist will face. Proper education and practice will adequately calm those fears and make the experience of lymphedema management successful for the therapist and patient.

MLD alone will not successfully treat and manage lymphedema. Patients may ask to only receive the MLD and try to forgo the compression bandaging. This scenario will yield unsuccessful results and be frustrating for both the therapist and the patient.

Diagnostic Imaging

A thorough physical evaluation, in addition to the patient's history and symptoms, is generally sufficient for the diagnosis of lymphedema.

Diagnostic imaging methods may be used if the diagnosis of lymphedema is unclear or if better definition for prognostic considerations (possible malignancies) is needed. Imaging methods may also be useful for investigational (research) purposes. It is recommended that these tests be performed by a clinical lymphologist or the patient be referred to a lymphologic center, if accessible.

Lymphoscintigraphy (isotope lymphography)

This method has largely replaced direct lymphography with oily contrast mediums for visualization of the lymphatic system. Lymphoscintigraphy, also called lymphangioscintigraphy (LAS), has not yet been standardized. A radioactive tracer is usually injected intradermally; mobile scanners in combination with computer equipment are used to visualize the rays, which are reflected by the radioactive tracer. LAS provides images and data on lymph vessels and nodes, lymph node uptake speeds, and rate of lymph (radiotracer) movement.

Conventional ("direct") Lymphography

Conventional lymphography has been the clinical standard for assessing problems with the lymphatic system. In the past 15 to 20 years this procedure has been phased out in favor of less invasive techniques. This technique is usually reserved for more complex conditions such as chylous reflux syndrome and thoracic duct injury. This procedure involves identifying a lymph collector on the dorsum of the foot or hand (using blue dye) and injecting an oily contrast medium into this lymph collector. Radiographs are then taken to show the lymph collectors as well as the lymph nodes.

Complications are reported using this method, such as allergic reactions and inflammatory reactions of the lymphatic system in the area where the lymphography was performed. Pulmonary embolism has been reported, especially in patients with cardiac and pulmonary conditions. The oily contrast medium may damage intact lymph vessels, causing further reduction of lymph flow.

Indirect Lymphography

By this method, normal lymph vessels, which are so fine that they cannot be punctured for direct lymphography, can be demonstrated in the healthy skin of hands and feet. A water-soluble contrast medium is injected intracutaneously. The agent is then absorbed into the lymph capillaries and continues to flow into precollectors and collectors. The radiograph shows the superficial lymph vessel system (including the initial lymph vessels) over a distance of up to 23 inches (60 cm). Regional lymph nodes cannot be identified using this method.

Fluorescent Microlymphangiography

This method is used primarily for research purposes. A fluorescent agent (if exposed to light radiation, certain substances have light-emitting properties, usually ultraviolet) is injected intracutaneously, normally in the area of the medial malleolus. This method allows observing the cutaneous lymph vessel plexus and other functions of the lymphatic system. A fluorescent microscope and a camera are used to record the diffusion of the fluorescent substance.

Magnetic Resonance Imaging

This noninvasive visualization method is very costly and primarily used in tumor diagnosis. The body is placed in a magnetic field, which enables imaging without the use of any radiation or radioactive agents.

Computed Tomography

This imaging method provides cross-sectional views of body segments and is often used to identify abdominal and retroperitoneal tumors. The density of tissues can be analyzed, which is helpful to distinguish between fatty tissue and accumulations of protein-rich fluid. Two- and three-dimensional measurements of edema volumes are possible.

Venous Doppler

This noninvasive technique uses ultrasound to assess blood flow in the deep venous system. It is primarily used to supplement or complement the evaluation of lymphedema and determines any venous involvement in the swelling.

Therapeutic Approach to Lymphedema

Therapeutic approaches to lymphedema range from ignorance ("You have to live with it") to numerous surgical procedures. Between these two extremes are several conservative treatments.

Complete decongestive therapy (CDT) is the therapy of choice for the vast majority of patients suffering from primary and secondary lymphedema. In addition to CDT, there are various treatment approaches that may be used to supplement CDT. Some of them will be discussed in the following section; others, such as ultrasound and electrotherapy, will be included in Chapter 4.

Complete Decongestive Therapy

> Because there is currently no cure for lymphedema, the goal of any therapy must be to reduce the swelling and to maintain the reduction; that is, to bring the lymphedema back to a stage of latency.

The only physiological way to achieve this goal is to remove the excess plasma proteins from the tissues via lymph vessels and tissue channels. For a majority of patients, this can be achieved by the skillful application of complete decongestive therapy. CDT shows good long-term results in both primary and secondary lymphedema. The components and techniques of CDT will be described in detail in Chapter 4.

Numerous studies have proven the effectiveness of this therapy, which has been well established in European countries since the 1970s. Although CDT has been practiced in the United States in one form or another since the 1980s, this therapy became accepted only after definitive guidelines and all components of CDT were included in the teaching curricula of schools providing training in lymphedema management in the 1990s.

CDT is applied in two phases. In phase 1, the goal is to mobilize the accumulated protein-rich fluid and to initiate the reduction of fibrosclerotic tissues (if present). The duration of this intensive phase varies and averages 2 to 3 weeks for patients with upper extremity lymphedema and 2 to 4 weeks for patients with lymphedema of the lower extremity. Ideally, the treatment is performed daily, 5 days a week (Table 3–5).

Another important goal in this first phase is to instruct the patient in techniques designed to maintain and improve the achieved success of the treatment (proper skin care, correct application of bandages, wearing of compression garments, etc.).

The first phase of the therapy is immediately followed by phase 2, which is aimed to preserve and improve the success achieved in phase 1. This phase for the most part is continued by the patient. With good patient compliance, the volume reduction not only can be maintained but also improved by progressive reduction of fibrosclerotic tissues in this second phase.

In more severe cases of lymphedema, it may become necessary to repeat phase 1; if lymphedema is associated with other conditions, the individual steps of CDT are modified accordingly.

CDT not only has been proven to be effective, with excellent long-term results, it is also noninvasive and safe, that is, without any known side effects to the patient, provided the patient is an appropriate candidate for CDT.

CDT is also cost effective in that it transfers the care from the medical professional to the patient and/or the patient's family. It significantly reduces the risk factors of developing cellulitis attacks, and improves or reduces lymph cysts, lymphatic fistulas, varicose lymphatics, and fungal infections.

Massage

Massage traditionally has been used to treat edema, but it is not recommended to manage lymphedema. The differences between edema and lymphedema are outlined in Chapter 2, Insufficiencies of the Lymphatic System.

Table 3–5 Stages of Lymphedema and Therapeutic Approach

Stages	Duration of Treatment	CDT–Phase I	CDT–Phase II
Latency		Patient Instruction	
Stage 1	2–3 weeks	◆ MLD daily ◆ Short-stretch bandages ◆ Skin care ◆ Decongestive exercises ◆ Patient instruction	◆ MLD if necessary ◆ Compression garments ◆ Skin care ◆ Decongestive exercises
Stage 2	3–4 weeks	◆ MLD daily ◆ Short-stretch bandages ◆ Skin care ◆ Decongestive exercises ◆ Patient instruction	◆ MLD as needed ◆ Compression garments ◆ Bandages at night ◆ Skin care ◆ Decongestive exercises ◆ Repeat phase I if necessary
Stage 3	4–6 weeks	◆ MLD daily ◆ Short-stretch bandages ◆ Skin care ◆ Decongestive exercises ◆ Patient instruction	◆ MLD as needed ◆ Compression garments (if necessary in combination with bandages) ◆ Bandages at night ◆ Skin care ◆ Decongestive exercises ◆ Repeat phase I if necessary ◆ Plastic surgery (if indicated)

CDT, complete decongestive therapy; MLD, manual lymph drainage

The meaning of the word *massage* is "to knead" and is used to describe forms of "classic" or "Swedish" massage, to include such techniques as effleurage, petrissage, tapotement, vibration, and friction.

The word *massage* is frequently misused to describe the techniques of manual lymph drainage (see Chapter 4). MLD includes no kneading elements in its strokes and has nothing in common with traditional massage techniques.

> Traditional massage can have negative effects on lymphedema, including active hyperemia, due to the release of histamine from mast cells in skin areas where those techniques are applied.

Active hyperemia results in an increase of blood capillary pressure and a subsequent increase in capillary filtration. This results in more water accumulating in the interstitial spaces, overloading an already stressed or impaired lymphatic system.

Superficial lymphatics are vulnerable to external pressure. Traditional massage techniques can cause focal damage on anchoring filaments and the endothelial lining of lymph vessels. Massage techniques also increase the lymphatic load of water (and often cells) and may further decrease the transport capacity of the lymphatic system by causing additional damage to lymph vessels. The application of traditional massage is therefore contraindicated in extremities (and their ipsilateral trunk quadrants) at risk for lymphedema and in extremities affected by lymphedema.

Thermo Therapy

Ice, heat, thermal ultrasound, hydrotherapy (hot packs), saunas, contrast baths, and paraffin are all contraindicated for the involved limb and the ipsilateral trunk quadrant in lymphedema management. Basic and advanced physiology identifies that active hyperemia occurs with any of the aforementioned modalities. Vasodilation increases blood capillary pressure, and in turn will increase the lymphatic load of water. Any modality that causes vasodilation to the involved limb, or "limb at risk," and/or ipsilateral trunk quadrant should be avoided.

Elevation

Simple elevation of an extremity affected by lymphedema may help reduce the swelling. This may be the case particularly in stage 1 lymphedema. If the lymphedematous limb decreases by elevation, the effect should be maintained by wearing appropriate compression garments.

Pneumatic Compression Pump

The use of pumps for lymphedema management and decongestion continues to be a topic of discussion. Compression pumps consist of either a single-chambered or a multichambered sleeve that uses rubber tubing to connect to a pump that moves compressed air into the sleeve. Single sleeves fill uniformly, whereas multichambered sleeves fill sequentially from distal to proximal. No particular pump appears to be more effective than another; newer versions of compression pumps offer on/off cycles with variation.

> Pumps are effective in removing water from the interstitial spaces, but they do not remove proteins. It must be stressed that the primary goal in lymphedema treatment is the removal of excess plasma proteins from the interstitial tissues (lymphedema is a high-protein edema). Proteins that remain in the tissues continue to attract fibroblasts and generate new connective tissue, which creates more scar tissue.

By reducing the water content in the lymphedematous limb, the extremity will initially become smaller with the application of pneumatic compression. However, if the interstitial water content is reduced, but the accumulated protein molecules remain in the tissue, the interstitial fluid colloid osmotic pressure (COP_{IP}) increases. This will result in more water leaving the blood capillaries, exacerbating the swelling.

There are several disadvantages of compression pump therapy for lymphedema management:

◆ Remaining/intact functioning lymph collectors may be destroyed.
◆ Trunk quadrants previously not swollen may fill with fluid.
◆ External genitalia may swell.
◆ Moves water from the distal to the proximal extremity, where it accumulates.
◆ Moves water but not protein.
◆ Pumps have no effect on softening of fibrotic tissue and may worsen fibrosis.
◆ Application time is long and questionable (minimum of 4 hours; some protocols suggest 8).
◆ Patients are immobile during pump sessions.
◆ No standardized settings.

In 2002, Segers et al investigated multichambered pumps to determine if the pressure set on the dial was the actual pressure produced by the chamber on the skin. The authors found that even though the dial was set at 30, 60, 80, and 100 mmHg, respectively, the pressure applied to the skin in each chamber actually reached 54, 98, 121, and 141 mmHg.

Boris, Weindorf, and Lasinski in 1998 performed a retrospective analysis and found that 53 of 128 lower extremity lymphedema patients used a compression pump during their course of treatment for lymphedema. It was not stated if the pump was used during the initial decongestive stages of therapy, but the authors noted that 23 of the 53 patients who used the pump developed genital edema and that only 2 of the 75 patients who did not receive pump therapy experienced genital edema. This study concluded that the "incidence of genital edema after pump therapy was unaffected by age, sex, grade or duration of lymphedema, whether lymphedema was primary or secondary, whether a single or sequential pump was used, the pressure level applied or duration or hours per day of pump therapy. Compressive pump therapy for lower limb lymphedema produces an unacceptably high incidence of genital edema."

In 2001, Miranda et al performed a prospective, blind study protocol with sequential intermittent pneumatic compression (SIPC). The study evaluated 11 patients who underwent an isotope lymphography before SIPC and 48 hours following a 3-hour session of SIPC. Measuring the lower extremities at six designated points revealed there was a significant reduction of circumference after SIPC below the knee, but not in the thigh. Conclusion: "Compression increased transport of lymph fluid (e.g., water) without comparable transport of macromolecules (e.g., protein). Alternatively, SIPC reduced lymphedema by decreasing blood capillary filtration rather than by accelerating lymph return, thereby restoring the balance in lymph kinetics responsible for edema in the first place."

Some patients who attempt to use pneumatic compression eventually realize the transitory or limited benefits and discontinue its use. A survey conducted by the Greater Boston Lymphedema Support Group in 1998 revealed that 48 (78%) of their 56 members who had used a pump discontinued the pump for the following reasons: negative effects caused by pumping, no further results were gained, pain or soreness increased in adjacent areas to the involved limb, swelling of previously uninvolved areas began, and/or negative impact on lifestyle.

At the 1993 International Congress of Lymphology, it was determined that, if pumps were used at all, the adjacent trunk area and base of the involved limb should be cleared first using CDT.

Pumps were first manufactured and used in Germany, where they were advertised as a "modern alternative for manual lymph drainage." After some time it became evident that the swelling in lymphedema worsened with the sole use of pumps in the treatment of lymphedema. Today, pump manufacturers in Germany (basically the same models as those used in the United States) include in their brochures that "in primary and secondary lymphedema, the device can only be used in combination with manual lymph drainage." The use of pneumatic compression pumps is not reimbursed by health insurance in Germany.

Pneumatic compression pumps should be used, if used at all, only in combination with complete decongestive therapy.

Nutritional Aspects

There is no special diet for lymphedema. There are also no vitamins, food supplements, or herbs that have been proven to be effective in the reduction of lymphedema. In the United States, dietary supplements are regulated as food, not drugs. Premarket approval by the Food and Drug Administration (FDA) is not required unless specific disease prevention or treatment claims are made. Because there is no requirement to review dietary supplements for manufacturing consistency, and no specific standards for dosage or purity exist, there may be considerable variation from lot to lot for all products marketed as dietary supplements. Patients with lymphedema willing to experiment with these products should consult with their physician and/or lymphedema therapist and use common sense and caution, especially if these products are taken in large quantities.

> It is important to understand that lymphedema cannot be reduced by the limitation of protein ingestion. An accepted approach is to follow a low-salt, low-fat diet, which positively contributes to weight control. It is also important not to limit fluid intake. Good hydration (water) is essential for basic cell function.

As discussed earlier, obesity generally worsens the symptoms of lymphedema.

Medication

◆ **Diuretics.** Most experts agree that the use of diuretics in the management of uncomplicated lymphedema is ineffective and may lead to the worsening of symptoms. Diuretics are able to remove the water content of the edema, while the protein molecules remain in the tissue spaces. These proteins continue to draw water to the edematous area as soon as the drug loses its effectiveness. Diuretics result in a higher concentration of proteins in the edema fluid and may cause the tissue to become more fibrotic.

The 2003 Consensus Document of the International Society of Lymphology states:

"Diuretic agents are occasionally useful during the initial treatment phase of CDT. Long-term administration of diuretics, however, is discouraged for it is of marginal benefit in treatment of peripheral lymphedema and potentially may induce fluid and electrolyte imbalance. Diuretics may be helpful to treat effusions in body cavities (e.g., ascites, hydrothorax) and with protein-losing enteropathy. Patients with peripheral lymphedema from malignant lymphatic blockage may also derive benefit from a short course of diuretic drug treatment."

Diuretics are also indicated in those cases where lymphedema is associated with other conditions that necessitate the application of these drugs.

◆ **Benzopyrones.** These drugs include coumarin and flavonoids and have been shown to stimulate macrophage activity and to promote the breakdown of proteins in the lymph fluid. The limited beneficial effects in reduction of some symptoms associated with lymphedema manifests so slowly that their practical usefulness is questionable. It may take 6 months or longer for the drugs to show some effects. Benzopyrones have been used in Australia and Europe since the 1980s, but they do not have FDA approval for use in the United States.

The 2003 Consensus Document of the International Society of Lymphology states:

"Oral benzopyrones, which are thought to hydrolize tissue proteins and facilitate their absorption while stimulating lymphatic collectors, are neither an alternative nor substitute for CDT. The exact role for benzopyrones as an adjunct in primary and secondary lymphedema treatment including filariasis is still not definitively determined, including appropriate formulations and dose regimens. Coumarin, one such benzopyrone, in higher doses has been linked to liver toxicity."

Surgery

The best summative statement about surgical attempts to "repair" the lymphatic system and surgical correction for lymphedema is from Goldsmith and De Los Santos (1967): "The large number of operations devised for improving lymphatic drainage from a chronically lymphedematous limb indicates the lack of a surgical procedure which is consistently effective." Various types of surgical repairs for the lymphatic system include lympholymphatic repair, lymphovenous repair, collector replacement, and enteromesenteric bridge, to name a few.

To date, the surgical attempts to increase the transport capacity of the lymphatic system have failed. Földi asserts,

"The use of prosthetic material (e.g., nylon threads) with hopes of re-establishing lymph flow simply disregards the fact that the propulsive force of the lymph flow is furnished by the pulsation of the lymph angions. A blood vessel may readily be replaced by a tube because the heart pumps the blood through it, but there is no force that could propel lymph through an artificial, valve-less tube."

◆ **Debulking.** In debulking procedures, the excess skin and the subcutaneous tissue of the lymphedematous limb are surgically removed. Together with the tissue, the subcutaneous lymph vessels are also removed. This seriously interferes with any later attempt to treat the limb with CDT.

Debulking procedures do not prevent the reaccumulation of lymph fluid, and they do nothing to repair or improve the function of a compromised lymphatic system. Today, these operations are not as common as they were in the late 1980s and early 1990s. The surgical removal of excess skinfolds after successful decongestion of the swollen limb may be useful.

◆ **Liposuction.** Liposuction removes the suprafascial fatty tissues and destroys any remaining intact lymph collectors; lymphatic microcirculation is significantly disturbed. Lymphedema can still recur if the extra fatty deposits are removed.

The long-term effect of liposuction in patients with lymphedema is still an enigma.

Brorson supports the use of liposuction to correct a "physical and psychological handicap" for post–breast cancer patients. He advocates the use of liposuction combined with compression over the use of compression alone to reduce the size of the involved limb. Brorson notes that "liposuction does not improve lymphatic system function, but [it] did increase skin microcirculation."

Clinically, liposuction is considered a major surgery for some patients. It can be costly and very invasive. There are other, less invasive options with minimal to no side effects to effectively manage lymphedema.

◆ Chronic Venous and Lymphovenous Insufficiency

Definition of CVI

Chronic venous insufficiency (CVI) is an advanced stage of venous disease in which the veins and the muscle pump activity become incompetent, causing blood to pool in the legs and feet. The condition may be caused by repeated damage to the veins due to superficial (severe varicose veins) or deep venous pathology, or a variety of other vein-related conditions, such as the congenital absence of venous valves. CVI is characterized by an increased venous pressure during walking.

Venous insufficiencies directly affect the lymphatic system. Insufficient venous return results in an elevated blood capillary pressure, causing an increase in net filtrate. The lymphatic system reacts with its safety factor as an active edema protective mechanism.

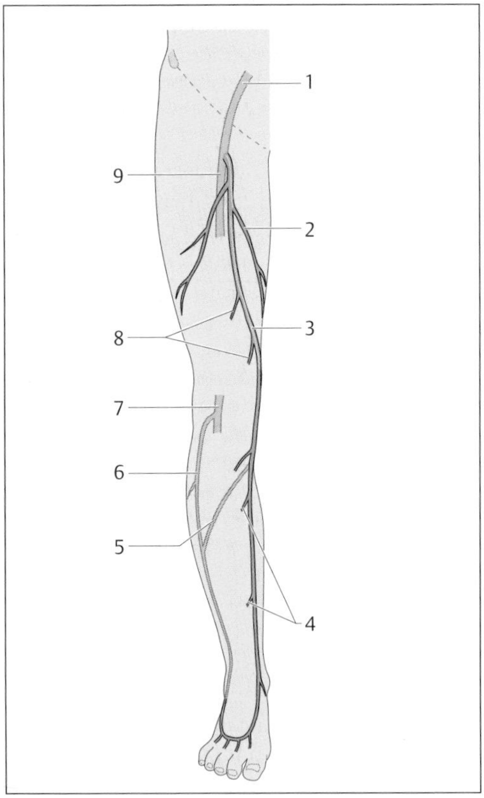

Post-thrombotic Syndrome

One of every three patients with deep venous thrombosis (DVT) in the lower extremities or the pelvic area will develop post-thrombotic sequelae within 5 years. Most episodes of post-thrombotic syndrome will occur within 2 years of the thrombosis. Individuals who have had thrombosis more than once (recurrent thrombosis) are at higher risk for post-thrombotic syndrome (PTS).

PTS is one of the most common causes of CVI, and if therapeutic measures are not initiated in early stages, it is characterized by edema, pigmentation, superficial varicosis, lipodermatosclerosis, ulceration, and pain, especially after ambulation. The long-term effects of PTS are caused by deficient function of the venous valves. DVT typically occurs at the valvular section of the veins, causing irreversible damage and/or obstruction of the deep veins with ambulatory venous hypertension (see Pathophysiology of CVI later in this chapter)

Venous Dynamics in the Lower Extremities

As with the lymphatic system, the venous system is divided into a superficial (cutaneous) and deep layer, both separated by fascia. The superficial layer communicates with the deep veins, which usually accompany deep arteries, by veins perforating the fascia (perforating veins). A major part of the blood volume, ~60%, is contained within the venous system, and for this reason veins are sometimes referred to as capacity vessels (Fig. 3–23).

Venous return to the heart occurs along relatively small pressure gradients. As explained in Chapter 2, Heart and Circulation, the blood pressure value decreases continuously between the arterial and the venous end of the systemic circulation. In the veins near the heart, the pressure amounts to only 1.5 to

◁ **Figure 3–23**   Superficial and deep veins on the lower extremity. 1. External iliac vein; 2. Accessory saphenous vein; 3. Great saphenous vein; 4. Perforating veins; 5. Transverse connection; 6. Small saphenous vein; 7. Popliteal vein; 8. Perforating veins; 9. Femoral vein.

4 mmHg. The effect of gravity additionally retards venous return.

A sufficient venous return from the lower extremities would not be possible without the help of the muscle and joint pumps (primarily the calf musculature), diaphragmatic breathing, the suction effect of the heart during the diastole, and the pulsation of adjacent arteries enclosed by the same sheath. Together with a functioning valvular system, which prevents retrograde flow, these supporting mechanisms propel the blood within the deep venous system back to the heart. During the relaxation phase of the muscle pump, venous blood from the superficial system reaches the deep veins via the perforating veins.

The normal blood pressure value in venous vessels on the foot amounts to ~10 mmHg in the supine position. When upright and standing motionless (orthostasis), the thin-walled veins dilate, and due to the hydrostatic pressure of the column of blood in the veins below the level of the heart, blood will collect or pool in the feet and legs. The pressure in the foot veins will subsequently increase to ~100 mmHg. During ambulation, pooling is avoided by the muscle and joint pumps, which help propel the venous blood back to the heart. The venous pressure in the same veins on the foot will decrease during ambulation by 70% to roughly 30 mmHg, provided the valves are sufficient.

Pathophysiology of CVI

The deficient venous valves in CVI fail to prevent retrograde flow of venous blood during muscle pump activity. In the ambulatory phase, the muscle pump forces the venous blood in the deep veins not only toward proximal but also toward distal and via the perforating veins into the superficial venous system (*blow-out syndrome*). This condition is called *ambulatory venous hypertension*, which is thought to cause CVI by the following sequence of events: Increased venous pressure transcends the venules to the capillaries, impeding the flow rate. Low-flow states within the blood capillaries cause leukocyte trapping. Trapped leukocytes release proteolytic enzymes and oxygen free radicals, which damage capillary basement membranes. Plasma proteins, such as fibrinogen, leak into the sur-

rounding tissues, forming a fibrin cuff. Interstitial fibrin and resultant edema decrease oxygen delivery to the tissues, resulting in local hypoxia with possible subsequent inflammation and tissue necrosis. High intracapillary pressure causes blood capillary endothelial cells to be stretched away from each other (*stretched-pore phenomenon*). Erythrocytes subsequently leave the blood capillaries, causing the skin to become reddish brown due to hemosiderin deposits.

Effects of CVI on the Lymphatic System

Ambulatory venous hypertension and the subsequent increase in blood capillary pressure results in an increase in net filtration. By activation of its safety factor, the lymphatic system is able to drain the additional amount of water (and protein) for some time. However, without adequate treatment (elevation, compression), the lymphatic system will eventually develop a dynamic insufficiency with subsequent edema, which in most cases will initially recede with elevation and rest.

Over time and without treatment, damage to the lymphatic system, combined with reduction in transport capacity, is unavoidable. The lymphatic system may develop a mechanical insufficiency caused by the constant strain. Due to high intralymphatic pressure and subsequent seepage of proteins into the wall structure, the walls of the lymph angions become fibrotic (mural insufficiency). In addition, the inflammatory process in the deep venous structures may involve adjacent lymph vessels, further reducing the transport capacity.

This condition, described in Chapter 2, Combined Insufficiency (reduced transport capacity in combination with an increase in lymphatic loads), has serious consequences and contributes to the signs and symptoms of CVI described in the following section.

Stages of CVI

Without treatment, the symptoms associated with chronic venous insufficiency and ambulatory venous hypertension will gradually worsen, and the condition will progress through the following stages (Table 3–6).

Table 3–6 Stages of Chronic Venous Insufficiency and Therapeutic Approach

Stage	Symptoms	Effects on the Superficial Lymphatic System				Therapeutic Approach
		Lymphatic Load of Water	Lymphatic Load of Protein	Status Lymph Vessels	Pathology Lymph Vessels	
O	None	High	Normal	Normal	LTV increased, lymphatic safety factor	Compression therapy, elevation, exercises
I	Mild (edema)	High	Normal	Normal	Phlebolympho-dynamic insuffi-ciency	Compression therapy, elevation, exercises
II	Moderate (pigmentation, varicosis, pain)	High	High	Morpho-logical changes	TC reduced, phlebolympho-static insuffi-ciency	CDT
III	Severe (hypoxia, necrosis, pain)	High	Very high	Morpho-logical changes	TC reduced, severe phle-bolymphostatic insufficiency	CDT and wound care

CDT, complete decongestive therapy; LTV, lymph time volume; TC, transport capacity

Subclinical Stage (Stage 0)

The lymphatic system activates its safety factor as an active edema protective mechanism. It responds to an increase in lymphatic load of water with an increase in lymph formation on the lymph capillary level and with an elevated contraction frequency in lymph collectors and trunks.

> As long as the healthy lymphatic system is able to compensate for the increase in lymphatic load of water resulting from venous hypertension, passive vasodilation, and subsequent increase in net filtrate, the individual remains free of edema.

Stage 1

The lymphatic system is still healthy but fails to drain the elevated lymphatic water load. Edema develops during the course of the day as a result of dynamic insufficiency of the lymphatic system. This stage is also referred to in the literature as *phlebolymphodynamic insuffi-ciency*. Initially, the swelling tends to decrease

or completely recede during rest at night. Venous pressure and net filtrate return to normal values in the supine position, providing the lymphatic system with a chance to "catch up" with the excess water in the interstitial tissue.

Stage 2

Blood capillaries and lymph collectors with elevated pressure values that remain without treatment for extended periods of time will eventually suffer damage as described in the section Pathophysiology of CVI. The combination of this damage and possible inflammatory processes causes the lymphatic system to develop a mechanical insufficiency, which, with the elevated loads of water and protein, presents as a combined insufficiency. Lymphedema will develop as a result of the venous pathology, and its symptoms are exacerbated by the symptoms associated with CVI (varicosis, pigmentation, pain). Stage 2 of CVI (CVI and lymphedema) is also referred to in the literature as *phlebolymphostatic insufficiency*.

The lymphedema in the early stage appears initially smooth and is pitting. Without treatment it will progress into a more fibrotic stage (see Stages of Lymphedema previously in this chapter). Regardless of genesis, lymphedema is always a progressive condition.

Stage 3

Typical for this stage are severe changes in the skin associated with the phlebolymphostatic edema. The interstitial fibrin cuff that forms as a result of plasma protein leakage in combination with the increased diffusion distance associated with the swelling decreases oxygen and nutrient delivery to the tissues. This results in local hypoxia and necrosis. Also typical for this stage is *lipodermatosclerosis*. These characteristic skin changes in the lower extremities include capillary proliferation, fat necrosis, and fibrosis of skin and subcutaneous tissues. Pain, especially after ambulation, is present.

Lymphedema resulting from prolonged CVI may show signs and symptoms of elephantiasis. It is important to understand that extremity volume is not considered within the different stages of lymphedema (and phlebolymphedema; see also Grading of Lymphedema Based on Severity previously in this chapter).

> Ulcerations, pigmentation, varicosis, lipodermatosclerosis, and pain may develop in extremities that show minimal swelling.

Complications

The elevated venous pressure in CVI, as well as the delayed clearance of venous blood from the legs, produces a high risk of recurrent thrombophlebitis. Blood clots in the deep veins of the legs are dangerous because they can break free and travel to the lungs. This problem, called pulmonary embolism (PE), can be fatal. It is important that patients and therapists understand the signs and symptoms of pulmonary embolism. Should those signs present, the individual must contact a doctor immediately (see Thrombophlebitis in Deep Veins later in this chapter).

Thrombophlebitis in Superficial Veins

Thrombophlebitis is a blood clot that forms at a certain point in a superficial vein due to irri-

tation or injury to the vein at that point. For example, thrombophlebitis may occur in a vein after an intravenous injection or infusion has been given in that vein. It also may occur as a result of irritation to a varicose vein.

> Symptoms of thrombophlebitis include redness, swelling, and heat in the area of the vein that has been irritated or injured. A vein close to the surface of the skin may appear more noticeable than usual or may feel like a hard piece of rope or cord upon palpation. Pain or discomfort over the involved area as well as fever may be present.

Treatment options for thrombophlebitis may include anti-inflammatory medication (non-steroidal), antibiotics if an infection of the vein is involved, rest and elevation of the extremity, and the application of moist, warm compresses in the involved area. If lymphedema is associated with thrombophlebitis, the application of warm compresses may supersede the possibility of active hyperemia (vasodilation) and its negative effects on lymphedematous tissue; however, caution should be taken.

Because the blood clot that forms usually stays stuck to the wall of the vein, thrombophlebitis in the superficial veins in most cases is not considered to be a serious condition unless an infection develops. The body will gradually absorb the blood clot as the thrombophlebitis clears up over a period of 1 to 2 weeks. On occasion, however, the blood clot that occurs as a result of thrombophlebitis can contribute to the development of a larger blood clot extending into one of the subfascial veins. This is a more serious condition because the blood clot or a piece of the blood clot in a deep vein may break off and travel to the lungs, causing pulmonary embolism.

Thrombophlebitis in Deep Veins

In deep venous thrombosis, a blood clot forms in a subfascial vein. These clots most often occur as a result of poor or sluggish blood flow through the veins as in CVI, or sitting/standing for long periods of time without moving around, periods of prolonged bed rest, or wearing clothing that interferes with the blood flow. Blood clots may also form as a result of hypercoagulability of the blood (recent surgery, liver

Chronic Venous and Lymphovenous Insufficiency

77

diseases, taking oral contraceptives, severe infections, etc.).

Symptoms of thrombophlebitis in deep veins on extremities include

◆ Redness, swelling, and heat in the area over the path of a deep vein

◆ A deep vein feeling like a hard piece of rope or cord

◆ Pain or discomfort over the path of a deep vein (usually in the middle of the calf)

◆ Discoloration or ulceration of the skin over a deep vein

◆ Pain in the involved extremity, which increases with coughing, sneezing, or pressing

◆ Cramps, which intensify over several days

Treatment options for thrombophlebitis in deep veins may include restricting activity if there is a danger of the clot traveling to the lungs, elevating the extremity, taking anticoagulants, and wearing compression garments. Patients should be careful not to rub the affected area as clots may be broken off or dislodged, causing pulmonary embolism.

Many patients with PE have a vague sense that something is wrong but have difficulty describing or defining the problem.

The most common warning signals of pulmonary embolism are

◆ Unexplained shortness of breath

◆ Chest discomfort, usually worse with deep breathing or coughing

◆ Anxiety or nervousness

◆ Lightheadedness or blacking out

> Should any sign or symptom of thrombophlebitis in the deep veins or symptoms of pulmonary embolism develop, the patient must see a doctor immediately, and any treatment must be interrupted until the condition is resolved.

Ulcerations

Venous stasis ulcers are the most common form of ulcerations and appear predominantly in the distal third of the lower extremity (usually around the malleoli). Ulcerations generally are persistent and are known to heal slowly (or not at all) if the surrounding environment is edematous. Ulcerations are also a frequent cause for infections in the swollen extremity.

The most important goals in the treatment of venous ulcers is to make sure that the wounds are clean (i.e., free of necrotic tissue, bacteria, yeast, and fungi), that exudate is absorbed while maintaining a moist wound base, and that a normal arterial and venous blood supply is reestablished (decongestion, no constrictive dressings).

Evaluation

The physician's assessment of venous reflux and/or venous occlusion generally consists of noninvasive tests, such as duplex ultrasonography. The evaluation in the lymphedema clinic includes history, inspection, and palpation, as described in Diagnosis and Evaluation of Lymphedema previously in this chapter.

A major issue in the evaluation of phlebolymphostatic edema is to check skin integrity. Compromised skin integrity requires additional padding under the compression bandage and meticulous skin care. If ulcerations are present, it is imperative to communicate with the patient's physician or wound specialist to synchronize dressing and wound care issues. It is often more productive if wound care is performed in the lymphedema clinic as part of the treatment protocol.

Therapists should carefully check for any signs and symptoms of superficial or deep thrombophlebitis.

Therapeutic Approach

Prevention

Knowing certain risk factors for venous thrombosis can greatly reduce the likelihood of developing DVT. Maintaining ideal body weight with a healthy nutritional program and exercise regimen, avoiding inactivity or immobility, or wearing support stockings and elevating the legs as often as possible reduces the risk of developing thrombosis. Patients on oral contraceptives who experience symptoms of venous insufficiency should discuss alternatives with the physician due to an elevated risk for DVT.

If signs and symptoms of CVI are present, it is important to prevent it from progressing through its stages by constantly wearing compression stockings prescribed by the physician and by performing meticulous skin care. In the early stages of CVI, it is sufficient to apply compression during the daytime only.

Complete Decongestive Therapy

If CVI remains without adequate treatment (in most cases, compression), the active and passive edema protective mechanisms (Chapter 2, Safety Factor of the Lymphatic System) of the body will not be able to compensate for the elevated levels of water resulting from ambulatory venous hypertension.

Patients with deficient function of the venous valves in postthrombotic syndrome without visible swelling (CVI stage 0) are able to avoid the clinical onset of swelling by the application of daily compression with either bandages or compression garments, provided the compression does not present a contraindication. (Refer to Chapter 4 for contraindications in compression therapy.) The application of cold water on the affected extremity and other noninvasive preventive measures described earlier also assist in preventing the onset of edema (Table 3–6).

If treatment starts in stage 1 of CVI, decongestion of the extremity by elevation precedes the application of compression bandages and/or garments. In some cases, a physician may choose a one-time application of a diuretic to decongest the limb. Because the lymphatic system is healthy (normal TC), although overwhelmed in this stage of the venous pathology, manual lymph drainage is not indicated.

> The presence of lymphedema in stages 2 and 3 of CVI necessitates the application of the complete spectrum of complete decongestive therapy, including manual lymph drainage. The goal of the therapy, as in the treatment of uncomplicated lymphedema, is to bring the lymphedema back to a stage of latency. Decongestion of the extremity greatly increases the tendency of venous stasis ulcers to heal.

The treatment protocol of the lymphedema associated with CVI corresponds with the protocol for primary lymphedema.

◆ Wounds and Skin Lesions
(by Teresa Conner-Kerr, P. T.)

Individuals with lymphedema may present with a variety of skin lesions. These lesions may be directly related to the dysfunctional lymph vascular system or to other comorbid conditions. They can result from trauma, allergies, or therapeutic procedures, such as surgery and radiotherapy. These lesions range from simple excoriations to complex wounds with multiple etiologies. Skin lesions in individuals with lymphedema may be classified according to the level of tissue involvement and state of the wound (i.e., acute or chronic).

Depending on the location of the dysfunctional lymphatics and coexisting morbidities, individuals may be at greater or lesser risk for particular lesion types. For example, individuals presenting with lower extremity lymphedema often copresent with venous insufficiency and are at increased risk for lesions related to extremity swelling. Likewise, individuals who have undergone mastectomy with concurrent radiotherapy are at risk for skin breakdown due to radiation burns. Lesions that occur in individuals with lymphedema due either to the disease process itself or to related conditions are listed in Table 3–7.

Skin Lesions Often Associated with Lymphedema

Vascular Ulcerations

It is estimated that as many as 3.2 million Americans have lower extremity ulcerations due to vascular insufficiency. Vascular ulcerations may result from arterial, venous, or lymphatic dysfunction or a combination thereof. Vascular ulcerations are most commonly observed in the lower extremity and are associated with long-term vascular compromise. Research indicates that 80 to 90% of these ulcerations have a venous etiology. The prevalence of venous ulceration is ~0.16, or 1% of the general population over 70 years of age; this rate of occurrence increases exponentially with age. The incidence of venous ulceration is also increased in females (62%).

In comparison, skin lesions due to arterial insufficiency account for ~5 to 20% of lower extremity ulcers, with as many as 15% of these

Table 3-7 Possible Skin Lesions with Lymphedema

Lesion Type	Characteristics		
	Wound Bed	**Location**	**Periwound**
Vascular			
Venous	Shallow, irregular	Anteromedial leg	Hemosiderin staining; scaly, weepy, warm skin
Arterial	Round, deep, necrotic, or pale base	Lateral leg/foot, tips of toes	Tissue pallor; dry, scaly skin; cool to the touch
Mixed	Characteristics of both venous and arterial lesions		
Inflammatory			
Vasculitis	Small, dark base	Anywhere; common malleolar area	Raised, palpable purpura
Pyoderma	Irregular, jagged necrotic base	Mostly leg or trunk	Violaceous wound border, erythema
Fungating	Raised, necrotic; bleeds easily; extremely malodorous	Anywhere; chest	Lip of tissue at wound margin
Radiation	Exposed dermis; superficial	Skin in treatment field	Erythema; dark black coloration
Minor trauma			
Excoriations	Linear, shallow	Anywhere	Local or advancing erythema
Skin sears	Shallow, linear flap	Arms, hands commonly	Ecchymosis
Failed surgical site	Partial or full thickness, necrotic base	Site of incision	Erythema, edema
Fistulas	Pathological openings between organs/body cavities and the skin	Site of abscess	Opening in wound beds presenting with drainage organs and tissue cavities

lesions having both an arterial and a venous component. Lesions due solely to lymphedema are poorly discussed in the literature. Other less commonly seen vascular ulcers include those with an underlying genetic or inflammatory etiology.

Venous Ulcerations

Venous ulcerations result from an insufficiency of the venous system, as described previously. They present most often on the anteromedial aspect of the lower leg and ankle, with a high preponderance immediately above the medial malleolus. These ulcerations are typically superficial in nature and are described clinically as being of partial thickness (down to but not through the dermis). Venous ulcers have irregular borders and exhibit moderate to heavy exudate. The wound bed often has a ruddy or granular surface that is dull red in appearance. The wound bed is also commonly covered with yellow and/or grayish white slough. Black eschar or necrosis may also be present in the wound. Venous wounds often have strong odors that can be described as foul or putrid. These odors are a result of high numbers of bacteria found in necrotic tissue.

Due to the accumulation of blood vascular fluids in the surrounding tissues and the presence of chronic inflammation, the periwound area as well as the entire lower limb typically presents with an increased temperature upon palpation. Other periwound characteristics include scaly skin and loss of skin appendages (hair, glands), with microulcerations or pinpoint openings that allow the passage of accumulated tissue fluids to the skin surface. The skin will often appear to be "weeping." The periwound area both immediately adjacent to and at varied distances from the wound bed is usually discolored (blue-purple or brown-black staining) due to the deposition of iron (hemosiderin staining). Hemosiderin staining results from the deposition of iron into the interstitial tissue spaces upon lysis of extravasated red blood cells.

◆ **Therapeutic Approach.** The key to successful treatment of wounds that result from the chronic accumulation of interstitial fluids such as that observed with venous insufficiency or lymphedema is reduction or clearance of the swollen tissues. Manual techniques such as MLD, along with the application of short-stretch bandaging for initial reduction of chronic fluid accumulation, followed by maintenance therapy with a compression garment, are necessary for clinical success. However, vascular status should be determined prior to any addition of compression therapy so that ischemic limbs are not treated inadvertently (see Arterial Ulcerations following here). If an active wound is present, advanced dressing technologies with sufficient fluid handling characteristics should be utilized to control exudates and facilitate autolysis of necrotic tissue. Enzymatic preparations may also assist with necrotic tissue reduction and facilitate wound healing. Newer antiseptic technologies that utilize slow-release iodine or silver preparations will help control wound bioburden, thus reducing malodor and enhancing wound closure. Charcoal-based dressings may also be applied over primary dressing to assist with odor control. Exercises that stimulate the muscle pumps also hasten reduction of tissue edema and enhance wound healing.

Arterial Ulcerations

Arterial or ischemic ulcerations also commonly present on the lower extremity but differ significantly in character from venous ulcerations. Arterial ulcerations typically are deep with even wound margins. They are located predominantly on the lateral side of the leg or foot, with lesions also occurring over the tips of the toes, between the toes, and over the phalangeal heads. The wound base is usually pale pink in coloration due to ischemic conditions. Arterial ulcers are most often dry and covered by a thickened black eschar. The periwound skin is thin, dry, and scaling, with an overt loss of skin appendages such as hair, sweat, and sebaceous glands because of tissue ischemia. The skin is blanched, especially with elevation of the limb, or purpuric when in a dependent position. Depending on the severity and extent of tissue ischemia, muscle and fat atrophy may also be present. Toenails are also usually dystrophic due to fungal infection.

◆ **Therapeutic Approach.** The key to successful treatment of ischemic wounds is revascularization. Revascularization can be achieved through graded exercise programs, medication, surgery, or a combination thereof. Prior to the initiation of therapy, vascular status of the involved tissues should be established. Without adequate blood flow, arterial wounds simply will not heal. Graded exercise programs have been shown to be successful in facilitating revascularization of an ischemic limb through induction of collateralization. Likewise, some success has been obtained with the use of the antiplatelet medication Pletal or Cilostazol. The therapeutic indication for Pletal is reduction of claudication or exercise pain related to tissue ischemia. Research has shown that walking distances and ankle/brachial indexes improve with Pletal therapy. Other interventions include percutaneous transluminal angioplasty, which entails introduction of a balloon-tipped catheter into a blocked artery for stretching the vessel wall and/or flattening plaques with subsequent placement of a stent to maintain vessel patency. Bypass grafting procedures may also be selected if the individual is not a candidate for the above therapies.

Noninvasive vascular tests can provide extremely useful data on the vascular status of individuals presenting with signs and symptoms of arterial insufficiency. These tests can be performed by most clinicians and do not require extensive equipment or space. Common noninvasive vascular testing involves obtaining peripheral pulses, ankle/brachial index, toe pressures, and transcutaneous oxygen pressures ($TcpO_2$). In the lower extremity, the femoral, popliteal, dorsalis pedis, and posterior tibial arteries should be evaluated via examination of pulses. Examination via Doppler ultrasound can give a more accurate picture because pulses may be difficult to detect in either an ischemic or a swollen limb. A variety of scales exist to rate the pulses. An example of these scales follows.

0 = no pulse
1+ = very shallow
2+ = decreased
3+ = normal
4+ = bounding

Toe pressures (systolic pressure of digital arteries) and local $TcpO_2$ (oxygen levels in the blood adjacent to the lesion) are useful as toe pressures less than 20 mmHg and TcpO$_2$ of less than 40 mmHg are associated with poor healing in lower extremity wounds. An ankle/brachial index (ABI) of less than 80 is also indicative of poor healing of lower extremity ulcerations.

An ABI is useful because it gives a picture of systolic blood pressure in the lower limb. The systolic blood pressure is determined at the brachial artery on the same side as the wounded lower limb. Both the systolic pressure from the dorsalis pedis and the posterior tibial artery should be used separately to calculate the ABI because they give a clinical picture of different regions of the lower limb and foot (see Chapter 4, Contraindications for Compression Therapy).

Systolic ankle pressures of less than 80 mmHg, along with toe pressures of less than 20 mmHg and TcpO$_2$ of less than 40 mmHg, are associated with poor healing.

Arterial ulcers that present with a stable, dry, adherent eschar on a distal extremity should not be disturbed unless an area of wet necrosis is detected. Ulcers with stable, dry eschars may heal by reepithelialization beneath the hardened eschar. A conservative approach to treatment of these intact eschars is warranted due to their poor prognosis for healing and the risks of infection and subsequent limb loss. On the other hand, wet necrosis can become rapidly infected in ischemic tissue due to poor immune surveillance. In this case, the wet necrosis should be removed as quickly as possible through either surgical or sharp debridement. As with venous ulcers, several advanced wound dressings with topical antiseptics are available along with the necessity of systemic therapy. When the wet necrosis has been effectively reduced, hydration of the wound bed may be necessary to facilitate wound closure. Moisture balance in a wet, necrotic arterial wound requires different interventions than a dry, clean wound bed. Hydration of desiccated wound bed tissues is required for cellular migration and subsequent wound closure. Hydrogels, amorphous or sheet, can provide the moisture required for wound healing processes to occur.

Vascular/Inflammatory Ulcerations

Although arterial and venous insufficiency ulcerations are the most commonly recognized vascular ulcers, other types do occur. These ulcerations are often painful and difficult to heal. Vascular ulcers that fall into this category include those associated with vasculitis of small or large vessels, pyoderma gangrenosum, and sickle cell anemia.

◆ **Vasculitis.** Vasculitis or angiitis of both small and large blood vessels is characterized by the onset of necrotizing inflammation with the subsequent necrosis of blood vessel walls. Evidence of this process is manifested in the development of skin lesions or ulcerations. Small vessel vasculitis involves the arterioles, capillaries, and venules. Clinical signs of small vessel vasculitis include urticaria, a palpable purpura (small red lesion or papule that does not blanch with pressure), and the development of nodules, bullae, or ulcers. Small vessel vasculitis is often associated with hypersensitivity disorders, Henoch-Schönlein purpura (self-limited inflammation of the vascular system), cryoglobulinemia (accumulation and precipitation of abnormal proteins-cryoglobulins in the blood vascular system), serum sickness (immunologic reaction to the administration of an antiserum), chronic urticaria (chronic itching due to an allergic response), connective tissue diseases, certain malignancies, and hepatitis type B infection. In comparison, large vessel vasculitis involves the small and medium-sized muscular arteries. Clinical signs of large vessel vasculitis include subcutaneous nodules, ulcers, and ecchymosis. Diseases associated with the onset of large vessel vasculitis include polyarteritis nodosa (a severe collagen-vascular disease associated with widespread inflammation of the small and medium-sized muscular arteries), Churg-Strauss syndrome (vasculitis associated with subcutaneous nodule formation and abnormal cellular changes), and giant cell arteritis (chronic inflammation of the small and medium-sized muscular arteries associated with abnormal cellular changes).

◆ **Therapeutic Approach.** Because vasculitic lesions are the result of inflammatory processes, anti-inflammatory or immunosuppressive therapies are required. Sharp debridement should not be used because it often leads to a worsening of the ulcerations. Autolytic or enzymatic debridement provides a gentler and more successful intervention. As with other wounds, bacterial numbers need to be controlled and exudate levels need to be balanced for healing to occur. Therefore, absorbent dressings that do not produce additional trauma to the wound upon removal are recommended. Any product applied to the wound or skin should also be free of common skin sensitizers as is true for most other wound types, particularly venous. Common skin sensitizers include lanolin, balsam of Peru, cetylsterol alcohol, parabens, rosins, latex, and neomycin.

◆ **Pyoderma Gangrenosum.** Another inflammatory condition that involves the skin and vascular system that can culminate in skin ulcerations is pyoderma gangrenosum (PG). PG is a chronic inflammatory disorder of unknown etiology that often evolves from a folliculitis and/or abscess. It may also be associated with a vasculitic condition. PG is associated with the following systemic diseases: inflammatory bowel syndrome, rheumatoid arthritis, systemic lupus erythematosus, AIDS, chronic active hepatitis among others. Lesions are typically found on the lower extremity but may occur elsewhere such as the thigh and trunk. Initially, Pyoderma gangrenosum begins as small, red, sensitive lesions. These lesions may present either as macules, papules, pustules, nodules, or bulla. As the lesion grows in size, the perilesion skin becomes dusky red and indurated. As the inflammatory process that underlies these lesions progresses, purulent, necrotic ulceration(s) develop with irregular, raised purple/red wound margins and an intense periwound erythema.

◆ **Therapeutic Approach.** Pyoderma gangrenosum can be one of the more challenging types of ulcers to treat. Response to therapy can be unpredictable and variable. However, similar to vasculitis, anti-inflammatory and immunosuppressive agents are used to control the underlying chronic inflammatory processes. As with the vasculitic lesion, additional trauma should be avoided. Autolytic and enzymatic debridements are preferred along with nontraumatic cleansing and dressing changes.

Exudate and pain control measures are also necessary with pyoderma gangrenosum wounds.

◆ **Sickle Cell Anemia.** An additional condition related to the vascular system that also results in the formation of ulcerations is sickle cell anemia. Sickle cell anemia, an incurable hemoglobinopathic or hemolytic anemia that occurs in individuals who produce an abnormal hemoglobin (S type), results in an alteration of the shape of red blood cells (RBCs) from the normal biconcave disk to a sickle shape. Because of this shape alteration, the RBCs become trapped in capillary beds of peripheral tissues such as skin and subsequently undergo cellular lysis. This premature destruction of red blood cells leads to a reduction of the overall oxygen-carrying capacity of the blood. As a result, tissues develop a hypoxic ischemia. Ulcerations are painful and tend to produce clinical signs similar to those of both arterial and venous insufficiency wounds.

Fungating Wounds/Malignant Ulcerations

Fungating ulcers evolve as a result of a malignant tumor invading the skin or a chronic ulcer site. These ulcers can develop either quite rapidly or over a more gradual course. Rapid onset or change in the wound bed is often associated with disease progression. When the disease is progressing more rapidly, physical changes are detectable on a daily basis. Another characteristic of fungating wounds is the exuberant development of capillaries in the wound bed. Because of this excessive formation of capillary beds in the wound base and the concomitant deficiency in platelets, the wound is often quite friable. This rapid and excessive formation of blood capillary beds is also associated with focal areas of necrosis. Other characteristics of fungating ulcers include extreme malodor due to tissue necrosis and infection and a distinct lip of tissue around the wound margin. Fungating wounds may also be associated with fistula development. Fistulas or passages from internal cavities and organs to the skin may occur in areas where malignant tumors give rise to fungating skin lesions. Retrograde drainage from the wound may lead to sepsis; likewise, drainage from internal organs may be carried into the ulcer.

◆ **Therapeutic Approach.** One of the hallmarks of a fungating lesion is malodor. Quality of life for the individual and family is certainly affected by this issue. Frequent wound cleansing, removal of necrotic tissue, and control of bacterial content and exudate levels are paramount to decreasing wound odor. However, depending on the size of the lesion, this can be a monumental task. Charcoal secondary dressings and topical antimicrobials such as metronidazole or antiseptic dressings that employ ionized silver or slow-release iodine provide some benefit. Wound cleansing with pulsatile lavage with suction, a power spray that is applied under pressure in a pulsatile fashion with concomitant aspiration of the delivered fluid on low settings, may also be indicated, depending on risk of further metastasis.

Radiation-Related Skin Changes

Acute skin reactions to radiotherapy may be mild to severe. Because radiotherapy targets rapidly dividing cells, the epidermis is at risk for damage due to an intrinsically high rate of cellular proliferation. Skin reactions are related to the dose and dosing schedule, location, total treatment area, radiation type, and individual skin differences. The appearance of radiation-induced skin changes is variable and may present in days or be delayed for months or years postexposure. Skin reactions to radiation can be divided into four categories that include erythema, dry desquamation, moist desquamation, and necrosis.

Necrosis, the most severe response of the skin to radiotherapy, results in severe discoloration of the skin with the development of a nonhealing, necrotic ulcer. In contrast, the mildest form of reaction is the development of an erythema with concurrent epidermal edema. Successive levels of damage include dry and moist desquamation. With dry desquamation, the epidermis begins to peel, as is evidenced by the presence of dry, scaly skin. Skin undergoing this reaction may either appear thin and atrophied if epidermal cells are not produced rapidly enough to replace dying and dead cells, or skin may take on a scaly appearance if new skin cells accumulate faster than dead ones can be shed. The third category of skin reaction that may occur is moist desquamation. Radiotherapy-related damage at this level leads to a robust erythema with subsequent loss of the epidermis and exposure of the dermis. This superficial, partial thickness lesion is associated with the production of exudates and an increased risk of infection. In addition, radiation-induced ulcers may be associated with fistula development, particularly in the area of an abscess.

◆ **Therapeutic Approach.** An acute inflammatory reaction may occur in skin over an area that has received radiotherapy. Skin areas that have undergone changes due to radiation and that are subject to trauma or moisture accumulation are at great risk for breakdown. Individuals should be educated about the risk for breakdown and encouraged to keep areas prone to excessive moisture buildup dry. Padding may be used to wick away moisture and to prevent injury due to frictional forces such as scrubbing by clothing. Maintaining a dry environment will also aid in preventing fungal infections. Areas that are prone to this excessive accumulation of moisture include the axillae and perineal area.

To maintain skin exposed to radiotherapy in the healthiest state possible, individuals should be encouraged to use mild soap for baths and to pat dry not to rub skin, as this may further traumatize tissue. Use of a basic skin cream that is free of sensitizers or allergens is also recommended so as to maintain skin hydration. Individuals should also be instructed to drink fluids, as this improves skin hydration.

Open skin areas that are dry may be treated effectively with amorphous or sheet hydrogels. Wounds that are producing excessive drainage may be treated effectively with alginates (sheets or ropes, depending on wound shape and depth), foams, or collagen-based wound dressings. Alginate or collagen-based dressings are also useful for establishing hemostasis, as these wounds are friable and hence prone to bleeding.

◆ **Minor Trauma.** Skin that is fragile due to aging, radiation treatment, chronic edema, lymphedema, and so on is at risk for traumatic injury. Minor traumatic injuries such as skin tears, excoriations, and erosions occur with everyday activities. Skin tears or excoriations result from mechanical injury that may result in either partial or full thickness injury. Because the synthesis of structural proteins and certain cellular organelles declines or becomes impaired with age or chronic disease, skin weakens and is more susceptible to mechanical injury. Excoriations typically are linear and shallow and result commonly from frictional forces such as scratching due to chronic irritation or medication-related side effects. Skin tears also are shallow in nature but may present either as a linear injury or as a skin flap that remains partially attached to the surrounding tissues.

◆ **Therapeutic Approach.** Employing several approaches may protect fragile skin. Hydration of the individual is prerequisite to maintaining the skin turgor. The dehydrated individual with dry skin appears to be at greater risk for skin tears. Use of creams rather than lotions will produce a longer lasting moisturizing effect. Arm pads, hydrocolloid, and thin film dressings also convey some level of protection from mechanical injury.

Excoriations can be prevented by use of oven mitts in the disoriented individual as well as encouraging fluid intake and the use of moisturizing cream. Frequency of baths may need to be decreased, as natural skin oils are stripped during bathing. Potential medication issues such as toxicity and side effects should be investigated.

Failed Surgical Sites

Failed closure of surgical incisions may be present due to debulking procedures, removal of tumor masses, implantation of medical devices, or removal of lines and tubes. Wounds that are left to heal by secondary intention may result from infiltration of intravenous lines, dehiscence of sutured incision sites post-removal of a tumor, or debulking of skin from an edematous limb. Closed incisional sites commonly fail due to infection or overwhelming mechanical stress that results from accumulation of fluids in the operated tissues. Additionally, failure or reopening of these sites can be associated with fistula development due to abscess formation. Fistulas due to deep tissue abscess allow organs or body cavities to communicate with the skin. As a result, wound exudate may drain to these deep areas, causing sepsis, or bodily fluids such as urine or fecal material may drain to the wound, causing tissue injury and malodor.

◆ **Therapeutic Approach.** Dehisced surgical wounds may involve large tissue areas and produce significant amounts of drainage. This excessive drainage may result from deep tissue abscess or fistulas. Because of the factors described above, dehisced surgical wounds often benefit from negative pressure wound therapy. Negative pressure wound therapy utilizes a vacuum to facilitate wound healing by drawing the wound together and reducing exudate levels and bacterial numbers in the wound tissues. Negative pressure therapy is also particularly useful in allowing early return to functional activities because the wound can be stabilized by the vacuum.

Wound Management/Wound Bed Preparation

Wound bed preparation is a relatively new term that describes the basic principles of effective wound management. The three primary principles of wound bed preparation are removal of necrotic tissue, bacterial control, and exudate management. Many of these principles have been referred to in the preceding therapeutic approach sections.

Wound Necrosis

Removal of necrosis is necessary for wound healing to occur. The presence of necrosis in the wound bed acts as a harbor for microorganisms and impedes cellular migration. Several methods exist for the removal of necrosis from the wound bed, and the selection of the appropriate method is based on individual characteristics such as health status, pain tolerance, necrosis type, and vascular status. Four primary methods of debridement: surgical or sharp, enzymatic, autolytic, and mechanical. Another category that is not included but that is seeing increased utilization is biotherapy or the use of chemically sterilized maggots. Sterilized maggots have the benefit of delivering the most selective debridement available.

Surgical or sharp debridement is the most rapid means of removing nonviable tissue. If large amounts of tissue need to be removed quickly and pain is an issue, then surgical debridement should be utilized. If the individual is not a candidate for surgery and cannot tolerate the pain associated with sharp debridement, then autolytic, enzymatic, or biotherapy-mediated debridement may be utilized. Of the enzymes available, the papain/urea-based enzymes have been shown to more quickly debride wounds. However, their rapid action is not without a drawback because these enzymes are associated with wound pain (burning upon application).

Mechanical debridement via pulsatile lavage for cleansing and removal of both large and small particulates may be used singly or in conjunction with the other debridement procedures. In fact, many of these procedures can be effectively mixed and matched. However, reimbursement is typically tied to only one procedure.

Bacterial Control

Bacterial control is another necessary component of advanced wound management. High wound bioburden may be a factor in nonhealing or chronic wounds and certainly is a major factor in the development of malodorous wounds. Currently, the definition of wound infection is being revised. Wound infection in the past has been defined as the presence of 10^5 organisms/gram of tissue. This definition is being revisited to include not only bacterial dose but also virulence of the microorganism and state of the host or individual's resistance. The relationship among these factors is described by the following equation:

$$\text{Risk of tissue infection} = \frac{\text{Bacterial dose} \times \text{Virulence}}{\text{Host resistance}}$$

The importance of the individual's immune response in fighting tissue infection and the virulence of the offending organism must be fully considered. The above equation points to the fact that the presence of a small number of organisms that are highly virulent may produce a tissue infection in a normal individual just as a high number of relatively nonvirulent organisms may produce infection in an immunocompromised individual. Other factors such as tissue anoxia and impaired circulation also play a role in determining host resistance and as such are important in individuals with conditions such as peripheral vascular disease, diabetes, lymphedema, and venous insufficiency, just to name a few.

When tissue infection is suspected, the clinician is faced with confirming the diagnosis. The value of culturing wounds versus the use of clinical signs and symptoms in diagnosing wound infection is undergoing serious study. Research indicates that the following signs of local infection are good predictors of localized infection: delayed healing, wound bed color changes, friable granulation tissue, absence or aberrant granulation tissue, strong odor, increased drainage, and increased wound tissue pain. The role of the wound culturing methods biopsy and swab are also being debated, and evolving thought indicates that both may be useful, especially in determining the best antibiotic for spreading tissue infection.

Individuals with lymphedema are at increased risk for cellulitis or acute tissue infection due to tissue hypoxia and a compromised immune system as the result of radiation or chemotherapy. *Streptococcus aureus* is commonly the offending wound pathogen. However, *S. pyogenes* often produces a more superficial form of cellulitis (erysipelas) that presents in the papillary or upper layer of the dermis. Individuals with lymphedema may be placed on penicillin prophylatically because of their propensity for erysipelas.

Other therapies that are useful in controlling wound infection either singly or in combination with antibiotic therapy for deeper infections include the newer antiseptic preparations described in the therapeutic approach sections, pulsatile lavage with suction, cold quartz ultraviolet (UVC), electrical stimulation, and topical antibiotics such as Bactroban Cream.

Moisture Balance

The third critical component of wound bed preparation is moisture balance. Wounds can be either too wet or too dry, so the challenge is to balance the moisture content at the appropriate level for optimizing healing. Wounds such as those that occur due to venous insufficiency and/or lymphatic dysfunction are typically wet in nature and require absorptive dressing with good fluid handling characteristics. A variety of dressings are available that can provide absorption, including foams, alginates, supra-absorbants, and combination dressings. These dressings have different abilities to contain and remove excess fluid from the wound bed while preventing maceration of the surrounding tissue. Vertically wicking dressings control wound exudates while protecting the periwound from excessive moisture. Additionally, using negative pressure therapy may effectively control large volumes of wound fluid.

◆ Lipedema

Lipedema is rarely discussed in medical textbooks. Many clinicians are unfamiliar with this condition, which is the reason why it is often misdiagnosed as bilateral primary lymphedema, extreme "cellulitis," or morbid obesity.

Definition

Allen and Hines first used the term *lipedema* in 1940.

> Lipedema is a chronic disease, which is marked by a bilateral and symmetrical swelling of the lower extremities, caused by extensive deposits of subcutaneous fatty tissue.

The proliferated adipose tissue is generally located between the iliac crest and the ankles; the feet are uninvolved. Flaps of fatty tissue overhang the ankles in many cases. Occasionally the upper extremities are affected, in which case the swelling extends to the wrist area; when the patient elevates the arm, a massive fold of fatty tissue is often visible on the posterior upper arm.

Lipedema almost exclusively affects females. According to the literature, it is usually associated with massive hormonal disorders or liver dysfunctions if present in males.

Etiology and Natural History

The underlying etiology of lipedema remains unknown; it is often associated with hormonal disorders and can be hereditary. In most cases, lipedema develops during puberty or a few years later.

Many younger patients try to reduce the fatty tissue associated with this condition by diet and athletic activities. For reasons unknown, it is not possible to significantly reduce the fatty tissue with these measures, which often results in frustration. Subsequently, the patients become more sedentary and start to put on weight. This often results in obesity, and the fatty tissue tends to become harder (liposclerosis). These changes, along with the fact that lipedema is often associated with venous disorders and other vascular diseases, may lead to the development of lymphedema (lipolymphedema). According to Földi, lipolymphedema develops on a statistical average of 17 years after the manifestation of lipedema. Reliable epidemiological studies on lipedema and lipolymphedema are unavailable at this time.

Pathology and Pathophysiology of Lipedema

The proliferated subcutaneous fatty tissue compresses the lymph collectors of the superficial lymphatic system. Lymphangiographic imaging shows that the lymph collectors within the excess fatty tissue have a coiled or corkscrew-like appearance rather than passing fairly straight toward the lymph nodes as in healthy tissue. This results in a decreased transport capacity of the lymphatic system in the affected area.

The diminished tissue resistance in fatty tissue will cause (without compression) ambulatory venous hypertension, which in turn results in more water leaving the blood capillaries, adding lymphatic load. This, along with the added problem of increased fragility (frequent hemorrhages) and permeability toward protein of the blood capillaries of the fatty tissue, explains the development of pitting edema in the later parts of the day in orthostatic-ambulatory positions. Constant overload of the lymphatic system (dynamic insufficiency) can result in additional morpho-

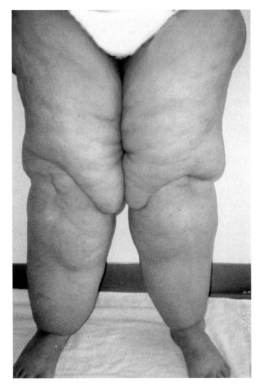

Figure 3–24 Lipolymphedema.

logic and functional damage to the lymph collectors, as explained in Chapter 2, Mechanical Insufficiency. Lymphedema develops in addition to lipedema (lipolymphedema). Without treatment, lymphedema will progress through its stages as outlined earlier in this chapter.

Stages

Some authors have divided lipedema in three stages. In stage 1, which may last for several years, the skin surface is normal, and the tissues exhibit a smooth nodular texture. The skin color is normal, and the tissue has a soft rubber-like feel. In stage 2, the skin surface becomes more uneven and is described as "orange peel" skin. Large fatty lobules begin to form, especially on the medial knee, the proximal thigh (laterally), and the medial and lateral ankles just above the malleoli. Pitting edema is common in the second half of the day. During stage 3, large contour-deforming lobular fatty deposits are observed in the same areas described in stage 2. These lobuli often

rub against each other when ambulating and interfere with normal gait. Changes in skin color often occur in the lower leg, which are indicative of lymphedema.

Evaluation

There are several significant clinical differences between pure lipedema and lipolymphedema, which in most cases can be easily identified during basic evaluation.

In lipedema, the swelling is always bilateral and symmetrical, the feet (and hands) are uninvolved, and the Stemmer sign—see Stage 3 (Lymphostatic Elephantiasis) previously in this chapter—is negative. The tissues are often painful upon palpation, feel rubbery, and tend to become harder over time (liposclerosis), with typical hard nodules palpable in the tissue. The natural skinfolds generally are not deepened. Pitting edema typically develops in the second half of the day, which is relieved by prolonged elevation of the extremities overnight.

In pure lymphedema, the swelling is usually unilateral; if it appears bilateral, as in lipolymphedema, it is almost always asymmetrical. The dorsum of the feet and hand become involved in the swelling, and the Stemmer sign is positive. The tissues in lipolymphedema are painful to pressure (not painful in pure lymphedema) and have a more firm and fibrotic feel. The natural skinfolds are deepened (Fig. 3–24).

> If lipolymphedema remains untreated, it will progress through the same stages as pure lymphedema. Deep pitting is present in earlier stages of lipolymphedema and becomes more difficult to induce in later stages.

Therapeutic Approach

General

If lipolymphedema is associated with obesity, nutritional guidance must be provided to reduce the weight and avoid further weight gain. Patients should be physically active and exercise regularly. Any hormonal imbalance should be corrected through medical management.

Complete Decongestive Therapy

Complete decongestive therapy shows good long-term results in lipolymphedema. However, the patient needs to understand that, although the lymphedematous component responds well and relatively fast to CDT, the lipedema itself responds more slowly, and sometimes not at all.

The treatment protocol of lipolymphedema corresponds with that for primary lymphedema. However, the pain and hypersensitivity may mandate lighter pressures in manual lymph drainage and compression techniques during the initial treatment sessions. In some cases, it may be necessary not to apply a compression bandage in the first few treatments. Patients often require more padding under the compression bandages, particularly in the anterior tibial area, and generally do not tolerate denser materials, such as Komprex or chip bags (see Chapter 5, Required Materials). The pain typically diminishes after several treatments.

After the decongestion of the lymphedematous component during the intensive phase of CDT, the patient should be fitted with a compression garment, which in the majority of cases needs to be custom made. The preferred garment is a pantyhose type of a higher compression class.

According to several authors, reduction of the excessive fatty tissue in lipedema is possible if the compression garments are worn constantly and if short-stretch compression bandages are applied at night.

Invasive Modalities

Several groups have studied the effects of liposuction and lipectomy on lipedema and lipolymphedema. The fact that fatty tissue cannot be removed without additional damage to the lymphatic system makes it understandable that these invasive procedures can worsen the lymphedematous component of the condition and cause additional problems in these patients.

◆ Traumatic Edema

As discussed earlier in this chapter, physical trauma may cause a reduction of the transport capacity of the lymphatic system to a level below the normal amount of lymphatic load. If the lymphatic system was healthy before the traumatic event, severe trauma with excessive scarring is usually necessary to cause post-traumatic secondary lymphedema. In a lymphatic system with an already reduced transport capacity (and functional reserve), as is the case in congenital malformations, the balance between lymphatic loads and transport capacity is often very fragile. Even minor trauma can cause the onset of post-traumatic primary lymphedema in these cases.

Swelling after traumatic events should be distinguished from general edema or post-traumatic lymphedema.

Definition

Traumatic events (surgery, blunt trauma, burns) result in inflammatory reactions accompanied by high-protein edema. The majority of these soft tissue swellings are temporary, and the tissue returns back to normal over time, but it is also possible that the inflammatory process causes permanent damage to the lymphatic system with long-lasting results.

The purpose of the following sections is to discuss inflammatory processes and their possible damaging effects on the tissues and the lymphatic system.

Pathophysiology

Inflammation is a nonspecific, localized immune response elicited by physical trauma with destruction of tissues. This process serves to destroy injured cells and to repair the damaged tissues.

Inflammation is characterized in the acute form by the classical signs of rubor (redness), calor (heat), dolor (pain), tumor (swelling), and functio laesa (functional disorder) with rapid onset (Fig. 3–25). In its chronic form,

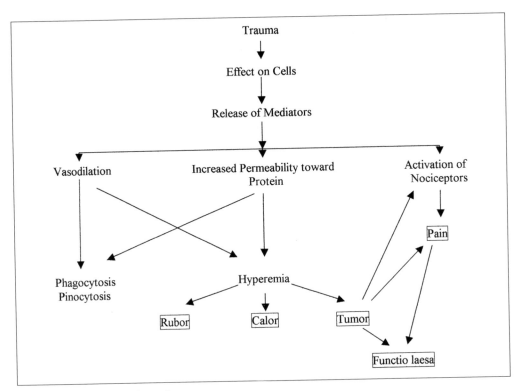

Figure 3-25 Pathophysiology of trauma.

these signs are usually less intense and have a prolonged duration. Increased leukocytes, pain, and low-grade fever may also present in chronic inflammation.

The initial step in the inflammatory process is a local vasodilation, which increases the blood flow, followed by an increase in the permeability of the blood capillaries toward plasma protein. These reactions cause redness, heat, and swelling, as well as pain secondary to pressure on nerve endings. Often clotting of the interstitial fluid occurs due to large amounts of fibrinogen and other proteins leaving the blood capillaries. White blood cells (neutrophil granulocytes) and monocytes leave the blood capillaries into the injured tissues. The neutrophils and tissue cells release mediators (histamine, kinin, serotonin), which continue the inflammatory response. Within a few hours, macrophages devour the damaged tissue cells. Tissue repair starts after the damage is controlled.

Whereas these inflammatory processes are important for tissue healing, they may also cause secondary damage to the tissues. Macrophages may further injure the still living tissue cells and surrounding structures. The lymphatic system may become involved in the inflammatory process or may be otherwise damaged due to a proliferation of macrophages in a localized area.

There are three possible results from the inflammatory process: complete healing, chronic inflammation, or additional tissue damage.

Effects of Inflammation on the Lymphatic System

The increased amount of lymphatic load of water (as well as protein and cells) triggers an increase in lymph time volume of the lymph collectors in the affected area (lymphatic safety factor). Either the lymphatic system is able to drain the excess fluid without the visible onset of edema, or it develops a dynamic insufficiency. Because of the increased amount of proteins leaving the blood capillaries in inflammation, the swelling resulting from the dynamic insufficiency is protein-rich.

> Involvement of the lymphatic system in the inflammatory process (lymphangitis) and spasms of the smooth musculature in the lymph collectors caused by pain (lymphangiospasm) are factors that may contribute to permanent damage to the lymphatic system.

The vicious pain cycle includes lymphangiospasm, increased swelling, and further pain (in combination with immobility), which can greatly exacerbate the symptoms.

The transport capacity may also be permanently reduced by the development of valvular and mural insufficiencies due to the constant strain, especially in chronic inflammations.

The consequence of the transport capacity of the lymphatic system falling below the normal amount of lymphatic load (mechanical insufficiency) as a result of inflammation is a combined insufficiency (increased lymphatic loads, decreased TC) of the lymphatic system (see Chapter 2, Combined Insufficiency).

Therapeutic Approach

The goals of treatment in traumatic edema are to eliminate edema and to support wound healing.

Traumatic edema results in increased tissue pressure and an extended diffusion distance between the blood capillaries and tissue cells, with the following negative effects:

- ◆ Lack of oxygen and nutrients in the traumatized area
- ◆ Impeded drainage of wound components from the traumatized area, causing delay in the healing process
- ◆ Irritation of pain receptors
- ◆ Delayed scar healing and/or increased scar formation

Manual lymph drainage in combination with other modalities improves lymph vessel activity proximal to the trauma and in the traumatized area itself, thus reducing the swelling. The subsequent decrease in diffusion distance improves local oxygenation and nutrition, thereby accelerating the drainage and elimina-

tion of wound components. Decongestion reduces tissue pressure and subsequently the pain associated with the inflammation.

Complete Decongestive Therapy in Blunt Trauma

CDT applied early following blunt trauma improves absorption of edema fluid and accelerates wound healing. These are important aspects especially in athletic care, where quick resolution and return to performance are of importance.

Severe injuries, such as fractures or compartment syndrome, must be ruled out before manual lymph drainage can be initiated. The individual must consult a doctor if severe pain or dizziness is present.

Cryotherapy (ice) and compression: Ice packs can be made by placing ice cubes or crushed ice in a self-closing plastic bag or by using a commercial frozen gel pack. Ice should be applied as soon as possible following the traumatic event. Long-term cooling decreases local metabolism, disengages nociceptors to reduce pain, and promotes vasoconstriction. Cryotherapy also reduces the muscle spindle activity responsible for mediating local muscle tone. Peripheral nerve injury and local frostbite secondary to prolonged cryotherapy have been reported, emphasizing the need for monitoring during the use of cryotherapy. To avoid frostbite, ice packs should not be placed directly on the skin, they should be placed over a wet washcloth or towel. To decrease filtration and to promote reabsorption, ice should be applied in combination with compression bandages for a minimum of 15 minutes over a period of 3 to 4 hours (refer to Chapter 4, Contraindications for Compression Therapy). An additional effect of compression bandages is stabilization and immobilization of the traumatized area.

Manual lymph drainage: MLD is applied with the ice/compression bandage in place and the individual placed in a comfortable position, promoting venous and lymphatic return during the treatment. MLD is applied to the regional lymph nodes and the lymph vessels proximal to the trauma. In the case of an injury below the knee, the treatment includes the inguinal lymph nodes and basic MLD techniques on the antero-medial thigh and knee. Following MLD (duration of the treatment is ~ 15–20 minutes), the ice/compression bandages are renewed. MLD may be repeated 2 to 3 hours after the initial treatment, if necessary. If edema is still present, the treatment should be followed by a padded compression bandage (no ice).

Postsurgery Application of Complete Decongestive Therapy

In addition to the effects of manual lymph drainage outlined above, scar management plays an important role in the early treatment of postsurgical conditions.

In 1989, Hutzschenreuther and Bruemmer showed in an experimental study that manual lymph drainage applied in the area of fresh scars promotes lympholymphatic regeneration of interrupted lymph vessels in scar tissue. The connective tissue fibers seem to be more organized, and the consistency of the scar tissue treated with manual lymph drainage seems to be softer than in untreated scars.

Manual lymph drainage: To avoid any disturbance of the wound healing process, it is important to apply MLD techniques in the first 5 to 7 days postoperatively only proximal to the scar tissue. For example, after knee surgery, the inguinal lymph nodes are stimulated, and basic techniques on the anterior, medial, and lateral thigh are performed. It is important to observe a safe distance from the scar tissue to avoid any tension on the edges of the scar. After 5 to 7 sessions, the general scar area may be carefully incorporated into the treatment area. It is important not to disturb the approximation of the wound edges; therefore, only mild pressure should be applied. Gentle stationary circles using the distal phalanges of the fingers or thumb can be applied directly around the scar tissue after the sutures are removed (usually after 1–2 weeks). Stationary circles are directed away from the wound edges, but again, to avoid disturbance of wound healing, only very light pressure should be applied. Pretreatment of the regional lymph nodes and the thigh precedes scar treatment.

General considerations: As always in postsurgical care, signs and symptoms of DVT and PE should be observed. During the treatment the extremity is placed in a comfortable position, promoting venous and lymphatic return. Mild compression using padded short-stretch bandages or compression stockings may be applied with the physician's permission. Sterile gloves should be worn while working in the area of the scar.

◆ Inflammatory Rheumatism

Definition

Inflammatory rheumatism or rheumatoid arthritis is a chronic, systemic, inflammatory disease that mostly affects the synovial membranes of multiple joints.

Because of its systemic nature, there are many extra-articular symptoms of rheumatism, or rheumatoid arthritis (RA), such as fever, loss of energy, loss of appetite, and anemia. RA can attack any synovial joint in the body. The small joints of the hand (excluding the distal interphalangeal joints), wrist, and foot are the most commonly affected joints. Joints that are actively involved with the disease are usually symmetrically tender and swollen and demonstrate reduced motion. To better understand the effects of RA on a joint, a brief anatomic review of a synovial joint follows.

Anatomy of a Synovial Joint

A synovial joint has the following components: The *joint capsule*, which isolates the joint cavity from the surrounding tissue, is composed of an outer fibrous layer and an inner synovial layer. The outer layer is poorly vascularized but contains a large number of joint receptors; the opposite is true for the synovial layer (Fig. 3–26A). In addition to a large number of blood vessels, the synovial layer contains lymph vessels (Fig. 3–26B). The joint capsule forms the *joint cavity* containing synovial fluid. Synovial fluid is the medium by which nutrients are carried to, and waste products are removed from, the avascular hyaline (articular) cartilage. Synovial fluid is secreted by the synovial layer and not only is responsible for carrying oxygen and nutrients but also serves as a lubricant for the joint. The *hyaline cartilage* covers and protects the ends of long bones participating in the

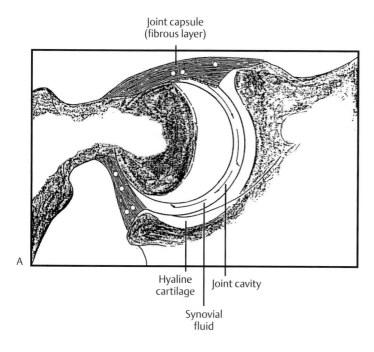

Joint capsule
(fibrous layer)

Hyaline
cartilage

Joint cavity

Synovial
fluid

A

Figure 3–26   A. Cross section through the hip joint. B. Cross section through the joint capsule (the arrows indicate the diffusion distance between the blood capillaries and the synovial membrane cells).

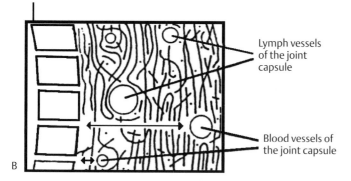

Synovial membrane cells

Lymph vessels of the joint capsule

Blood vessels of the joint capsule

B

joint and minimizes friction and wear between the opposing joint surfaces during movement. It also dissipates the forces on the joint over a wider area, thus decreasing stress on the joint surfaces.

Pathophysiology

Despite many years of intensive investigation, the etiology of rheumatoid arthritis remains unknown. Metabolic and nutritional factors, the endocrine system, and geographic, psychological, and occupational data have been studied extensively without conclusive find-ings. It appears that an unknown antigen initiates the autoimmune response; that is, the body's immune system attacks healthy joint tissue and initiates a process of inflammation and joint damage, resulting in RA.

Early in the course of RA several changes in joint structures occur. Inflammation of the synovial layer, with the typical signs of heat, redness, swelling, pain, and loss of function, is present (inflammatory phase). Additionally, changes in the ends of the bones forming the joint (osteoporosis) may occur early in the disease process. As the disease progresses, the synovial layer may grow considerably larger, eventually forming tissue called *pannus*. Pannus can be considered the most destructive element affecting joints in the patient with rheumatoid arthritis. It attacks and destroys articular cartilage (destructive phase). Pannus can also destroy the soft subchondral bone, after the protective articular cartilage is gone. The destruction of bone eventually leads to laxity in tendons and ligaments. Under the strain of daily activities and other forces, these alterations in bone and joint structure result in the deformities frequently seen in patients with rheumatoid arthritis.

Effects on the Lymphatic System

In addition to the effects of inflammatory processes on the lymphatic system as described earlier in this chapter (see Pathology and Pathophysiology of Lipedema), including the vicious cycle of pain generated by these effects, additional problems contribute to the swelling associated with RA.

Lymphangiographic imaging has shown that clotted fibrin obliterates channels in the tissues through which the protein-rich tissue fluid reaches the initial lymph vessels, thus inhibiting lymph formation. The lymphatic system in rheumatoid arthritis is involved in both the inflammatory and the chronic phases of the disease; therefore, lymphedema can be associated with RA.

Therapeutic Approach

The significance of a systemic disease like RA is that it is pervasive, leaving almost no part of the patient's life untouched. Attempting to maintain one's lifestyle while dealing with the effects of a chronic disease can be difficult. The financial burdens placed on patients with RA magnify the emotional and physical stress. Yet, with appropriate, accurate guidance from health care practitioners, many patients with RA can live the lifestyle of their choice for many years.

To cover all aspects of physical therapy (mobilization, thermotherapy, etc.) in RA would extend beyond the scope of this text. The following covers the role of complete decongestive therapy as an adjunct to other modalities used in the treatment and management of rheumatoid arthritis.

Complete Decongestive Therapy in the Treatment of Rheumatoid Arthritis

The goal of manual lymph drainage is to reduce the intra- and extra-articular swelling, thereby interrupting the vicious pain cycle previously described. With the reduction of pain, the patient is able to move the affected joints more freely, thus improving nutrition and oxygenation of the articular cartilage.

If possible, manual lymph drainage should be applied daily in the subacute phase of RA and should be avoided in the inflammatory phase. Basic MLD stroke sequences are used to treat the regional lymph nodes and the extremity, including the affected joints. For example, if RA is present on the hand and wrist, the therapist should utilize the axillary lymph nodes, collectors of the upper arm, elbow, and forearm, as well as wrist, hand, and finger techniques. As always, during the treatment the extremity should be placed in a comfortable position for the patient, promoting venous and lymphatic return.

Mild compression bandages may be applied in this stage with physician's approval and should be worn only for short time periods (several hours, if possible). Bandages must not cause pain or considerably restrict movement. If the RA is located on the fingers/wrist, padded bandages are applied on the hand and arm; fingers are bandaged unpadded.

Complete Decongestive Therapy in the Treatment of Lymphedema Associated with Rheumatoid Arthritis

The goals of the therapy—to reduce the swelling and to maintain the reduction—correspond with those outlined in uncomplicated primary or secondary lymphedema (refer to Chapter 4).

In the case of a combination of lymphedema and RA in the subacute stage, the treatment protocol in the intensive phase of CDT is modified in such a way as to accommodate the considerations and guidelines outlined above (the bandages must never cause pain or discomfort and should only be worn for short time periods). Compression garments of a lighter compression class are recommended for lymphedema patients with a combination of RA. If possible, treatments should be provided daily for maximum benefit.

If lymphedema is associated with chronic RA, special padding is necessary under the compression bandages to accommodate areas of deformity, muscle atrophy, or possible tendon ruptures.

In most cases of RA, the patient has remissions and exacerbations of the symptoms; therefore, it is important to observe any signs or symptoms of increased disease activity or worsening of symptoms (flare-ups or flares).

◆ Reflex Sympathetic Dystrophy

Definition

Reflex sympathetic dystrophy (RSD), also known as complex regional pain syndrome, is most often initiated by trauma to a nerve, neural plexus, bone, or soft tissue. It is one of the most frequent complications after surgery to extremities. RSD includes other medical diagnoses, such as causalgia, Sudeck's dystrophy, shoulder-hand syndrome, and post-traumatic osteoporosis.

Its five components are pain, edema, autonomic dysfunction, movement disorder, and trophic changes. If not treated, RSD can cause stiffness and loss of use of the affected part of the extremity.

Pathology and Stages

RSD occurs from a disturbance in the sympathetic nervous system affecting all tissue levels—skin, subcutaneous tissue, fascia, muscle, synovial layer, and bone. The disease shows simultaneous involvement of nervous tissue, skin, muscle, blood vessels, and bones. The only common denominator in all patients is pain, which is often described as burning in nature. It should be noted that RSD is a condition that affects not only adults but children as well.

The condition evolves in stages that progress insidiously over time. Some patients remain in one stage or another for many months or even years. They may never progress, or they may progress quickly through the stages.

Stage I (acute or inflammatory) may last up to 3 months. During this stage, the symptoms include severe pain closely localized to the site of injury and more severe than would normally be expected from the injury, localized pitting edema, increased warmth in the affected body part/limb, and excessive sweating. There may be faster than normal nail and hair growth and joint pain, as well as muscle spasms during movement of the affected area.

Stage II (dystrophic or degenerative) can last 3 to 12 months (usually 3–6 months). The edema spreads and becomes firmer, skin wrinkles disappear, and the skin temperature becomes cooler. The fingernails become brittle and cracked. The pain is more severe and more widespread. Hand or foot dryness becomes prominent, and atrophy in skin, subcutis, and muscle tissue develops. Stiffness develops, and there may be diffuse osteoporosis.

In stage III (atrophic), the pain spreads proximally, involving the entire limb. Although it may diminish in intensity, pain remains the prominent feature in this stage. The skin of the affected area is now pale, dry, tightly stretched, and shiny. Atrophy of muscle tissue and contractures in flexor tendons may also be present. Subluxations in interphalangeal joints are occasionally produced. Edema is absent, and deossification of bone tissue has now become marked and diffuse. Flare-ups may occur spontaneously.

Lymphatic Involvement

The lymphatic load of water (and protein) exceeds the transport capacity of the lymphatic system, resulting in dynamic insufficiency (stages I and II). Accumulation of protein-rich fluid affects the subcutaneous tissues but may also be present in muscle tissue, tendons, and joint cavities.

Therapeutic Approach

After the diagnosis of RSD is established, several therapeutic approaches that have been proven helpful are available. RSD is treated by neural blockage (surgically or chemically), drug therapy, thermotherapy, and electrotherapy. Physical therapy shows good results, particularly in children.

Goals of treatment include controlling and minimizing the pain. Studies have shown that breaking through the pain cycle early precipitates a better outcome, preventing progression of the disease, restoring function of the limb affected by RSD, and improving the patient's quality of life.

Complete Decongestive Therapy in RSD

MLD is applied in stages I and II of RSD. The goal of the therapy is to reduce the pain and to increase lymphatic drainage, thereby reducing or eliminating the swelling associated with the early stages of RSD. The resulting decrease in diffusion distance improves the trophic situation.

The extremity is placed in a comfortable and elevated position to promote venous and lymphatic return. The treatment must never cause or increase pain. Treatments should be given daily (if possible) and include basic MLD stroke sequences on the regional lymph nodes and the extremity to the proximal joint. If RSD is present on the hand, strokes on the axillary lymph nodes, upper arm, and elbow should be utilized. The forearm may be included in later treatments and only if comfortable for the patient. The application of compression bandages is contraindicated in the treatment of RSD.

◆ Cyclic Idiopathic Edema

Cyclic idiopathic edema is a syndrome characterized by soft (pitting) symmetric edema and weight gain. The cause of this condition is unclear. It occurs in menstruating females (not present before the menarche or after the menopause) and in the absence of cardiac, renal, or hepatic disease. The swelling involves the entire body and appears in cycles (premenstrual syndrome), or the edema is constantly present and varies in volume. In premenstrual syndrome, the swelling starts with the ovulation and recedes spontaneously after the beginning of the menstruation.

With orthostatic-ambulatory cyclic idiopathic edema, the swelling is dependent on gravity. The face and hands are swollen in the morning, and lower extremities and trunk, including the often painful mammary gland, become involved during the day.

Many women experience excessive weight gain during the day in the edema phase, with heat and orthostasis aggravating the symptoms. Altered vascular permeability may also be part of the disorder

Cyclic idiopathic edema is often associated with other conditions, such as lipedema, chronic venous insufficiency, and lymphedema. The symmetric involvement of the swelling in cyclic idiopathic edema makes it difficult to distinguish this from other conditions in which CDT may be contraindicated (cardiac edema).

Complete Decongestive Therapy

In the edema phase, MLD should be applied daily, if possible. The treatment involves the neck, face, thorax (including axillary lymph nodes), and legs (including inguinal lymph nodes), using basic stroke sequences. Following the MLD treatment, compression bandages are applied on the lower extremities and the abdomen.

Patients should be fitted with a compression garment (pantyhose style), which should be worn continuously. In premenstrual syndrome, the compression garment is worn between the ovulation and the beginning of the menstruation. Compression garments increase the tissue pressure, which results in reduced net filtration. Compression garments reduce, or may even prevent, the onset of swelling in the edema phase of this condition. If lymphedema is associated with cyclic idiopathic edema, the treatment protocol for lymphedema has priority.

Recommended Reading

Lymphedema

1. Breast Cancer Dig April 1984;78
2. Brennan MJ. Lymphedema following the surgical treatment of breast cancer: a review of pathophysiology and treatment. J Pain Symptom Manage 1992; 7(2):110–116
3. Erickson VS, Pearson ML, Ganz PA, et al. Arm edema in breast cancer patients. J Natl Cancer Inst 2001;93(2): 96–111
4. Földi E. Preventions of dermatolymphangioadenitis by combined physiotherapy of the swollen arm after treatment for breast cancer. Lymphology 1996;29:48–49
5. Földi E, Földi M, Weissleder H. Conservative treatment of lymphedema of the limbs. Angiology 1985;36(3): 171–180

6. Földi E. Massage and damage to lymphatics. Lymphology 1995;28:1–3
7. Földi M. Treatment of lymphedema [editorial]. Lymphology 1994;27:1–5
8. Getz DH. The primary, secondary, and tertiary nursing interventions of lymphedema. Cancer Nurs 1985; 8(3):177–184
9. Greenlee R, Hoyme H, Witte M, Crowe P, Witte C. Developmental disorders of the lymphatic system Lymphology 1993;26:156–168
10. Herpertz U. Das Lipödem. Lymphologie 1995;19:1–7
11. Horsley JS, Styblo T. Lymphedema in the postmastectomy patient. In: Bland KI, Copeland EM, eds. The Breast: Comprehensive Management of Benign and Malignant Diseases. Philadelphia: Saunders; 1991: 701–706
12. Kim DI, Huh S, Hwang JH, Kim YI, Lee BB. Venous dynamics in leg lymphedema. Lymphology 1999;32(1): 11–14
13. Markowski J, Wilcox JP, Helm PA. Lymphedema incidence after specific post-mastectomy therapy. Arch Phys Med Rehab 1981;62(9):449–452
14. Mortimer PS, Bates DO, Brassington HD, et al. The prevalence of arm edema following treatment for breast cancer. Q J Med 1996;89:377–380
15. Petrek JA, Lerner R. Diseases of the Breast. Philadelphia: Lippincott-Raven; 1996
16. Petrek JA, Senie RT, Peters M, et al. Lymphedema in a cohort of breast carcinoma survivors 20 years after diagnosis. Cancer 2001;92(6):1368–1377
17. Rosenfeld RG, Tesch LG, Rodriguez-Rigau LJ, et al. Recommendations for diagnosis, treatment and management of individuals with Turner syndrome. Endocrinologist 1994;4:351
18. Stanton AW, Levick JR, Mortimer PS. Cutaneous vascular control in the arms of women with postmastectomy edema. Exp Physiol 1996;81(3):447–464

Surgical Procedures
1. Arnold DK, Tran KN, et al. Lessons learned from 500 cases of lymphatic mapping for breast cancer. Ann Surg 1999;229(4):528–535
2. Edwards MJ, Whitworth P, Tafra L, McMasters KM. The details of successful sentinel lymph node staging for breast cancer. Am J Surg 2000;180(4):257–261
3. Kissin MW, Querci della Rovere G, Easton D, et al. Risk of lymphedema following the treatment of breast cancer. Br J Surg 1986;73(7):580–584
4. Kwan W, Jackson J, Weir LM, et al. Chronic arm morbidity after curative breast cancer treatment: prevalence and impact on quality of life. J Clin Oncol 2002;20(20):4242–4248
5. Mackay-Wiggan J, Ratner D. Suturing techniques. Available at: http://emedicine.com. Accessed 2003
6. National Cancer Institute Website. A collection of material about sentinel lymph node biopsy. Available at: http://www.cancer.gov/clinicaltrials/digestpage/sentinel-node. Accessed August 18, 2004

Filariasis
1. Information on filariasis. Available at: http://www.filariasis.net. Accessed August 18, 2004

Diagnostic Imaging
1. Bräutigam P, Földi E, Schaiper I, Krause T, Vanscheidt W, Moser E. Analysis of lymphatic drainage in various forms of leg edema using two compartment lymphoscintigraphy. Lymphology 1998;31(2):43–55
2. Partsch H, Urbanek A, Wenzel-Hora B. The dermal lymphatics in lymphedema visualized by indirect lymphography. Br J Dermatol 1984;110(4):431–438
3. Pecking A, Behar A, et al. In vivo assessment of fluid and fat component in lymphedematous skin. Paper presented at: International Society of Lymphology Congress; 2001; Genoa, Italy
4. Svensson WE, Mortimer PS, Tohno E, et al. Colour Doppler demonstrates venous flow abnormalities in breast cancer patients with chronic arm swelling. Eur J Cancer 1994;30A(5):657–660
5. Szuba A, Shin WS, Strauss HW, Rockson S. The third circulation: radionuclide lymphoscintigraphy in the evaluation of lymphedema. J Nuc Med 2003;44(1)

Complete Decongestive Therapy
1. Boris M, Weindorf S, Lasinski B, Boris G. Lymphedema reduction by noninvasive complex lymphedema therapy. Oncology 1994;8(9):95–106
2. Eliska O, Eliska M. Are peripheral lymphatics damaged by high pressure manual massage? Lymphology 1995;28:21–30
3. Hocutt JE Jr. Cryotherapy. Am Fam Physician 1981; 23(3):141–144
4. Hutzschenreuter P, Ehlers R. The effect of manual lymph drainage on the autonomic nervous system. Zeltschrift Lymphologie 1986;19:58–60
5. Hutzschenreuther P, Bruemmer H, Silberschneider K. Die Vagotone Wirkung der Manuellen Lymphdrainage nach Dr. Vodder. LymphForsch 2003;7(1):7–14

Pneumatic Compression Pumps
1. Bock AU. Prinzipielle Überlegungen zur Apparativen Intermittierenden Kompressionstherapie. LymphForsch 2003;7(1):27–29
2. Boris M, Weindorf S, Lasinski B. The risk of genital edema after external pump compression for lower limb lymphedema. Lymphology 1998;31(1):15–20
3. Dini D, Del Mastro L, Gozza A, et al. The Role of Pneumatic Compression in the Treatment of Postmastectomy Lymphedema: A Randomized Phase III Study. Boston: Kluwer Academic Publishers; 1998
4. Lynnworth M. Greater Boston Lymphedema Support Group Pump Survey. Natl Lymphedema Network Newsletter 1988;10:6–7
5. Miranda F, Perez MC, Castiglioni ML, et al. Effect of sequential intermittent pneumatic compression on both leg lymphedema volume and on lymph transport as semi-quantitatively evaluated by lymphoscintigraphy. Lymphology 2001;34(3):135–141
6. Bernas MJ, Witte CL, Witte MH. Draft Revision of the 1995 Consensus Document of the International Society of Lymphology. Lymphology 2001;34:84–91
7. Richmand DM, O'Donnell TF, Zelikovski A. Sequential pneumatic compression for lymphedema: a controlled trial. Arch Surg 1985;120(10):1116–1119
8. Segers P, Belgrado JP, Leduc A, Leduc O, Verdonck P. Excessive pressure in multichambered cuffs used for sequential compression therapy. Physical Therapy 2002;82(10):1000–1008
9. Weissleder H. Stellenwert der Apparativen Intermittierenden Kompression—Literaturueberblick. LymphForsch 2003;7(1):15–18

Medication
1. Bassett ML, Dahlstrom JE. Liver failure while taking coumarin. Med J Aust 1995;163(2):106
2. Casley-Smith J, Morgan R, Piller N. Treatment of lymphedema of the arms and legs with 5,6-benzopyrone. N Engl J Med 1993;329(16):1158–1163

3. Consensus document of the International Society of Lymphology: diagnosis and treatment of peripheral lymphedema. Lymphology 2003;36:84–91
4. Cox D, O'Kennedy R, Thornes RD. The rarity of liver toxicity in patients treated with coumarin (1,2-benzopyrone). Hum Toxicol 1989;8(6):501–506
5. Faurschou P. Toxic hepatitis due to benzopyrone. Hum Toxicol 1982;1(2):149–150
6. Fentem JH, Fry JR. Species fifferences in the metabolism and hepatotoxicity of voumarin. Comp Biochem Physiol C 1993;104(1):1–8
7. Casley-Smith JR. Lymphedema, the poor and benzopyrones: proposed amendments to the consensus document. Lymphology 1996;29:137–140
8. Loprinzi CL, Kugler JW, Sloan JA et al. Lack of effect of coumarin in women with lymphedema after treatment for breast cancer. N Engl J Med 1999;340(5):346–350
9. Loprinzi CL, Sloan J, Kugler J. Coumarin-induced hepatotoxicity. J Clin Oncol 1997;15(9):3167–3168
10. Morrison L, Welsby PD. Side-effects of coumarin. Postgrad Med J 1995;71(841):701

Surgery for Lymphedema
1. Goldsmith HS, De Los Santos R. Omental transposition in primary lymphedema. Surg Gynecol Obstet 1967;125:607–610
2. Miller TA. Surgical approach to lymphedema of the arm after mastectomy. Am J Surg 1984;148(1):152–156
3. O'Brien BM, Khazanchi RK, Dumar PAV, Dviv E, Pederson WC. Liposuction in the treatment of lymphedema: a preliminary report. Br J Plast Surg 1989;42:530–533
4. Olszewski W. Risk of surgical procedures in limbs with edema (lymphedema). Lymph Link 2003;15(1)

Chronic Venous Insufficiency
1. Brand FN, Dannenburg AL, Abbott RD, Kannel WB. The epidemiology of varicose veins: the Framingham study. Am J Prev Med 1988;4:96–101
2. Eliska O, Eliskova M. Morphology of lymphatics in human venous crural ulcers with lipodermatosclerosis. Lymphology 2001;34:111–121
3. Földi M, Idiazabal G. The role of operative management of varicose veins in patients with lymphedema and/or lipedema of the legs. Lymphology 2000;33:167–171
4. Goldhaber SZ, Morrison RB. Pulmonary embolism and deep vein thrombosis. Circulation 2002;106:1436–1438
5. Griffin JH, Motulsky A, Hirsh J. Diagnosis and treatment of hypercoagulable states. Ed Prog of the Am Soc Hematology 1996:106–111
6. Harris JM, Abramson N. Evaluation of recurrent thrombosis and hypercoagulability. Am Fam Phys 1997;56(6):1591–1596
7. Hobson J. Venous insufficiency at work. Angiology 1997;48(7):577–582
8. Johnson MT. Treatment and prevention of varicose veins. J Vasc Nurs 1997;15(3):97–103
9. Kim DI, Huh S, Hwang JH, Kim YI, Lee BB. Venous dynamics in leg lymphedema. Lymphology 1999;32(1):11–14
10. Silverstein MD, Heit JA, Mohr DN, et al. Trends in the incidence of deep vein thrombosis and pulmonary embolism: a 25-year population-based study. Arch Intern Med 1998;158(6):585–593

11. Vanhoutte PM, Corcaud S, de Montrion C. Venous disease: from pathophysiology to quality of life. Angiology 1997;48(7):559–567

Wounds and Skin Lesions
1. Alvarez OM, Fernandez-Obregon A, Roger RS. Interim analysis of a prospective, randomized clinical trial of papain-urea and collagenase for the debridement of pressure ulcers. Paper presented at: Symposium on Advanced Wound Care;1999; Dallas, TX
2. Andersson E, et al. Leg and foot ulcer prevalence and investigation of the peripheral arterial and venous circulation in a randomized elderly population: an epidemiological survey. Acta Derm Venereol Suppl (Stockh) 1984;64:227
3. Barton P, Parslow N. Malignant wounds: holistic assessment and management. In: Krasner DL, Rodeheaver GT, Sibbald RG, eds. Chronic Wound Care: A Clinical Source Book for Healthcare Professionals. 3rd ed. Wayne, PA: HMP Communications; 2001:699–710
4. Bozeman PK. Arterial ulcers. In: Milne CT, Corbett LQ, Dubuc DL, eds. Wound, Ostomy, and Continence Nursing Secrets. Philadelphia: Hanley & Belfast; 2003:168–172
5. Callam MJ, Harper DR, Dale JJ, et al. Arterial disease in chronic leg ulceration: an underestimated hazard? Lothian and Forth Valley leg ulcer study. BMJ 1987;294:929–931
6. Capeheart J. Chronic venous insufficiency: a focus on prevention of venous ulceration. J Wound Ostomy Contin Nurs 1996;23(5):227–234
7. Corbett LQ, Burns PE. Venous ulcers. In: Milne CT, Corbett LQ, Dubuc DL, eds. Wound, Ostomy, and Continence Nursing Secrets. Philadelphia: Hanley & Belfast; 2003:163
8. Kunimoto BT. Management and prevention of venous leg ulcers: a literature guided approach. Ostomy Wound Manage 2001;47(1):36–49
9. Myers BA. Wound Management: Principles and Practice. Upper Saddle River, NJ: Prentice Hall; 2004:201–228
10. Naylor W, Laverty D, Mallet J. Handbook of Wound Management in Cancer Care. London: Blackwell Sciences; 2001:73–122
11. Nelzen O, Bergqvist D, Lindhagen A, et al. Venous and nonvenous leg ulcers: clinical history and appearance in a population study. Br J Surg 1994;81:182–187
12. Orsted HL, Radke L, Gorst R. The impact of musculoskeletal changes on the dynamics of the calf muscle pump. Ostomy Wound Manage 2001;47(10):18–24
13. Patterson GK. Vascular evaluation. In: Sussman C, Bates-Jensen BM, eds. Wound Care: A Collaborative Practice Manual for Physical Therapists and Nurses. Gaithersburg, MD: Aspen Publications; 2001:177–193
14. Reichardt L. Venous ulceration: compression as the mainstay therapy. J Wound Ostomy Contin Nurs 1999;26(1):39–47
15. Sibbald RG, Williamson D, Orsted HL, et al. Preparing the wound bed-debridement, bacterial balance and moisture balance. Ostomy Wound Man 2000;46(11):14–35
16. Slachta PA, Burns PE. Inflammatory ulcerations. In: Milne CT, Corbett LQ, Dubuc DL, eds. Wound, Ostomy, and Continence Nursing Secrets. Philadelphia: Hanley & Belfast; 2003:193–197
17. Young JR. Differential diagnosis of leg ulcers. Cardiovasc Clin 1983;13:171–193

Lipedema

1. Brorson H. Liposuction gives complete reduction of chronic large arm lymphedema after breast cancer. Acta Oncol 2000;39(3):407–420
2. Brorson H, Svensson H. Complete reduction of lymphedema of the arm by liposuction after breast cancer. Scand J Plast Reconst Surg. 1997;31:137–143
3. Brorson H, Svensson H. Liposuction combined with controlled compression therapy reduces arm lymphedema more effectively than controlled compression therapy alone. Plast Reconstr Surg 1998;102(4):1058–1067
4. Brorson H, Svensson H, Norrgren K, Thorsson O. Liposuction reduces arm lymphedema without significantly altering the already impaired lymph transport. Lymphology 1998;31(4):156–172
5. Földi M, Idiazabal G. The role of operative management of varicose veins in patients with lymphedema and/or lipedema of the legs. Lymphology 2000;33:167–171
6. Harwood C, Bull RH, Evans J, Mortimer PS. Lymphatic and venous function in lipoedema. Br J Dermatol 1996;134:1–6
7. Lerner R. Understanding lipedema. NLN Newsletter 10(2)
8. Rudkin GH, Miller TA. Lipedema: a clinical entity distinct from lymphedema. Plast Reconstr Surg 1994;94(6):841–847
9. Zelikovski A, et al. Lipedema complicated by lymphedema of the abdominal wall and lower limbs. Lymphology 2000;33:43–46

Traumatic Edema

1. Hutzschenreuther P, Bruemmer H. Die Manuelle Lymphdrainage bei der Wundheilung mit Ecollment—eine experimentelle Studie. Lymphologica Jahresband 1989:97–100
2. Wingerden. Eistherapie-Kontraindiziert bei Sportverletzungen? Leistungssport 1992;2:5–8

Rheumatoid Arthritis

1. Földi M, Földi E. Der rheumatische Formenkreis—allgemeine lymphologische Gesichtspunkte. In: Lehrbuch der Lymphologie. 3rd ed. Stuttgart: Gustav Fischer Verlag; 1993:374
2. Klippel J, Crofford L, Stone J, et al. Primer on Rheumatic Diseases. 10th ed. 1993
3. Schoberth H. Der entzuendliche Rheumatismus. In: Lehrbuch der Lymphologie. 3rd ed. Stuttgart: Gustav Fischer Verlag; 1993:375–378

Reflex Sympathetic Dystrophy

1. Cantwell-Gab K. Identifying chronic peripheral arterial disease. Am J Nurs 1996;96(7):40–46
2. Clodius L. Das Sudeck Syndrom: lymphologische und funktionelle Aspekte. In: Lehrbuch der Lymphologie. 4th ed. Stuttgart: Gustav Fischer Verlag; 1999:393–395
3. Kemler MA, Rijks CP, De Vet HC. Which patients with chronic reflex sympathetic dystrophy are most likely to benefit from physical therapy? J Manipulative Physiol Ther 2001;24(4):272–276
4. Mucha C. Ergebnisse einer prospektiven Beobachtungsreihe zur funktionellen Therapie des Sudeck-Syndroms. Z Phys Therap 1993;14(5):329–333
5. Rockson S, Cooke J. Peripheral arterial insufficiency: mechanisms, natural history, and therapeutic options. Adv Intern Med 1998;43:253–277

4

Complete Decongestive Therapy

Complete decongestive therapy (CDT) is a non-invasive, multicomponent approach to treat lymphedema and related conditions. Numerous studies have proven the scientific basis and effectiveness of this therapy, which has been well established in European countries since the 1970s. CDT has been practiced in the United States in one form or another since the 1980s; it became accepted after definitive guidelines and all components of CDT were included in the teaching curricula of schools providing training in lymphedema management in the 1990s.

◆ History and Background

The following serves as a selective overview to describe the history of the discovery of the lymphatic system and the development of complete decongestive therapy.

Discovery of the Lymphatic System

Compared with other developments in the history of medicine, the lymphatic system was discovered relatively late. *Hippocrates* (460–377 BC) described vessels containing "white blood," and *Aristotle* (384–322 BC) later spoke of vessels holding "a colorless fluid." Physicians of the Alexandrian school were also aware of the lymphatic system; they described the lymph vessels as ductus lactei (milklike vessels). This knowledge was forgotten for almost 2000 years, probably because the Catholic Church considered anatomical studies to be sinful. The lymphatic system was rediscovered during the European Renaissance.

Gaspare Aselli, also spelled Asellio (1581–1626), an Italian physician, discovered the lacteal vessels during a vivisection of a dog in 1622.

The cisterna chyli was first described by *Jean Pecquet* (1622–1674), a medical student from Dieppe, France, in 1651. He also described the presence of valves within the lymphatics and the communication of the thoracic duct with the left subclavian vein.

Olof Rudbeck (1630–1708) from Sweden, one of Uppsala University's most outstanding figures throughout the centuries, was credited with the first complete description of the lymphatic system in the human body.

Thomas Bartholin (1616–1680), a Danish physician, also claimed to have produced the first complete representation of the lymphatic system, which he published in a book in 1652 (or 1653). He was the first to call the lymph vessels vasa lymphatica and the fluid carried by these vessels lympha (from the Latin *limpidus*, meaning "clear" or "transparent"). Bartholin and Rudbeck had animated discussions about who really delivered the first complete description.

It was because of great improvements in the art of dissection and injection and the invention of new and better instruments that anatomists attained a vast knowledge of the human lymphatic system. *Anton Nuck* (1650–1692), a Dutch anatomist, in 1692 first employed the technique of intralymphatic injection of mercury to outline the lymphatic system. *Mascani* (1787), *Cruikshank* (1789), and *Gerota* (1896) devised modifications of this technique.

Marie P. C. Sappey (1810–1896), a French anatomist, used the injection technique to conduct comprehensive topographical studies of the human lymphatic system to demonstrate the beauty of the vessels; he published his work in 1885. Mercury, or quicksilver, was used as an injection medium on cadavers for filling the lymphatic vessels. The injecting instruments included the lymphatic injecting tube and pipe, which were made of either glass or brass. Sappey's work was continued by another French anatomist named *Henri Rouviere* (1875–1952). Rouviere published a book on the human lymphatic system (*L'anatomie des lymphatiques de l'homme*) in 1932.

Modern technologies (computed tomography, lymphographic imaging techniques, etc.) have made it possible to gain a detailed view and complete understanding of the lymphatic system. Research pioneers such as *M. Földi, A. Gregl, E. Kuhnke* (Germany), *S. Kubik* (Switzerland), and *J. Casley-Smith* (Australia), among others, contributed to the field of lymphology and established the groundwork for current research.

Development of Complete Decongestive Therapy

Many clinicians have used this newly found knowledge and have incorporated it into the treatment of various conditions. *Alexander von Winiwarter* (1848–1917), a surgeon from Austria, successfully treated swollen limbs with elevation, compression, and a special massage technique. After Winiwarter's death, his approach was not developed further.

Emil Vodder (1896–1986), a massage therapist and doctor of philosophy from Denmark, lived and worked in France between 1928 and 1939. Vodder "intuitively" manipulated the swollen lymph nodes of some of his patients who suffered from chronic colds and sinus infections. He reported that his therapy was successful and that individuals treated with his techniques felt better. He continued to develop his treatment method and moved to Paris to do further research on the lymphatic system. Vodder called his technique "lymph drainage massage" and introduced it during an international health fair as *le drainage lymphatique*. During this time, the medical community did not accept Vodder's technique, and he continued to train primarily cosmetologists throughout Europe.

In 1963, *Johannes Asdonk* (1910–2003), a German physician, learned about Vodder's technique while working in Essen, Germany, and decided to meet personally with Vodder. Asdonk was impressed with the results Vodder achieved and decided to learn his hands-on technique. Asdonk established the first school for manual lymph drainage (MLD) in 1969 in Germany, with Emil Vodder and Vodder's wife, Astrid, as instructors.

With a more detailed knowledge about the anatomy and physiology of the lymphatic system and the expanding list of indications for this treatment, it was necessary to add new techniques and to modify Vodder's existing techniques. Vodder and Asdonk had differing opinions regarding the technical aspects of the MLD strokes and subsequently ended their partnership in 1971. Vodder moved to Austria to start his own school, and Asdonk remained in Germany, where he continued his extensive research on the effectiveness of manual lymph drainage and its effects on the lymphatic system.

Based on Asdonk's work, MLD as a treatment for lymphedema became reimbursable by national health insurance in Germany in 1974. Together with Kuhnke, Földi, Gregl, and others, Asdonk founded the German Society of Lymphology in 1976. The cooperation between these scientists within the society led to the development of a new therapy concept, which enabled the successful treatment of edemas of different geneses with the addition of various and new intervention techniques. The combination of these techniques is known today as complete decongestive therapy (CDT). Földi founded his own school for lymphology and phlebology in Freiburg, Germany, in 1981.

Kuhnke's work in the development of limb volume measurement techniques provided evidence of the effectiveness of CDT and helped to further establish this therapy in the treatment of lymphedema and other related conditions. Accurate measurement of limb volumes also provided the objective data to prove that the combination of various treatment approaches known as CDT in the treatment of lymphedema is far more effective than the treatment of lymphedema with manual lymph drainage as the sole therapeutic approach.

Most schools providing lymphedema training throughout the world today teach all components of CDT, which includes the advanced version of Vodder's manual lymph drainage.

◆ Goal of Complete Decongestive Therapy

Currently, there is no cure for lymphedema; the main goal of the treatment, therefore, is to return the lymphedema to a stage of latency, utilizing remaining lymph vessels and other lymphatic pathways. The normal or near normal size of the limb should be maintained, and reaccumulation of lymph fluid should be prevented. Additional goals are prevention and elimination of infections and the reduction and removal of fibrotic tissues.

◆ Components of Complete Decongestive Therapy

Complete decongestive therapy consists of a combination of manual lymph drainage, compression therapy, decongestive exercises, and skin care. Each component will be discussed individually.

Manual Lymph Drainage

Manual lymph drainage (MLD) is a gentle manual treatment technique that is based on the four basic Vodder strokes: the "stationary circle," "pump," "rotary," and "scoop." The common denominator in all strokes is the working phase and the resting phase.

In the working phase of a stroke, stretch stimuli are applied to the subcutaneous tissues, resulting in the manipulation of anchoring filaments of lymph capillaries and the smooth musculature in the wall of lymph angions. The light directional pressure in the working phase also serves to move lymph fluid in the appropriate direction. The pressure in this phase should be sufficient enough to stretch the subcutaneous tissue against the underlying fascia to its elastic capacity. It is not necessary to apply high pressure to achieve this goal. In fact, too much pressure could damage anchoring filaments or other lymphatic structures, or cause lymphangiospasm in lymph collectors. The pressure should also be light enough to avoid vasodilation (active hyperemia). The amount of pressure is sometimes described as the pressure applied while stroking a newborn's head. However, more pressure is needed if fibrotic tissue is present.

The pressure is released during the resting phase, in which the elasticity of the skin moves the therapist's hand passively back to the starting position. In this pressure-free phase, initial lymph vessels absorb tissue fluid from the interstitial spaces.

To achieve maximum results, each working phase should last about 1 second and should be repeated five to seven times in the same area in either a stationary or a dynamic pattern.

Massage should not be confused with the techniques of manual lymph drainage. The word *massage*, meaning "to knead" (from the Greek *massain*), is used to describe the techniques employed in "Swedish" or "classic" therapies. To achieve the desired effects on musculature, tendons, and other structures, massage is generally applied with considerably more pressure than MLD. There is no "kneading" in manual lymph drainage.

Effects of Manual Lymph Drainage

The most common effects of manual lymph drainage are the following:

◆ Increase in lymph production: stretch on the anchoring filaments of lymph capillaries stimulates the intake of lymphatic loads into the lymphatic system.

◆ Increase in lymphangiomotoricity: (1) mild perpendicular stimuli of the smooth musculature located in the wall of lymph collectors results in an increased contraction frequency of lymph angions; (2) increased lymph production results in an increase of the volume of transported lymph fluid. The subsequently elevated intralymphatic pressure results in increased contraction frequency of lymph angions.

◆ Reverse of lymph flow: in the treatment of lymphedema, MLD moves lymph fluid in superficial lymph vessels opposite its natural flow patterns. Lymph fluid is rerouted via collateral lymph collectors, anastomoses, or tissue channels.

◆ Increase in venous return: the directional pressure in the working phase of MLD strokes increases the venous return in the superficial venous system. Deeper and more specialized techniques of MLD, especially in the abdominal area, affect the venous return in the deep venous system.

◆ Soothing: the light pressures used in MLD decrease the sympathetic mode and promote the parasympathetic response.

◆ Analgesic: because of accelerated drainage of nociceptive substances from the tissues, light pressure used in MLD provides a stimulus for the "gate-control theory" of Melzack and Wall (1996), promoting pain control.

The goal of manual lymph drainage in the treatment of lymphedema and related conditions is to reroute the lymph flow around blocked areas into more centrally located healthy lymph vessels, which drain into the venous system.

The techniques of MLD include the manipulation of healthy lymph nodes and lymph vessels, which generally are located adjacent to the area with insufficient lymphatic drainage. The resulting increase in lymphangiomotoricity in the healthy areas creates a "suction effect," which enables accumulated lymph fluid to move from an area with insufficient lymph flow into an area with normal lymphatic drainage. To stimulate the return of lymph fluid into the venous system, the lymph nodes on the neck are manipulated. Depending on the location of the damage to the lymphatic system, the thorax, abdominal area, and ipsilateral and contralateral axillary or inguinal lymph node groups may be included in the treatment. The extremity itself is treated in segments (e.g., the proximal aspect of the affected extremity is decongested prior to expanding the treatment to the more distal aspects).

Basic Strokes

◆ **Stationary Circles.** This technique consists of an oval-shaped stretching of the skin with the palmar surfaces of the fingers or the entire hand; it may be applied with one hand or bimanually (alternating or simultaneously). Stationary circles are used on the entire body surface, but mainly on the lymph node groups, the neck, and the face.

Working phase: The pressure increases and decreases gradually in the direction of lymph drainage for about half of a circle, using either radial or ulnar deviation in the wrist. In the first portion of the working phase, the stretch is applied perpendicular to the lymph collects; in the second portion, parallel to the lymph collectors. The full elasticity of the skin should be used to apply the stretch.

Resting phase: The working hand relaxes and maintains contact with the patient's skin. The pressure is completely released, and the elasticity of the skin moves the therapist's hand passively back to the starting position (Fig. 4–1A).

"Thumb" circles represent a variation of stationary circles. This technique is applied with the palmar surface of the thumb and is used primarily on the hand and foot, in the area of joints, and in the treatment of infants (Fig. 4–1B).

◆ **Pump.** This stroke applies a circle-shaped pressure operating within almost the full range between ulnar and radial deviation. The entire palm and the proximal phalanges are used in this technique, which is applied primarily on the extremities. Pumps are dynamic strokes (i.e., the working hand moves from distal to proximal), and they can be applied with one hand or bimanually (alternating).

Working phase: The hand is placed on the skin with ulnar deviation and wrist flexion, the fingers are extended, and the thumb is in opposition to the fingers. In this starting position, the radial aspect of the thumb and index finger, as well as the web space between these two phalanges, is in contact with the skin. The pressure increases and decreases gradually during the transition to radial deviation and wrist extension and reaches its maximum stretch when the entire palm has made contact. Pressure is applied in the drainage direction.

Resting phase: When the skin is stretched to its maximum elasticity and the hand is in radial deviation, the transition to the resting phase begins, in which the elasticity of the skin carries the therapist's hand back to the starting position. To reach the starting point of the next working phase, the hand glides without pressure approximately half a hand width in the proximal direction (Fig. 4–2).

◆ **Scoop.** Scoops are applied on extremities (mainly the distal parts) and consist of a spiral-shaped movement. A transitional movement between ulnar deviation with forearm pronation, moving into radial deviation with forearm supination, is used in the application of this technique. This dynamic stroke is applied with one hand or bimanually (alternating).

Working phase: The hand is placed in ulnar deviation and pronation onto the skin (perpendicular to the pathway of lymph collectors). The web space between the index finger and the thumb is in contact with the body surface at this point. The working phase starts

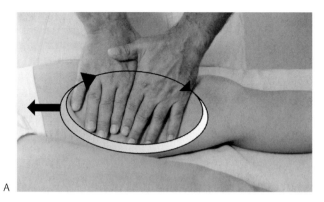

A

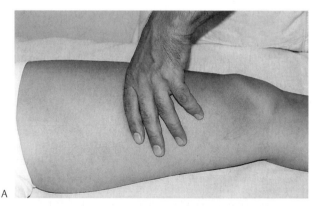

B

Figure 4-1 A. Stationary circles working phase (white half circle) and resting phase of stationary circles. B. Thumb circles on the dorsum of the hand.

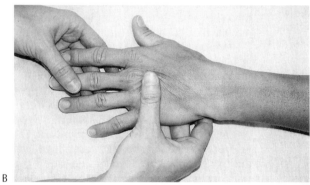

A

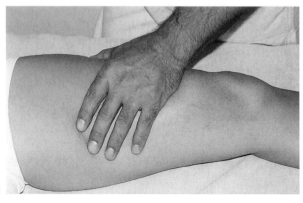

B

Figure 4-2 A. Pump stroke at the beginning of the working phase. B. Pump stroke at the end of the working phase.

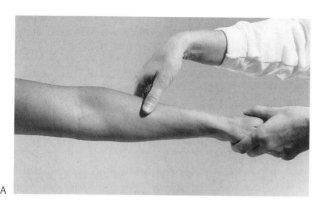

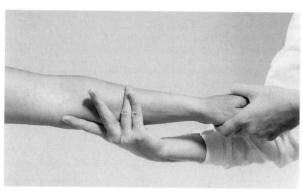

Figure 4–3 A. Scoop at the beginning of the working phase. B. Scoop during the working phase.

A

B

with the hand gliding over the skin in a spiral-like movement in the proximal direction. During the gliding phase, the pressure increases gradually, and the palm and the palmar surfaces of the fingers come in contact with the skin. The pressure reaches its maximum value when the palm is in complete contact with the body surface. With the palm in contact, the fingers glide over the skin in a fanlike pattern until they are aligned parallel with the extremity. During this phase, the pressure gradually decreases again.

Resting phase: After the hand and fingers are parallel with the extremity, the hand does not return to the starting position. It returns to ulnar deviation and pronation, approximately one hand width further proximal, where the next working phase starts (Fig. 4–3).

◆ **Rotary.** This dynamic technique is used on large surface areas—primarily on the trunk, but also on lymphedematous extremities—and can be applied with one hand or bimanually (at the same time or alternating).

Working phase: The hand is placed on the body surface in an elevated position and paral-lel to the pathway of the lymph collectors. The wrist is in flexion, the finger joints (except the thumb) are in a neutral position, and the thumb is ~90 degrees abducted. All fingertips are in contact with the skin. The working phase is initiated as the palm is placed on the skin in an elliptical movement (over the ulnar side). At the same time, the thumb slides to abduction. In this phase, the subcutaneous tissues are stretched against the fascia and perpendicular to the flow of lymph. When contact is established with the full hand and palmar surface, the skin is stretched toward the drainage area with gradually increasing pressure. While the hand stretches, the thumb is adducted until aligned with the hand. The pressure decreases again, the elasticity of the skin moves the hand back to the starting position, and the hand relaxes.

Resting phase: The hand moves back into wrist flexion until it is elevated again. The fingers slide at the same time without pressure (but in skin contact) in drainage direction, until the thumb reaches ~90 degrees of abduction. The sequence continues in this position with the next working phase.

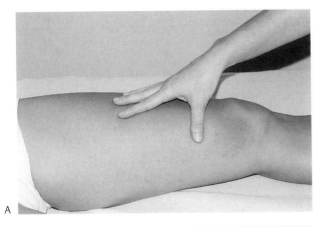

A

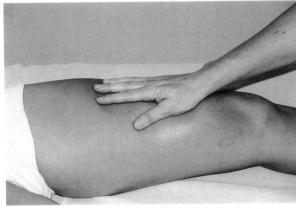

B

Figure 4–4 A. Rotary at the beginning of the working phase. B. Rotary at the end of the working phase.

During the working and the resting phase, the fingers remain in neutral position (Fig. 4-4).

Additional Techniques

◆ **Deep Abdominal Technique.** This technique primarily stimulates deep lymphatic structures, such as the cisterna chyli, the abdominal part of the thoracic duct, lumbar trunks and lymph nodes, pelvic lymph nodes, and certain organ systems. Manipulation of these lymphatic structures, particularly the thoracic duct, accelerates lymph transport toward the venous angles. This results in improved lymphatic drainage from structures distal to the thoracic duct, including the lower extremities. The manipulation of deep veins located in the same area also improves venous return to the heart.

The considerable decongestive effects on the lymphatic and the venous systems make deep abdominal techniques a valuable tool in the treatment of lower extremity swelling.

To reach the deeper structures of the lymphatic system, it is necessary to apply more pressure than with the basic MLD techniques. Therefore, the following cautionary measures must be observed:

◆ Deep abdominal technique must never cause pain or discomfort.

◆ Contraindications listed later in this chapter must be observed.

◆ To reduce the tone and resistance of the abdominal musculature, the head and legs should be elevated during the application.

◆ To avoid hyperventilation and dizziness, these techniques are not repeated five to seven times, as in basic MLD applications. Instead, the sequence of hand placements is applied only once.

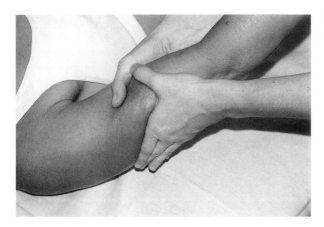

Figure 4–5 Edema technique (superficial) on the upper arm.

The deep abdominal technique is applied on five different locations (for a total of nine strokes) and combined with diaphragmatic breathing. The different hand placements are discussed in Chapter 5, Abdomen (Superficial and Deep Manipulations). The therapist coordinates the technique with the patient's breathing rhythm. The flat and soft hand follows the patient' exhalation into the abdominal cavity, where it remains until the next inhalation (at this point, it is important to note the patient's response to the pressure). A brief period of moderate resistance is applied during the initial inhalation phase. The resistance is released to allow full inhalation. During this phase, the therapist's hand moves to the next location. The full and soft hand then follows the next exhalation phase; this procedure is repeated for all nine strokes.

◆ **Edema Technique.** The goal of this specialized technique is to mobilize the free protein-rich and sluggish edema fluid in extremities toward the drainage area. Edema strokes should be applied only after the drainage area proximal to the application was previously cleared with basic MLD strokes, the ipsilateral trunk quadrant is free of edema, and the extremity has at least begun to decongest.

Edema techniques are administered with increased pressure and prolonged duration (5–8 seconds) in the working phase, and the hands move dynamically from distal to proximal to cover a certain portion of a limb. Edema techniques are immediately followed by reworking techniques (explained in the Chapter 5) and the application of compression bandages.

Two different variations of edema technique may be used. The less intensive technique consists of bimanual pump techniques, which are applied simultaneously on opposing sides of the extremity. This technique can be used on the entire limb (Fig. 4–5).

The deeper and more effective variation is administered circumferentially with the radial surface of both hands. The hands move simultaneously into the subcutaneous tissue and proceed to move the lymph fluid toward proximal. This technique is applied on the lower leg and foot and the hand and forearm.

This more intense technique cannot be used with the following conditions: painful lipedema or lipolymphedema, if pain is present in swellings of other genesis, patients with hemophilia, patients on anticoagulants, and with varicose veins or deep venous thrombosis. Other contraindications listed later in this chapter must be observed (Fig. 4–6).

◆ **Fibrosis Technique.** This modality is used to soften and break up lymphostatic fibrosis and should be used only if the extremity has begun to decongest. Fibrosis techniques are applied directly in the area of lymphostatic fibrosis with more intensity and prolonged duration than the basic techniques of MLD; these techniques may cause local vasodilation. To optimize the fibrinolytic effect, compression bandages (preferably in combination with special foam applications) should be applied directly following fibrosis techniques.

Two different variations of the fibrosis technique may be used. With the "kneading" technique, the fibrotic tissue is lifted softly from

109

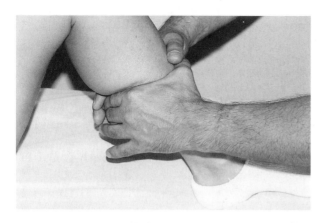

Figure 4–6 Edema technique (deep) on the lower leg.

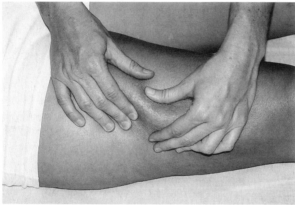

Figure 4–7 Fibrosis technique ("kneading" technique) on the thigh.

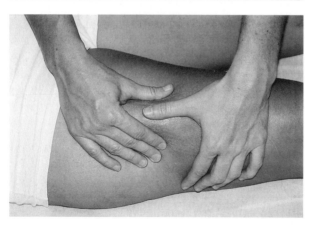

Figure 4–8 Fibrosis technique ("thumb" technique) on the thigh.

the underlying tissue with the flat finger pads. The skinfold is then softly and slowly moved using an S-shaped manipulation between the thumb of one hand and the fingers of the other hand. This treatment can be compared with kneading strokes used in massage techniques (Fig. 4–7).

In the other, more intense technique, the fibrotic tissue fold is lifted softly with the flat fingers of one hand. The flat thumb of the other hand manipulates the skinfold by pressing down on it.

Fibrosis techniques are contraindicated in the area of radiation fibrosis. Other contraindications include the same as discussed in edema technique (Fig. 4–8).

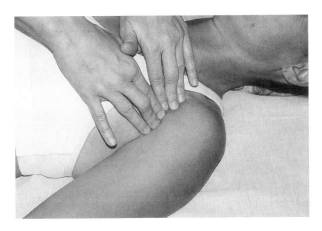

Figure 4–9 Vasa vasorum technique (cephalic vein).

◆ **Vasa Vasorum Technique.** This technique uses and optimizes the drainage pathways of the plexus-like lymph vessels in the adventitia of larger blood vessels (veins). These structures serve as additional drainage pathways in the treatment of lymphedema (Fig. 4–9).

Contraindications for Manual Lymph Drainage

General contraindications for MLD include the following:

◆ Cardiac edema: there is no therapeutic benefit of MLD/CDT in the treatment of swellings caused by decompensated cardiac insufficiency. If cardiac edema is combined with lymphedema, MLD may be indicated, but cardiac and pulmonary functions need to be closely monitored by the referring physician.

◆ Renal failure

◆ Acute infections: the application of MLD may exacerbate the symptoms.

◆ Acute bronchitis: the parasympathetic effect of MLD may exacerbate the symptoms in the acute phase by producing contractions of the smooth bronchial musculature.

◆ Acute deep vein thrombosis: MLD/CDT is contraindicated on the affected extremity and the abdominal area.

◆ Malignancies: close cooperation with the referring physician is necessary. MLD/CDT may be indicated as palliative treatment. To date there is no scientific evidence that the application of MLD (or other manual treat-ment techniques) would accelerate the spread of malignant cells to other parts of the body or contribute to the growth of malignant tumors.

◆ Bronchial asthma: because of the parasympathetic stimulation, MLD may cause the onset of an asthma attack. In lymphedema patients with a combined diagnosis of bronchial asthma, MLD generally can be applied safely if the treatment time is incrementally increased, starting at ~20 minutes of initial treatment time. If no negative reactions are noted during or after the therapy, the treatment time may be increased by 5 to 10 minutes until reaching normal treatment time values.

◆ Hypertension: MLD/CDT may be applied if cardiac functions are monitored.

Local contraindications on the neck include the following:

◆ Carotid-sinus syndrome: hypersensitivity of pressure receptors on the carotid bifurcation may cause cardiac arrhythmia.

◆ Hyperthyroidism: manipulation on the neck may accelerate the release of thyroid hormones and/or medications into the blood.

◆ Age: with patients over 60 years of age, there may be an increased risk of atherosclerosis in the neck arteries.

Local contraindications for the abdominal area include the following:

◆ Pregnancy

◆ Dysmenorrhea

◆ Ileus

◆ Diverticulosis

◆ Aortic aneurysm (also palpation of strong aortic pulse)

◆ Recent abdominal surgery

◆ Deep vein thrombosis

◆ Inflammatory conditions of the small and large intestines: Crohn's disease, ulcerative colitis, diverticulitis

◆ Radiation fibrosis, radiation cystitis, radiation colitis

◆ Unexplained pain

◆ Compression Therapy

The elastic fibers of the cutaneous tissues are damaged in lymphedema. This is true for lymphedema in its pure appearance (primary and secondary), as well as in lymphedema combined with other pathologies. Although lymphedema may be reduced to a normal or near normal size utilizing proper treatment techniques, the lymphatics are never normal again after lymphedema is present, and the skin elasticity may never be regained completely. The affected body part is always at risk for a reaccumulation of fluid. External support of the affected extremity/body part is therefore an essential component of lymphedema management. The primary goal in compression therapy is to maintain the decongestive effect achieved during the MLD session; that is, to prevent reaccumulation of fluid into the tissues. Without the benefits provided by compression therapy, successful treatment of lymphedema would be impossible.

Based on the phase of the treatment (see The Two-Phase Approach in Lymphedema Management later in this chapter), compression therapy is applied by specific bandage materials, so-called short-stretch bandages, or by compression garments, or a combination of both modalitities.

Effects of Compression Therapy

The following effects are achieved with compression bandages and garments:

◆ Increases the pressure in the tissues itself, as well as on the blood and lymph vessels contained in these tissues

The tissue pressure plays an essential role in the exchange of fluids between the blood capillaries and the tissues. The beneficial effects of increased tissue pressure are especially important during airplane travel (see Chapter 5, Lymphedema and Air Travel).

◆ Improves venous and lymphatic return

External compression forces these fluids in the proximal direction; it also improves the function of the valves contained in these vessels.

◆ Reduces net filtration [blood capillary pressure (BCP) – interstitial fluid pressure (IP)]

To determine the fluid value leaving the blood capillary, it is necessary to subtract the inward forces (IP) from the outward forces (BCP) on the capillary (see Chapter 2, Filtration and Reabsorption).

◆ Improves the effectiveness of the muscle and joint pumps during activity

The activity of skeletal musculature is an important factor in the return of fluids within the venous and lymphatic system. Together with other supporting mechanisms, the muscle and joint pump activity propels these fluids back to the heart and ensures an uninterrupted circulation. External compression provides a sufficient counterforce to the working musculature, thus improving its efficiency.

◆ Prevents the reaccumulation of evacuated lymph fluid and conserves the results achieved during MLD

Compression therapy compensates for the elastic insufficiency of the affected tissue.

◆ Helps to break up and soften deposits of connective tissue and scar tissue

This effect is especially beneficial in the treatment of lymphostatic fibrosis and can be increased by the use of special foam materials in combination with compression therapy.

◆ Provides support for those tissues that have lost elasticity

◆ Depending on the materials used (compression garments, short-stretch bandages), it provides for a high working pressure and a low resting pressure (see Compression Bandages later in this chapter).

Laplace's Law

The value of pressure achieved on a body part by use of external compression is generally measured in millimeters of mercury (mmHg). To achieve the desired effects in compression therapy, it is imperative that the pressure value decreases gradually from distal to proximal. Bandages and compression garments achieve this effect if they are applied correctly. Complications are common if the measurements or compression classes of compression garments are faulty or if short-stretch bandages are applied incorrectly.

> The Laplace's law can be used to explain the importance of graded compression using elastic materials. This law states that if the radius (r) of a cylinder (extremity) is increased, the tension (T) needs to be increased to achieve the same pressure (P). This means that if compression is applied on a cylinder using equal tension, the pressure is greatest where the radius (of the cylinder) is the smallest.

A normal extremity can be compared with a cylinder. If compression therapy is applied on a leg, using the same tension (T) between the distal and the proximal end of the extremity, the pressure (P) in the ankle area (smaller radius) would be greater than the pressure on the calf (greater radius), and the pressure on the thigh would be lower than the pressure on the calf.

This law can be applied in a true cylindrical or cone-shaped extremity. In the area of bony prominences (ankles, wrists, or the medial and lateral circumferences of the hand and foot), the pressure is higher due to the smaller radius and the greater tension of the compressive medium, whereas the pressure is lower in concave areas (behind the ankles).

These issues and the fact that swollen extremities generally lose their cone shape make it necessary to use foam materials for padding in combination with compression bandages to "construct" a cylinder.

Padding is usually not necessary in compression garments. Because of the manufacturing process of these materials, a compression gradient is built into the garments.

Compression Bandages

Short-stretch compression bandages are primarily used in the decongestive phase of CDT. These bandages are textile-elastic; the braided cotton fibers used in the production process are woven to achieve a certain degree of elasticity. In newly manufactured short-stretch bandages, this interwoven pattern allows for ~60% extensibility of the bandage's original length. To understand the effects of various bandage materials on the tissues and the vascular systems embedded within the tissues, it is important to discuss the difference between short-stretch and long-stretch bandages.

Two different qualities of pressure can be distinguished in compression therapy: the working pressure and the resting pressure. Relevant in the determination of these pressure qualities are the type of bandage (long-stretch or short-stretch), the tension used during the application of the bandage, the number of layers, and the condition of the material (age). Bandages lose some of their elasticity over time and with repetitive use and cleaning.

Working pressure: The resistance the bandage sets against the working musculature determines the working pressure. This pressure is temporary; that is, it is active only during muscle expansion, and its value depends on the extent of muscle contraction. The active working pressure results in an increase of tissue pressure (TP), and the venous and lymphatic vessels in the superficial and in the deep systems are compressed. The return of fluids within these vessel systems is improved.

The lower the elasticity of a compression bandage, the higher the working pressure. Short-stretch bandages (up to 60% elasticity) exert a high working pressure on the tissues and form a strong support during muscle contraction.

Long-stretch bandages (Ace bandages) contain polyurethane and retain a low working pressure. Newly manufactured long-stretch bandages allow for an extensibility of more than 140% of the bandage's original length. This relatively high elasticity exerts a low resistance against the working musculature, and the decongestive effect on the venous and lymphatic system is minimal, especially in the deep systems.

Resting pressure: This is the pressure the bandage exerts on the tissues at rest, that is, without muscle contraction. The resting pressure is a permanent pressure, and its value depends on the amount of tension used during the application of the bandage. The higher the tension (or stretch), the higher the pressure the bandage exerts on the tissues. A bandage with a high extensibility will therefore result in increased pressure on the tissues during rest.

Long-stretch bandages exert a relatively high resting pressure, during which the venous and lymphatic vessels primarily in the skin (above the fascia) are compressed. This permanent compression may cause a tourniquet effect on the bandaged extremity.

Short-stretch bandages employ a very low resting pressure on the tissues and the vascular systems. The risk of a tourniquet effect is therefore relatively low as long as a specially trained individual applies the compression bandages correctly.

The high working and low resting pressure qualities of short-stretch bandages make them the preferred compression bandage in the management of lymphedema and swellings of other geneses.

Long-stretch bandages may constrict veins and lymph vessels at rest and provide minimal support of the tissues during muscle contraction. Long-stretch bandages are therefore not suitable for the treatment of lymphedema.

To avoid constriction of venous and lymphatic vessels and to achieve a compression gradient in the treatment of lymphedema, it is necessary to apply compression bandages in layers. Following the application of a suitable moisturizer on the skin (see Skin and Nail Care later in this chapter), a cotton stockinette is applied to absorb sweat and to protect the skin from the padding materials. As discussed earlier, the goal in the use of padding is to protect bony prominences and to bring the extremity into a cylindrical shape. Special soft foam materials or synthetic cotton bandages are used for this purpose. For the padding of concave areas (behind the malleoli, palm) or to increase the pressure over lymphostatic fibrosis or wounds, a more dense foam material is suitable. Short-stretch bandages of various widths are then applied in layers on the extremity. Tape should be used to affix the band-age material, not clips or pins. Sharp bandaging clips or pins may cut into the patient's skin and provide an avenue for infection.

> Only trained therapists or patients and their caregivers who have received instruction in the application of short-stretch bandages from a trained individual should apply compression bandages in the treatment of lymphedema.

Correctly applied compression bandages are safe and effective and represent an indispensable part of CDT. Bandage materials are used primarily during the decongestive phase of CDT and can be bulky. Most patients adjust to and tolerate the compression bandage well after a few applications. Patients should maintain their normal activity level and perform the decongestive exercise program (see Decongestive Exercises later in this chapter) while wearing the bandages.

Refer to Chapter 5 for detailed illustrations and guidelines for the application of short-stretch bandages (materials used in compression therapy are listed under Required Materials).

Compression Garments

Patients with lymphedema graduate from bandages to elastic compression garments once the limb is decongested (phase 2 of CDT). To preserve the treatment success achieved during the decongestion of the edematous limb, compression garments have to be worn throughout the patient's life. Because compression garments will not, by themselves, reduce swelling, they must not be worn on an untreated, swollen extremity.

To ensure the long-term benefits of compression garments described earlier in this chapter, it is important that only trained individuals with a full understanding of the pathology of lymphedema and its related conditions take the appropriate measurements and make an educated choice regarding the garment selection. Compression garments become a part of the patient's life, much like hearing aids or eyeglasses. Ill-fitted and ineffective compression garments not only produce poor results but also can be dangerous to the patient. Many potential problems and special needs of the individual patient must be

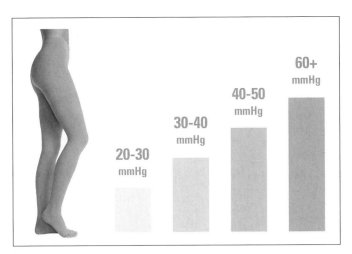

Figure 4-10 Compression levels (With permission from JUZO, Inc.).

addressed and solved to arrive at a comfortable yet supportive garment solution.

Compression garments are available as compression gauntlets, sleeves, and stockings and are made for specific body parts (e.g., brassieres or vests). They are manufactured in several sizes, variations (circular knit, flat knit), styles, compression levels (or classes), and materials, and they may be ordered in standard sizes or be custom made.

Compression Levels

Currently, an international standard for compression values in different compression levels is unavailable. The compression levels establish the compression value the garments produce on the skin surface and are measured in millimeters of mercury (mmHg). To ensure the benefits of compression, a gradient from distal to proximal is necessary. The pressure values within the different levels of compression are measured on the distal circumference of the extremity (on the leg at the ankles), where the pressure is highest. Most manufacturers in the United States use the following values:

Compression level I: 20 to 30 mmHg
Compression level II: 30 to 40 mmHg
Compression level III: 40 to 50 mmHg
Compression level IV: >60 mmHg (Fig. 4–10)

Values below 20 mmHg are not suitable in the management of lymphedema. These pressures are used in the support-stocking categories, which cover a lower level of compression ($\sim$8–15 mmHg) or a higher level of compression ($\sim$15–20 mmHg).

In some cases of lower extremity lymphedema, a compression of more than that available in compression level IV may be used. In these cases, a compression level III knee-high stocking may be worn in addition to a compression level III thigh-high stocking (or pantyhose). It is important to understand that the individual compression values of garments worn on top of each other do not double in values. Two level III stockings, for example, do not add up to a level VI; the resulting pressure would be somewhere between a level IV and V.

Physical limitations of the patient could be a rationale for a decision to combine two stockings. For example, an arthritic patient who requires a lower extremity garment of a higher compression level may have less difficulty donning a compression level III thigh-high with a compression level II knee-high stocking.

The average upper extremity lymphedema patient will use a compression level II arm sleeve, provided there are no contraindications that would require the use of a lower class compression, such as in the case of a partial, completely paralyzed, or flaccid limb. A patient with upper extremity lymphedema may require a compression level III arm sleeve if he or she is involved in a high-intensity and repetitive activity. For example, if a patient wishes to return to playing golf, a level III arm sleeve can be used on the involved extremity during play and a level II arm sleeve for daily activities.

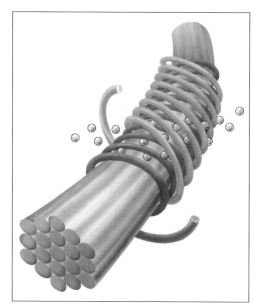

Figure 4–11 Covered compression threads used in compression garments (JUZO Fibersoft) (With permission from JUZO, Inc.).

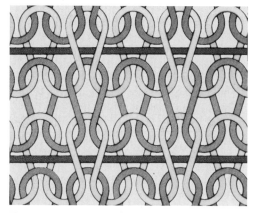

Figure 4–12 Two-way elasticity in compression garments (With permission from JUZO, Inc.).

Patients with lower extremity involvement will usually require a compression level III garment. Again, contraindications may be present that may require the use of a lower level of compression, and certain situations may require a higher level of compression.

Many factors must be considered, such as age, activity level, skin integrity, congestive heart failure, partial or complete paralysis, diabetes, and wound care issues, to determine the correct compression level for a patient.

If the patient has tolerated compression well during the decongestive phase, her or she may easily fit into the standard compression levels for the upper and lower extremities. It is important to consider the physical ability of the patient, as well as the patient's home support system, when choosing a compression garment. A 70-year-old patient with lower extremity lymphedema may not be physically able to don a level III garment; thus a level II garment may better serve the patient's needs.

Circular Knit and Flat Knit Garments

Compression garments are manufactured in either a flat knit or a circular knit method. Both types are knitted using threads made of some form of rubber (some manufacturers use nonsynthetic rubber). Either cotton or a synthetic material generally covers this elastomer, providing the garment with additional qualities (Fig. 4–11). Covered compression threads are more durable in that they limit or regulate stretch of the elastic fiber and protect it from sweat and skin ointments. The softer cover fibers make the garments more breathable and easier to apply. The manufacturing process provides compression garments with a two-way elasticity (Fig. 4–12). The more two-way stretch a compression garment provides, the more comfortable it is to wear.

Circular knit garments are manufactured on a cylindrical knitting machine, which allows them to be seamless. The same number of needles or meshes is used throughout the length of the garment. The size of the meshes, as well as the degree of prestretch of the inlay elastomer, provides for a smaller circumference on the distal and a larger circumference on the proximal portion of the garment.

In flat knit garments, the number of needles or meshes varies according to the patient's measurements, which provide these garments with the same density throughout their length. Flat knit garments can be custom manufactured in any shape or size and are available in various ready-made sizes. Compression levels of more than 50 mmHg are provided only in flat knit materials; however, flat knit garments are also available in lower compression levels.

The choice between flat or circular knit compression garments involves various considerations. Circular knitted materials are less expensive and cosmetically more attractive than flat knit garments, because they have no seam and are produced using finer and sheerer materials. Because of the manufacturing process of flat knit garments, these items are usually denser and more costly to produce. However, they produce a more perfect fit because the number of meshes is determined by the patient's circumferential measurements, provided that the measurements are taken correctly. This could be a determining factor for those patients with grossly deformed extremities.

Esthetic considerations are an important aspect in choosing the right compression garment. It is important to understand that compression garments are effective only if they are worn consistently. If the patient is unhappy with the garment and does not want to wear it, the therapeutic benefit is lost. Compression level IV can be provided by a singular flat knit garment, which would be able to provide a constant compression gradient throughout the extremity, or by wearing a compression level III thigh-high (or pantyhose) circular knit material in combination with a compression level II knee-high (or thigh-high) garment of the same material. Flat knitted stockings can be disguised by wearing a sheer (preferably dark) nylon stocking on top of them.

Custom-Made and Standard Compression Garments

Compression garments with a compression level of more than 50 mmHg are available only in custom-made materials. The high degree of compression requires the garment to be manufactured to the patient's exact circumferential measurements. As discussed earlier, custom-made garments are also a better choice for those individuals with extremely deformed extremities. Some manufacturers provide custom garments with zippers, which could be a choice for patients who may be physically unable to don a closed compression garment.

Standard or ready-made garments are available in compression levels I–III. Ready-made garments can be obtained from most manufacturers and in a large number of premade sizes and styles that can accommodate the vast majority of extremities.

Custom-made garments are very costly, and the production time for these garments is longer. Although some lymphedema patients benefit from custom-made garments, they are certainly not a necessity for all lymphedema patients. The availability of a large variety of standard garments helps to reduce the cost and allows patients to wear cosmetically more attractive compression garments.

Styles of Compression Garments

Custom-made and standard compression garments are available in different styles and lengths and can be ordered with a variety of fastening systems and integrated pressure pads. Refer to Figure 4–13 for a summary of available styles and lengths.

Fastening systems are designed to prevent the garments from sliding, which could create a tourniquet effect and thus make the compression garment uncomfortable to wear for the individual. These systems consist of garter belts (Fig. 4–14), hip attachments (Fig. 4–15), or fasteners that attach to shoulder straps or borders made of synthetic polymers (usually silicone dots or stripes) on the inside of the proximal end of the garments (Fig. 4–16).

Some manufacturers provide adhesive lotions, which can be used to prevent the garment from slipping.

Built-in pressure pads constructed of dense foam materials ensure an even distribution of pressure in concave areas, such as behind the malleoli or the palmar surface of the hand.

To ensure maximum therapeutic benefit, it is absolutely necessary that only individuals with a thorough understanding of the pathology of lymphedema, together with the patient, decide on the compression level, style, and length of the garment. Compression garments should be worn daily and applied first thing in the morning. They should be replaced every 6 months or sooner if the garments have lost their elasticity. Refer to Chapter 5,

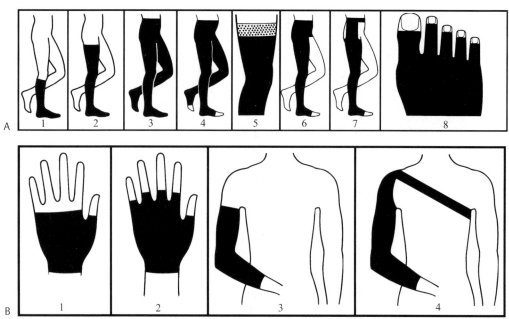

A

B

Figure 4-13 A. Compression styles. 1. Knee-high stocking. 2. Thigh-high stocking. 3. Pantyhose. 4. Pantyhose with highly elastic body part. 5. Thigh-high stocking with fastening border (silicone dots). 6. Thigh-high stocking with hip attachment. 7. Thigh-high stocking with garter belt. 8. Toe caps. B. Compression styles. 1. Compression gauntlet. 2. Compression gauntlet with finger stubs. 3. Arm sleeve. 4. Arm sleeve with shoulder cover and strap (With permission from JUZO, Inc.).

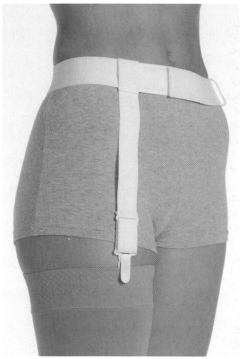

Measurements for Compression Garments, for measuring techniques.

Donning aids can be useful to help in the application of compression garments. Rubber gloves, slip-on/off aids, and nonslip mats are examples of donning systems, which also help to protect the garment from damage (Fig. 4–17).

Alternative Materials

In recent years several adjustable compression devices became available for patients with lymphedema and venous disorders. These devices provide gradient compression by use of nonelastic adjustable bands. Some of these devices use foam pads underneath the nonelastic material to provide additional padding, others may be combined with traditional compression garments (Fig. 4–18).

◁ **Figure 4-14** Thigh-high compression stocking with garter belt (With permission from JUZO, Inc.).

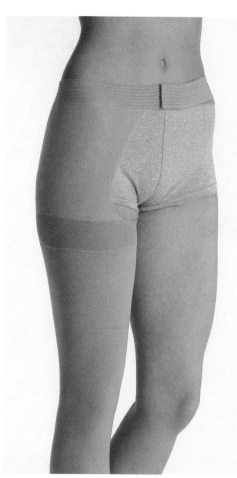

Figure 4–15 Thigh-high compression stocking with hip attachment (With permission from JUZO, Inc.).

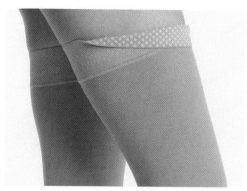

Figure 4–16 Thigh-high compression stocking with fastening border made of silicone dots (With permission from JUZO, Inc.).

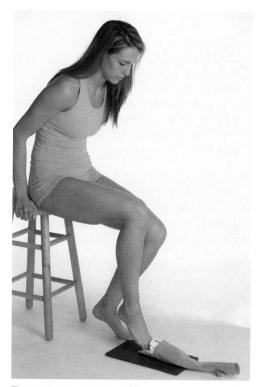

Figure 4–17 Donning aid for open-toe compression stockings (JUZO Slippie; With permission from JUZO, Inc.).

There is a broad consensus between clinicians that these devices should not be used to decongest a swollen limb. The application of short-stretch bandage materials in combination with appropriate padding allows customization of the compression in virtually unlimited variations. Nonelastic, adjustable compression may be used as an alternative to nighttime bandaging in the second phase of CDT, when the extremity has decongested to a normal or near normal size. Patients who are physically unable (or unwilling) to apply nighttime bandaging may choose this more costly alternative.

Contraindications for Compression Therapy

The application of compression on an extremity is absolutely contraindicated in the following cases:

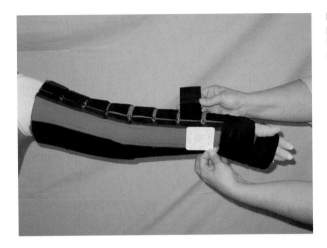

Figure 4–18 Padded gradient compression with nonelastic adjustable bands (CircAid Measure-Up; With permission from CircAid Medical).

◆ Cardiac edema

◆ Peripheral arterial diseases: compression therapy is contraindicated with an ankle/brachial index (ABI) of less than 0.8. Normal ABI values are 0.95 to 1.3; mild to moderate arterial disease, 0.5 to 0.8. ABI values of less than 0.5 are interpreted as severe arterial insufficiencies.

> The ankle/brachial index compares the systolic blood pressure of the ankle to that of the arm (brachial). These measurements are useful in the assessment, follow-up, and treatment of patients with peripheral vascular disease.

◆ Reflex sympathetic dystrophy (RSD)

◆ Acute infections (cellulitis, erysipelas)

The following is a summary of conditions in which compression therapy may be used with caution (relative contraindications). To determine which level of compression is appropriate, close cooperation with the referring physician is necessary:

◆ Hypertension

◆ Cardiac arrhythmia

◆ Decreased or absent sensation in the extremity

◆ Partial or complete paralysis, flaccid limbs

◆ Age

◆ Congestive heart failure

◆ Mild to moderate arterial disease (ABI values 0.5–0.95)

◆ Diabetes

◆ Malignant lymphedema

◆ Decongestive Exercises
(by Kim Leaird, P.T.)

The intensity and prescription of exercise has been a controversial topic in the field of lymphedema management. There is a general consensus that exercise is beneficial, but the primary question is, how much is too much? Another point of contention is adherence to a list of exercise precautions. Because of the benefits of exercise or activity in general, physicians are reluctant to caution patients about limiting activities without evidence-based research to support the precautions.

Some professionals contend that patients with lymphedema or a limb at risk for lymphedema should return to their daily activities (to include recreational activities) and "wait to see what happens." Although most patients who have undergone lymph node disruption (radiation or resection) will not develop lymphedema, it is difficult to specifically identify which patients will develop lymphedema. Prudent clinicians and therapists should educate their patients about risk factors and precautions in an attempt to prevent the onset of lymphedema and to facilitate patient fitness goals.

The lymphatic system maintains a state of homeostasis of body fluids and "sweeps" or filter the interstitial space to remove the lymphatic loads (water, cells, fat from the intestines, and proteins). This is a delicate balance, because the body continuously shifts water to maintain that state of homeostasis so that the body does not become too edematous or dehydrated. With a *dynamic insufficiency*, the lymphatic system attempts to remove excess interstitial fluid with an increase in lymph angiomotoricity. Slight swelling may occur, but with time a normal lymphatic system can compensate and remove the swelling. If the lymphatic system is impaired (*mechanical insufficiency*), morphological and functional changes inhibit the transport of the lymphatic loads, as well as any additional water accumulation in the interstitium.

Lymphedema occurs from the buildup of excess water and proteins in the interstitial space. It is the primary responsibility of the lymphatic system to remove proteins and other large macromolecules from the interstitium. Complicating this process is the fact that proteins are hydrophilic, that is, they attract water. A buildup of proteins in the interstitium will ultimately equate to an increase in water. An impaired lymphatic system is unable to remove water and proteins (and other lymphatic loads) and return them to the venous circulation.

Exercise is beneficial not only for the general population but also for patients with lymphedema. Some long-term benefits from exercise include improved muscular strength; a decrease in resting heart rate; improved strength in bone, tendons, and ligaments; and a decrease in body fat. During active exercise, there is an increase in blood capillary permeability, filtration, and the lymphatic load of water. Cellular responses along with other chemical reactions produce energy and provide adequate nutrition to meet muscular demands. Blood flow increases to supply the working muscles, which leads to the production of additional fluid (lymphatic loads) for transport via the lymphatic system. Under normal physiological conditions, an intact lymphatic system can handle this increase without difficulty.

Exercise is most beneficial for patients with lymphedema when compression (bandages or garments) is used on the affected limb during periods of exercise. Collectors of the superficial lymphatic system are located above the muscle and fascia and below the epidermis in the superficial fatty tissue. Compression provides a slight, forgiving resistance so that the musculature can act as an internal pumping mechanism. The rhythmic contraction and relaxation of the muscles against the garments or bandages will increase lymph angiomotoricity and limit filtration by providing an increase in tissue pressure. With compression, exercise can increase the uptake of fluid into the initial lymphatics and improve the pumping action of the lymph collectors.

Compression must be adequate to prevent reaccumulation of fluid in the involved extremity, but too much compression may undermine the positive effects of exercise. Also, too much compression may have a tourniquet effect on any residual functioning lymph collectors, thus impairing lymph flow.

There are no specific exercises that are better for lymphedema; in fact, all patients with lymphedema can benefit from some form of decongestive exercises. The patient's constraints and ability levels determined by an orthopedic evaluation will govern exercise prescription. The impact of exercise varies significantly between patients and is contingent on the status of the lymphatic system—the extent of residual functioning lymphatic vessels and/or the presence of lymph node fibrosis. Therefore, exercise prescription and guidance should be under the direction of a qualified clinician or therapist with knowledge of lymphedema risk factors, contraindications, and exercise progression.

An appropriate intensity to perform exercise could be described as the level where the activity can easily be sustained, allowing the patient to engage simultaneously in conversation. Light to moderate exercise allows the individual to reach a steady state and continue the activity for a given period of time with less risk of reaching fatigue. Strenuous exercise will cause an increase in plasma lactate and a systemic drop in blood pH levels, which inhibits the chemical reactions that promote muscle contraction. After fatigue is reached, the patient is less likely to continue the exercise.

The muscular soreness that follows excessive exercise is due to the microswelling and microtearing within the muscle fibers. This will lead to pain and stiffness, which may discourage participation in an exercise program.

Gradual progression is imperative when prescribing exercises or recommending the return to activities for patients with lymphedema or a limb at risk. Exercise programs should be comparable to the patient's fitness level, while trying to accomplish the ultimate goal—improve the flow of lymph—and not further stress an impaired lymphatic system. High-intensity and repetitive activities such as tennis, golf, bowling, running, and mountain biking may not be beneficial for patients to immediately return to at the end of phase 1 of therapy. If the patient was proficient at the activity prior to the onset of lymphedema, the individual may be able to return to some form of the activity, provided constant monitoring of the at-risk or involved limb shows no signs of exacerbation of symptoms. The patient with lymphedema will be at a lower risk of reaccumulation of fluid or exacerbation of symptoms if the involved extremity is compressed during exercise.

Strength training can be beneficial for most patients with lymphedema. An improved baseline of strength will allow daily tasks to be performed with less effort and possibly prevent muscular or ligament sprain or strain. Improved strength can prevent overuse syndrome and restore intramuscular balance and normal biomechanics to the involved limb and surrounding joints. When beginning a resistance program, weights should be light, with higher repetitions (initially 15–20 repetitions for 1–2 weeks, then progressing to 30 repetitions), as opposed to choosing the heaviest weight the patient can only lift one to three times. It cannot be stressed enough that a patient is unlikely to develop negative effects in terms of accumulation of fluid if exercise is performed with compression on the involved extremity.

In some instances, individuals may not tolerate exercises that isolate the involved extremity. For example, a patient with upper extremity involvement may be prescribed bicep curls, wrist flexion and extension, gripping exercises, and shoulder presses using a 1 or 2 pound weight for 15 repetitions. If the involved

limb responds adversely to these exercises, the patient may benefit from general, systemic activities such as light to moderate walking or biking. Walking and biking will stimulate diaphragmatic breathing, which will promote the return of lymph to the venous angle. Therapists should encourage patients not to swing their arms excessively when walking. The centrifugal forces created with forcefully swinging the upper extremities in the dependent position may actually pull fluid toward the distal ends of the extremities. A walking stick can be a valuable tool with walking. This will prevent forceful swinging of the arms, and if tall enough may allow the arm to be carried at or above heart level, combating the forces of gravity. Biking on a level surface in a high gear (easy to pedal) is preferred for lower extremity patients as opposed to biking against heavy resistance or in a lower gear.

Occasionally, there may be patients who think if some exercise is good, then more must be better. Others may find traditionally prescribed decongestive exercises (which can be any comfortable movements performed with compression of the involved extremity) not vigorous or intense enough. Again, how much is too much? With physical work, a cascade of events occurs to meet the demands of working muscles and remove metabolic buildup. The intensity of this exercise or work will determine how long the activity can be sustained and the effectiveness of nutritional supply and waste removal of the tissues (e.g., one can sprint only a given distance, and this varies with each individual). Regardless of the fitness level, exercise programs for patients with lymphedema should be progressed at a pace where the effects of exercise can be monitored and the program altered if needed.

Given that there is no method of predicting which individuals will develop lymphedema, each patient is considered at risk whether he or she is sedentary or physically fit. Exercise has several effects on the lymphatic system: it increases lymph angiomotoricity (by muscle contraction and pulsation of adjacent arteries), causes a fluctuation of the interstitial pressure, increases sympathetic tone, and provides a milking or suction effect on the thoracic duct (the thoracic duct travels through the diaphragm with the aorta at the aortic hiatus). To combat the potential negative effects of exercise on the involved extremity, it is recommended to use compression with exercise to prevent the accumulation of additional fluid in the interstitium and to encourage the uptake of fluid into the initial lymphatics. Structured, individualized exercise programs by a knowledgeable clinician will help improve lymphedema and help patients with their fitness goals.

◆ Skin and Nail Care

Patients suffering from lymphedema are susceptible to infections of the skin and nails. Meticulous care of these areas is essential to the success of CDT. Skin is usually impermeable to bacteria and other pathogens, but any defect in the skin, whether from trauma, heat, or other causes, can be an entry site for pathogens or infectious agents. Lymphedematous tissues are saturated with protein-rich fluid, which serves as an ideal breeding ground for pathogens. In addition, the local immune defense is low due to the increased diffusion distance, which hinders a timely response of the defense cells in the affected area. Lymphedematous skin can also become thickened and scaly, which increases the risk of skin cracks and fissures.

Streptococcus bacteria most commonly cause infections in patients with lymphedema. At a local level, *Streptococcus* is not highly toxic, and the body's defense reacts slow initially; therefore, the infectious bacteria can reproduce and migrate to other parts of the body. The process of inflammation may develop into a serious medical crisis and can make lymphedema much worse by accelerating the progression through its stages. The basic consideration in skin and nail care is therefore the prevention and control of infections.

Patients are instructed in proper cleansing and moisturizing techniques to maintain the health and integrity of the skin. This educational process includes how to inspect the skin for any wounds or signs of infection or inflammation. A checklist of precautions should be presented to the patient in the early stages of treatment. This list increases compliance and helps the patient to avoid situations and activities that may worsen the lymphedema or cause infections. A list of precautions and high- and medium-risk activities is provided in Chapter 5, Precautions.

Suitable ointments or lotions formulated for sensitive skin, radiation dermatitis, and lymphedema should be applied before lymphedema bandages while the patient is in the decongestive phase of the treatment. After the limb is decongested and the patient wears compression garments, moisturizing ointments should be applied twice daily. Ointments, as well as soaps or other skin cleansers used in lymphedema management, should have good moisturizing qualities, contain no fragrances, be hypoallergenic, and be formulated to be in either the neutral or acidic range of the pH scale (around pH 5.0). The acidity or alkalinity of the skin is measured on the pH scale, which ranges from 0 (extremely acidic, as in lemon juice) to 14 (extremely alkaline, as in lye). Level 7 on the pH scale represents a neutral value (as in water). Normal skin pH is around 5.0.

To identify possible allergic reactions to skin care products, they should be first tested on healthy skin before the initial application on lymphedematous skin.

Tight-fitting compression sleeves or stockings, as well as materials used in compression bandaging, may cause skin irritation. Some patients may be allergic to a certain material used for compression therapy. This situation usually can be remedied easily by switching to other materials.

In mosquito-infected areas, it is necessary to apply insect repellents to the affected extremity (some moisturizers contain natural repellents) to avoid bites, which could cause infections.

◆ The Two-Phase Approach in Lymphedema Management

Successful lymphedema management is performed in two phases. In phase 1, also known as the intensive or decongestive phase, the patient is seen on a daily basis, and treatments are given until the limb is decongested. It is imperative for the success of the treatment that treatments are given daily and that the patient is thoroughly informed about all components of complete decongestive therapy before treatment is initiated (see Chapter 3, Evaluation of Lymphedema). Patients unable or unwilling to present for daily treatments should not be admitted.

The duration of the intensive phase varies with the severity of the condition and averages 2 to 3 weeks for patients with upper extremity lymphedema and 2 to 4 weeks for patients with lymphedema of the leg. In extreme cases the decongestive phase may last up to 6 to 8 weeks and may have to be repeated several times.

> The end of the first phase of treatment is determined by the results of circumferential or volumetric measurements on the affected extremity.

When the measurements approach a plateau, the end of phase 1 is reached, and the patient progresses seamlessly into phase 2 of CDT, also known as the self-management phase.

Depending on the stage of lymphedema, the involved extremity or body part may have reached a normal size at the end of the intensive phase, or there may still be a circumferential difference between the involved and the uninvolved limb. If treatment is initiated in the early stage 1 of lymphedema, which is characterized by a soft tissue consistency without any fibrotic alterations, limb reduction can be expected to a normal size (compared with the uninvolved limb). If intervention starts in the later stages of lymphedema, where lymphostatic fibrosis in the subcutaneous tissues is existent, the edematous fluid will recede, and fibrotic areas may soften. However, in most cases the indurated tissue will not completely regress during the intensive phase of CDT. Reduction in fibrotic tissue is a slow process, which can take several months or longer, and is achieved mainly in the second phase of CDT.

In phase 2 of CDT, the patient assumes responsibility for managing, improving, and maintaining the results achieved in phase 1. To reverse the symptoms associated with later stages of lymphedema, good patient compliance is indispensable. Compression garments have to be worn daily, and bandages have to be applied during the night. This self-management phase is a lifelong process; regular checkups with the physician and the lymphedema therapist are necessary.

Intensive Phase

Components of this phase are skin and nail care, manual lymph drainage, compression therapy and decongestive exercises.

Skin and Nail Care

Before compression bandages are applied, appropriate moisturizers or lotions are used to cover the lymphedematous limb. During the intensive phase of CDT, patients are continuously instructed in proper cleansing and moisturizing techniques to maintain the health and integrity of the skin and to prevent infections (refer to Chapter 3, Wounds and Skin Lesions).

Manual Lymph Drainage

In the first phase of therapy, MLD is applied at least once a day, 5 days a week. The MLD portion of the treatment generally requires 30 to 60 minutes. The duration of individual treatments depends on the number of involved limbs and body parts, as well as on the severity of the symptoms.

The most important aspect of MLD in phase 1 is to identify drainage areas with sufficient and healthy lymphatics. These pathways and lymph nodes are used to reroute the accumulated protein-rich lymph fluid around the blocked areas from the swollen extremity or body part back to the venous system.

To discuss the basic procedural pattern of treatment, the example of a unilateral secondary upper extremity lymphedema shall be used (detailed treatment sequences for this and other pathologies are found in Chapter 5). The swelling in upper extremity lymphedema usually involves the ipsilateral truncal quadrant. Healthy lymphatics are generally found in adjacent truncal territories (e.g., the contralateral upper quadrant and the ipsilateral lower quadrant), as well as the lymph vessels and lymph nodes in the supraclavicular area of the same side. To maximize the therapeutic effect of MLD, the method of procedure can be broken down into the following steps.

Manipulation of lymph nodes and collectors located in the healthy adjacent quadrants as well as in the supraclavicular area on the ipsilateral side will increase lymphangiomotoricity and result in a "suction effect" on the protein-rich lymph fluid in the congested area. Following this initial preparation, the congested body quadrant is included in the treatment. The protein-rich lymph fluid located in this area is carefully moved across the watersheds toward the previously manipulated adjacent territories, using primarily the appropriate anastomoses (in this case, the anterior and posterior axillo-axillary and the ipsilateral axillo-inguinal anastomosis). Even though MLD is not directly applied to the swollen extremity during this period of the treatment, a volume reduction already occurs, which can be noted in a decrease of circumferential measurements in the affected extremity. This volume reduction is generally observed following a series of two to four treatments.

When the extremity starts to decongest, the initial preparation is reduced to the relevant lymph nodes (in this case, axillary lymph nodes on the contralateral side and inguinal lymph nodes on the ipsilateral side) and anastomoses. The treatment area is now expanded to include the affected extremity on a step-by-step basis. To avoid stress (e.g., overload of the healthy lymphatics in the drainage areas), it is suggested initially to include only the upper arm in the treatment protocol. In severe cases of lymphedema, it may be necessary to treat only parts of the upper arm. In the following treatments, the forearm, then the hand and fingers, are carefully included.

Patients should be instructed early in the course of treatment how to perform simple self-MLD techniques (see Chapter 5). These techniques are used to stimulate lymph drainage during the weekends in the intensive phase as well as in the self-management phase.

Compression Therapy

In the intensive phase of the treatment, compression therapy is administered using short-stretch bandages in combination with appropriate padding materials. Bandages are applied following MLD and skin care measures and worn by the patient until the next treatments

session, 23 hours a day. Patients should be instructed not to remove the bandages at home. It is important that the bandages are taken off in the treatment facility prior to the next treatment session for the following reasons: skin marks left by the bandages and padding materials give the clinician important clues as to where to apply more padding if necessary, or if bandage tension needs to be adjusted in specific areas. If bandages are removed several hours before the scheduled treatment time, lymph fluid will reaccumulate in the extremity, forcing the clinician to spend part of the treatment time to again remove this fluid.

Patients cover the bandaged extremity with cast covers, garbage bags, or the like during showers at home. The extremity is cleaned in the facility after the removal of the compression bandages using either a shower (if available) or a washcloth.

Time management is essential in the intensive phase of the therapy. Depending on the number of bandages and padding materials used, it may take experienced lymphedema therapists 10 to 20 minutes (in extreme cases, even longer) to apply a compression bandage. Novices in the field should set aside ample time for this essential part of the therapy.

An important aspect in this stage of the treatment is to instruct the patient, and preferably a family member, in self-bandaging techniques. This requires a lot of practice, which makes it necessary to initiate the patient instruction early on in the intensive phase. It is also necessary to reserve sufficient time during the treatment session to allow the patient to learn and practice the bandaging techniques under the supervision of the clinician. To preserve and improve the treatment success following the intensive phase, it is essential that patients and/or family members are proficient in the application of compression bandages. Self-bandaging techniques should therefore be monitored and critiqued regularly during the intensive phase.

Self-bandaging during the decongestive phase is necessary on weekends should the bandages slide. Many patients also require compression bandages during the night during the self-management phase.

Decongestive Exercises

The goal of the exercise program is to improve lymph circulation and to maximize functional ability. Exercises are performed at least twice a day for ~10 to 15 minutes wearing the compression bandages (see Decongestive Exercises previously in the chapter). To promote patient compliance, it is important to create an exercise protocol that is easy to learn and to perform. Short protocols should be taught and tailored to the individual needs and limitations of the patient. The patient should assume the primary responsibility for the exercise portion as early as possible in the treatment program. A specific time should be set aside for the exercise sessions so that the patient can establish a daily routine. The therapist should monitor the exercise program regularly.

In addition to the decongestive exercise program, beneficial recreational activities should be discussed with the patient. High-risk activities (see Chapter 5, Precautions) that could trigger a further decrease in lymphatic transport capacity should be avoided or kept at a minimum. A balanced program of recreational activities supports general well-being, improves lymph drainage, and controls weight.

> The vast majority of lymphedema patients will benefit from complete decongestive therapy, provided that a clinician thoroughly trained in all components of CDT administers the treatments. Patient adherence to the treatment program and compliance are also indispensable components to ensure treatment success.

A lack of progress during treatment may be caused by the following:

- Improper treatment techniques: if CDT is applied only in part (MLD as the only form of intervention, no MLD, or improper bandaging), inappropriate use of pneumatic compression pumps, or the therapist is poorly trained, the treatment is prone to failure.
- Poor patient compliance
- The patient suffers from malignant lymphedema: the referring physician decides if CDT (or parts of this intervention) is suitable for palliative care.

- The patient has self-induced lymphedema: this form of lymphedema is caused by self-mutilation. In most cases, a tourniquet is applied to an extremity, which causes reduced lymphatic and venous return and the onset of swelling. If a diagnosis of self-induced (artificial) lymphedema is established by the physician, a cast may be applied to the affected extremity to prevent further strangulation.
- The severity of the symptoms, especially lymphostatic fibrosis, may have an impact on the treatment progress. The results in these cases generally are less dramatic and take a longer time to establish.
- Associated conditions: certain pathologies (see Chapter 3, Complications in Lymphedema) may slow treatment progress.

Self-Management Phase

With proper compliance and thorough instruction by the clinician, the majority of patients are able to maintain and improve the treatment results achieved during the intensive phase of therapy. Many patients report that changes in body weight and climate can cause their symptoms to fluctuate. Female patients commonly report that the swelling tends to increase during the menstrual cycle. These situations usually can be remedied by following the self-management protocol more closely.

For those patients who are unable to maintain decongestion, or who experience an increase in swelling during the second phase of CDT, it is necessary to follow up with additional CDT sessions in the clinic. Individual circumstances determine if follow-up treatments are applied in weekly, biweekly, or monthly sessions or if another shortened intensive phase is necessary (see Chapter 3, Therapeutic Approach to Lymphedema).

The components in phase 2 of CDT are similar to those in phase 1. The emphasis in phase 2 is self-improvement and self-management.

Skin and Nail Care

Patients apply proper cleansing and moisturizing techniques learned during the intensive phase of the treatment. Appropriate skin moisturizers should be applied twice daily to maintain the health and integrity of the skin.

Self-Manual Lymph Drainage

To stimulate lymph drainage, the patient performs simple self-MLD techniques and breathing exercises at least twice daily (refer to Chapter 5, Self-MLD).

Compression Therapy

Compression in this phase of the treatment is applied by compression garments, which have to be worn during the daytime hours. Measurements for compression garments are taken at the end of the decongestive phase, when the maximum level of decongestion is achieved. Measurement techniques for medical compression garments are documented in Chapter 5, Measurements for Compression Garments. At this time, the patient should be thoroughly instructed in donning techniques and garment care. The condition of the compression garment is evaluated during regular checkups (at least every 6 months), and the patient's measurements are taken again to ensure proper fit. Compression garments should be replaced every 6 months or sooner if the material is damaged or has lost its elasticity. Patients should have at least two sets of compression garments—one to wear and one to wash.

As a general rule, the highest possible and most tolerable compression level should be used for lymphedema garments. In some cases of lower extremity lymphedema, it may be necessary to wear two compression garments on top of each other. As discussed earlier, the most important aspect is the patient's comfort level. In some cases, it may be necessary to select a compression garment of a lower pressure level to improve patient compliance. A compression garment that is worn inconsistently or not at all has no beneficial effect.

The severity and chronicity of the symptoms determine if a lymphedema patient continues to apply compression bandages during the night in this phase. Self-bandaging techniques are explained and illustrated in Chapter 5, Self-Bandaging.

Bandages may be applied on top of the compression garment during times with increased swelling or activities that may trigger the onset of swelling (airplane travel, standing over long periods of time, high-risk activities).

Decongestive Exercises

Patients should continue the exercise program to maintain and improve the treatment success. For maximum benefit, the compression garment or compression bandages should be worn during the exercise protocol. Patients are also encouraged to maintain the level of recreational activities discussed with the clinician during the intensive phase of the treatment. The exercise program and any recreational activities should be discussed and reevaluated during regular checkups with the physician and the lymphedema therapist.

Most patients are able to maintain and improve the results achieved during the intensive phase. The volume may continue to decrease and/or the tissue may continue to soften. A lack of progress, frequent relapses, or a permanent increase in limb volume during the second phase of CDT may be caused by the following:

- Lack of compliance, lack of hygiene
- Recurrence of cancer
- The severity of the symptoms (as discussed earlier, treatment progress may be slower in those patients with extreme lymphostatic fibrosis and sclerosis)
- Associated conditions (see Chapter 3, Complications in Lymphedema)

◆ Documentation Techniques for Lymphedema

Documentation is necessary for several reasons. It serves as proof of the effectiveness of the therapy, which may be required by some insurance carriers for reimbursement, and it records the patient's progress. A reduction in limb volume not only indicates that the treatment is successful but also encourages patient compliance.

Documentation values also determine the end of the decongestive phase and the beginning of the self-management phase.

Measures to use to determine the end of phase 1 and the beginning of phase 2 include photographic documentation, simple circum-

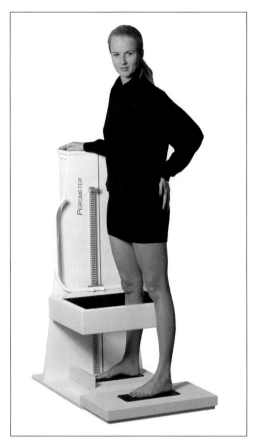

Figure 4–19 Perometer (With permission from JUZO, Inc.).

ferential, and volumetric measurements. Photographic documentation has the advantage of providing visual evidence of before and after effects of treatment, in addition to providing evidence of wound healing and changes in skin color. Simple circumferential measurements taken on defined areas of the extremity reflect a change in circumferential values of these areas. These values can be compared with the uninvolved extremity (in unilateral involvement) but do not provide limb volume values. Circumferential measurements are also used to determine the appropriate size of the compression garment.

A variety of methods have been used over the years to determine limb volume, ranging from sophisticated imaging techniques (magnetic resonance imaging), bioelectrical impedance analysis (BIA), computed tomography, and infrared photoelectronic perometer tech-

nique, to simple water displacement methods and geometrical calculations from limb circumference measurements using the truncated cone formula.

Each of these procedures has its advantages and disadvantages. Imaging techniques are costly and time consuming and generally require equipment not available in lymphedema treatment centers. Perometers are more commonly used by treatment centers throughout the United States (Fig. 4–19). These devices use infrared light transmitters to determine circumferential measurements, which are then used to calculate the volume of the limb using the truncated cone formula. The advantage of this device is that the measurements can be compared with built-in sizing charts of different compression garment manufacturers for upper and lower extremity garments. The sizing charts can also be customized to correlate with sizing charts of other garment manufacturers.

The water displacement method uses volumeters filled with water and equipped with an overflow spout and a beaker. The extremity is then partially or completely immersed in the water, and the displaced water is collected in the beaker. The amount of displaced water represents the extremity volume. Though theoretically an accurate and precise technique, the water displacement method cannot be used if wounds are present; furthermore, it is cumbersome to perform and provides no information on the shape of the extremity. However, the water displacement method provides a reliable modus to include hand and foot measurements into the total limb volume measurement.

Volume calculations using the truncated cone formula from girth measurements is a common and relatively precise method employed in lymphedema treatment centers. A swollen extremity can be viewed as a series of cones or cylinders. Circumferential measurements are made in intervals of typically 4 to 6 cm along the extremity (generally, the smaller the segments, the more accurate the geometrical values). The volume of each segment (or cone) is determined, and the total volume is calculated by summing the volumes of each individual segment. User-friendly computer programs for volumetric measurements are available from various sources.

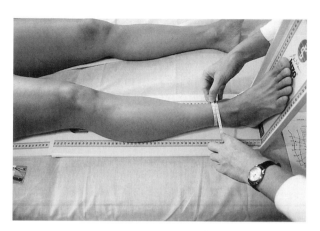

Figure 4–20 Measuring board.

General considerations: Accurate measurements are necessary to determine circumferential and volumetric values. If girth measurements are taken manually, the same examiner should take them each time. If several examiners are involved in measurements, a spring-loaded measuring tape should be used to maximize accuracy. Measurements should be taken on a measuring board (Fig. 4–20) to ensure the same body position between different measuring sessions.

Measurements are taken on the exact same points each time; it is therefore necessary to document each measuring point on the patient's chart.

Measuring levels for simple circumferential measurements: Seven measuring points are recommended for the upper extremity, one on the hand, one on the wrist, two points on the forearm, one measurement on the cubital fossa, and two measurements on the upper arm (Table 4–1). For the lower extremity, one point on the foot, one at the ankle area, two on the lower leg, one measurement in the popliteal fossa, and two on the thigh are recommended (Table 4–2). The location of the different measuring points should be determined by length measurements from the longest finger (in arm measurements) or from the heel/sole of the foot (in leg measurements) to ensure accuracy between measuring sessions.

Circumferential measurements to determine extremity volume: Incremental measurements of 3 cm should be used on the hand and foot (the water displacement method is usually a more reliable and easier to use method to determine hand or foot volumes). If hand or foot volumes are not included in the calculation, the circumferential measurements start at the wrist or ankle area and continue in increments of 4 cm along the extremity. The location of the initial measuring level is noted on the patient's chart.

Circumferential and/or volumetric measurements should be taken at least once a week to document treatment progress. Both techniques can be used for unilateral or bilateral involvement. In some cases, the uninvolved extremity shows some level of involvement in the swelling; in these cases, a reduction of the uninvolved extremity can be expected.

Table 4–1 Circumferential Measurement Chart for the Upper Extremity
PATIENT: JANE DOE DIAGNOSIS: Secondary UE Lymphedema.
AFFECTED LIMB

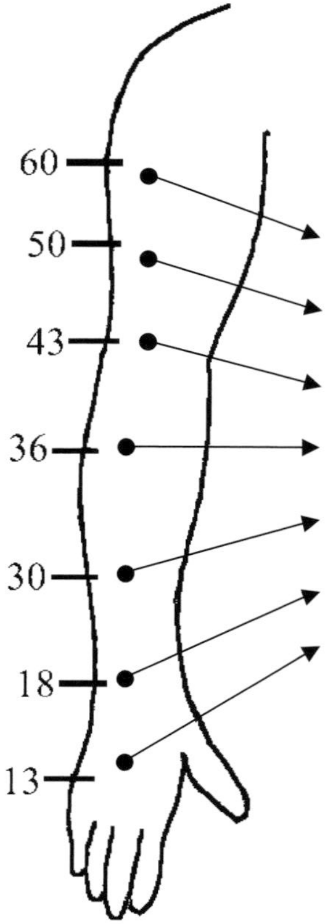

MEASUREMENTS	1/19		RIGHT ( ) 1/23	LEFT (X) 1/30	BOTH ( ) 2/6
	RIGHT	LEFT	L	L	L
	37	44	40.5	39.5	38
	36	42.5	38	37	37
	32	37	35	33.5	33
	30	34.5	31.5	31	31
	23	28.5	25	24.5	23.5
	19	24	21.5	20.5	20
	21	25.5	22.5	22	22

MEASUREMENTS ARE TAKEN IN CENTIMETERS 2.54 cm = 1 inch

WEIGHT
DATE WEIGHT

	1/23 196	1/30 193	2/6 193
198 lbs			

DATE MEASURED

60
50
43
36
30
18
13

Table 4–2 Circumferential Measurement Chart for the Lower Extremity
PATIENT: JANE DOE DIAGNOSIS: Primary LE Lymphedema.
AFFECTED LIMB RIGHT (X) LEFT () BOTH ()

	11/10 RIGHT	11/10 LEFT	11/14 R	11/17 R	11/21 R	11/24 R	11/28 R	12/1 R	12/4 R
MEASUREMENTS									
	127	59	110	116.5	86	89	81	79	79
	129	51	109.5	112	84	87	79	77	75.5
	82	38	71	68	53	51.5	47	47	46
	81.5	38	70.5	68.5	59	59	47.5	43.5	43
	69	30	59.5	58	49.5	47	40.5	39	38
	34.5	25	31.5	30.5	28.5	27.5	27	27.5	27
	33	25	30	30	30	30	27.5	27	27

MEASUREMENTS ARE TAKEN IN CENTIMETERS 2.54 cm = 1 inch

WEIGHT

DATE WEIGHT									
305 lbs.			11/14 294	11/17 298	11/21 290	11/24 292	11/28 288	12/1 284	12/4 287

DATE MEASURED

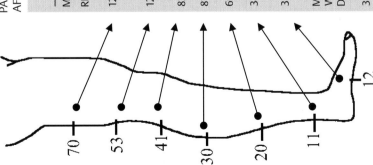

70
53
41
30
20
11
12

Recommended Reading

1. Bringezu G, Schreiner O. Die Therapieform Manuelle Lymphdrainage. Germany: Verlag Otto Haase; 1987
2. Camrath J. Physiotherapie—Technik und Verfahrensweise. Stuttgart: Thieme Verlag; 1983
3. Chikly B. Who discovered the lymphatic system? Lymphology 1997;30(4):186–193
4. Consensus document of the International Society of Lymphology: diagnosis and treatment of peripheral lymphedema. Lymphology 2003;36:84–91
5. Despopoulos A, Silbernagel S. Color Atlas of Physiology. 5th ed. New York: Thieme; 2003
6. Eliska O, Eliska M. Are peripheral lymphatics damaged by high pressure manual massage? Lymphology 1995;28:21–30
7. Földi E. Massage and damage to lymphatics. Lymphology 1995;28:1–3
8. Földi E, Földi M, Weissleder H. Conservative treatment of lymphedema of the limbs. Angiology 1985;36(3):171–180
9. Guyton A, Hall J. Textbook of Medical Physiology. 9th ed. Philadelphia: WB Saunders; 1996
10. Hutzschenreuter P, Ehlers R. The effect of manual lymph drainage on the autonomic nervous system. Zeltschrift fur Lymphologie 1986;19:58–60
11. Hutzschenreuther P, Bruemmer H, Silberschneider K. Die Vagotone Wirkung der Manuellen Lymphdrainage nach Dr. Vodder. LymphForsch 2003;7(1):7–14
12. Kuhnke E. Methodik der Volumenbestimmung menschlicher Extremitäten aus Umfangmessungen. Physiotherapie 1979;4
13. Kuhnke E. Ein vereinfachtes Verfahren zur Wirksamkeitskontrolle der Therapie bei Einseitigen Extremitätenödemen. Physik Th 1980;11(12)
14. Kurz I. Einführung in die manuelle Lymphdrainage nach Dr. Vodder: Therapie I/II. 3rd ed. Haug Verlag; 1984.
15. Lasinki B. Target: lymphedema, a closer look at the role of exercise. Adv Phys Ther PT Assist 2003;14(24)
16. Melzack R, Wall PD. The Challenge of Pain. 2nd ed. London: Penguin Books; 1996
17. Sander A, Hajer N, Hemenway K, Miller A. Upper-extremity volume measurements in women with lymphedema: a comparison of measurements obtained via water displacement with geometrically determined volume. Phys Therap 2002;82(12):1201–1212
18. Tierney S, Aslam M, Rennie K, Grace P. Infrared optoelectronic volumetry: the ideal way to measure limb volume. Eur J Vasc Endovasc Surg 1996;12:412–417
19. Vodder E. Die technischen Grundlagen der manuellen Lymphdrainage. Phys Therap 1983;4(1)

5

Treatment

◆ General Considerations

The techniques outlined in this chapter should not be substituted for the thorough instructions provided in comprehensive lymphedema management courses offered by qualified training centers. As with many manual techniques, the skills required to deliver adequate intervention using all components of complete decongestive therapy cannot be learned from reading a book, watching videotapes, or attending weekend classes. A high level of competency and skill is needed to master all components of CDT and to provide patients with a proper degree of intervention. The quality of training will have a great impact on the level of care the patients receive or do not receive.

CDT and its components have been practiced safely and effectively in Europe for many decades and became the standard of treatment for lymphedema in the 1970s, when the national health insurance system in Germany started to reimburse for lymphedema treatment. To ensure proper teaching standards, training centers in Germany have to comply with strict guidelines specified by professional organizations in the training and certification of lymphedema instructors as well as therapists. Certain organizations in the United States have acknowledged the need for certification programs in lymphedema management to ensure a base of knowledge considered fundamental in the treatment of lymphedema and related conditions.

◆ Application of Basic MLD Techniques on Different Parts of the Body

The four basic techniques of Dr. Vodder's manual lymph drainage (MLD)—stationary circle, pump, scoop, and rotary—their effects on the lymphatic system, and the contraindications for manual lymph drainage are discussed in Chapter 4. Additional techniques incorporated into MLD sequences are soft and rhythmic strokes known as *effleurage*. This method is adopted from more traditional massage techniques and is used to stimulate local sympathetic activity and to promote directional flow of lymph.

The techniques and sequences outlined in the following sections are applied in conditions where edema is present, but the lymph nodes are not removed or treated with irradiation. Examples include post-traumatic and postoperative swelling, lower extremity edema caused by pregnancy, swellings caused by partial or complete loss of mobility (pareses, paralysis), reflex sympathetic dystrophy (when swelling is present), migraine headache (swelling is present in the perivascular areas of intracranial blood vessels), cyclic idiopathic edema, and rheumatoid arthritis. Selected indications are cited in the appropriate subchapters.

Basic treatment sequences may also be used to accomplish a general increase in lymph circulation or to achieve a common soothing effect by decreasing sympathetic activity.

In the treatment of lymphedema, these techniques are used to improve lymph production and lymph angiomotoricity, as well as to promote the lymphatic return from the drainage areas described in Chapter 4 (Intensive Phase) to the venous system. In the lymphedematous extremity and/or body part, the treatment sequences are modified accordingly, as outlined later in this chapter.

Common denominators to all following techniques and sequences are the following:

◆ The hand positions of all basic strokes are adapted to the anatomy and physiology of the lymphatic system.

◆ Central pretreatment: the areas closest to the venous angles and regional groups of lymph nodes are stimulated first. This allows for drainage of the peripheral areas. At extremities, the stimulation begins proximal and is continued toward distal, in accordance with the direction of the lymph drainage.

◆ Stroke intensity: the applied pressure in individual strokes should be enough to utilize full elasticity of the skin and subcutaneous tissues, and to promote lymph formation and lymph angiomotoricity. Too much pressure may cause unwanted vasodilation and lymphangiospasm.

- Stroke sequence: each technique consists of a working and resting phase, during which the manual pressure increases and decreases gradually. The goal in the working phase is to promote lymph formation, lymph angiomotoricity, and directional flow by stretching the anchoring filaments and smooth musculature located in the wall of lymph angions. The suction effect created in the resting phase results in a refilling of lymph collectors with lymph fluid from more distal areas.

- Stroke duration: the relatively high viscosity of lymph fluid requires the working phase to last about 1 second. To ensure adequate reaction of the lymph collectors to the manual stimuli, the strokes should be repeated five to seven times in one area.

- Working direction of the strokes: the direction of the strokes depends on the anatomical actualities and generally follows the physiological patterns of lymphatic drainage. If surgery, radiation, or trauma results in an interruption of regular drainage pathways, it will become necessary to redirect the lymph flow around the blocked areas and toward regions with sufficient lymph flow patterns.

Lateral Neck and Submandibular Area

Selected indications: pretreatment for other drainage areas*; postsurgical (oral, dental, plastic surgery, etc.) and post-traumatic swellings (whiplash injury, others); migraine headache; partial treatment for primary head and neck lymphedema; general increase in lymph circulation, or to achieve a common soothing effect by decreasing sympathetic activity

Patient in supine position, therapist on the patient's side:
1. Effleurage, two or three times from the sternum to the acromion
2. Manipulation of the inferior cervical lymph nodes
   Stationary circles in the supraclavicular fossa (horizontal plane)

* An abbreviated sequence is used if the lateral neck serves as a pretreatment for other drainage areas. This shorter sequence consists of the first three techniques used in the complete sequence (see following page):

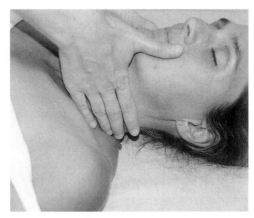

Figure 5–1 Stationary circles on the lateral cervical lymph nodes.

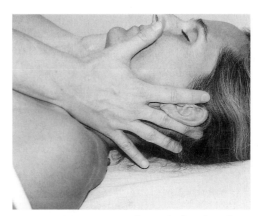

Figure 5–2 Stationary circles on the lymph nodes in front of and behind the ear.

3. Manipulation of the deep lateral cervical lymph nodes (Fig. 5–1)
   Stationary circles from the earlobe to the supraclavicular fossa in two hand placements, if necessary (sagittal plane)
4. Manipulation of the parotid and retroauricular lymph nodes (Fig. 5–2)
   Stationary circles with fingers in front of and behind the ear, followed by reworking the deep lateral cervical lymph nodes as in step 3 (both placements in sagittal plane)

Patient in supine position, therapist at the head-end of the patient:
5. Manipulation of submandibular lymph nodes (Fig. 5–3)
   Stationary circles with distal phalanges (2–5) from the tip of the chin in the direction of

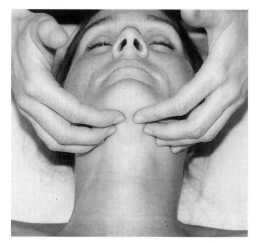

Figure 5–3 Stationary circles on the submandibular lymph nodes.

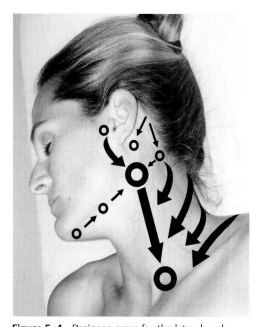

Figure 5–4 Drainage areas for the lateral neck.

the angle of the jaw (superior cervical lymph nodes). Two hand placements if necessary (phalanges in horizontal plane). This technique is followed by reworking the deep lateral cervical lymph nodes as in step 3.

Patient in supine position, therapist on the patient's side:
6. Manipulation of the shoulder collectors
   Stationary circles in two hand placements,

which should cover the area located cranial to the anterior and posterior upper horizontal watershed. First hand placement on the acromion, second hand placement on the medial shoulder (both placements in horizontal plane).
7. Effleurage (as in step 1)

Abbreviated Neck Sequence

Review Figure 5–4 for drainage areas on the lateral neck.

1. Effleurage, two or three times from the sternum to the acromion
2. Manipulation of the inferior cervical lymph nodes

   Stationary circles in the supraclavicular fossa (horizontal plane)
3. Manipulation of the deep lateral cervical lymph nodes (Fig. 5–1)

   Stationary circles from the earlobe to the supraclavicular fossa in two hand placements, if necessary (sagittal plane)

Posterior Neck and Occipital Area

Selected indications: postsurgical (oral, dental, plastic surgery, etc.) and post-traumatic swellings (whiplash injury, others); migraine headache; partial treatment for primary head and neck lymphedema; general increase in lymph circulation, or to achieve a common soothing effect by decreasing sympathetic activity (Fig. 5–5)
   Pretreatment: lateral neck

Patient in prone position, therapist at the head-end of the patient:
1. Effleurage, two or three times starting at the back of the head and following the descending trapezius muscle to the acromion
2. Manipulation of the deep lateral cervical lymph nodes
   Stationary circles starting at the angle of the jaw in the direction of the supraclavicular fossa (sagittal plane). Two hand placements if necessary.
3. Manipulation of the occipital and parietal region
   Alternating stationary circles in several tracks, starting on the posterior head toward the parietal area (frontal plane).

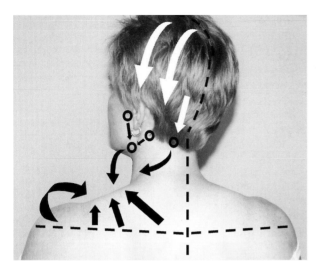

Figure 5–5 Drainage areas for the posterior neck and occipital area.

Working phase in the direction of the occipital and retroauricular lymph nodes.

4. Manipulation of the parotid and retroauricular lymph nodes
   Stationary circles with fingers in front of and behind the ear, followed by reworking the deep lateral cervical lymph nodes as in step 2 (both placements in sagittal plane).

5. Manipulation of the shoulder collectors
   Alternating pump techniques on both shoulders, starting at the acromion, following the upper trapezius muscle in the direction of the supraclavicular fossa.
   Both hands in horizontal plane.

6. Manipulation of the inferior cervical lymph nodes
   Bimanual thumb circles in the supraclavicular fossa (horizontal plane)

Patient in prone position, therapist on the patient's side:

7. Manipulation of the paravertebral lymph nodes and vessels
   Stationary circles paravertebrally with the finger pads (working deep)

8. Effleurage (as in step 1)

Face

Selected indications: postsurgical (oral, dental, plastic surgery, etc.) and post-traumatic swellings (whiplash injury, etc.); migraine headache; partial treatment for primary head and neck lymphedema; general increase in lymph

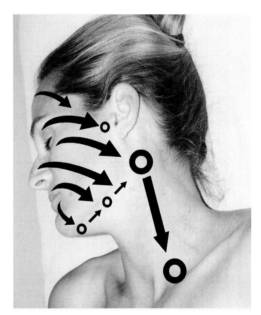

Figure 5–6 Drainage areas for the face.

circulation, or to achieve a common soothing effect by decreasing sympathetic activity (Fig. 5–6)

Pretreatment: lateral neck (posterior neck if necessary)

Patient in supine position, therapist at the head-end of the patient:

1. Effleurage, two or three times along lower jaw, upper jaw, the cheek, and the forehead in the direction of the angle of the jaw (following the pathway of the collectors)

137

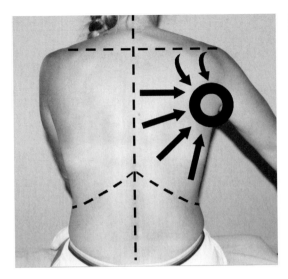

Figure 5–7 Drainage areas for the posterior thorax.

2. Manipulation of the submental and sub-mandibular lymph nodes (Fig. 5–3)
   Stationary circles with distal phalanges (2–5) from the tip of the chin in the direction of the angle of the jaw (superior cervical lymph nodes). Two hand placements if necessary (phalanges in horizontal plane). This technique is followed by stationary circles along the deep lateral cervical lymph nodes (sagittal plane).

3. Manipulation of the lower and upper jaw
   Alternating stationary circles working toward the submandibular lymph nodes. This technique is followed by stationary circles in the direction of the angle of the jaw and the supraclavicular fossa as described in step 2.

4. Manipulation of the lymph vessels in the area of the bridge of the nose and cheek
   Alternating stationary circles starting at the bridge of the nose, to include the lower eyelid, toward the cheeks. This technique is followed by the technique described in step 2, with the purpose of manipulating the lymph fluid toward the supraclavicular fossa.

5. Manipulation of the upper eyelid and eyebrows
   Alternating stationary circles (one or more fingers) in the direction of the preauricular lymph nodes (option: eyebrow roll)

6. Manipulation of the forehead and temporal area

Stationary circles starting at the middle of the forehead, traveling to the temple with the working phase directed toward the preauricular lymph nodes

7. Manipulation of the parotid and retroauricular lymph nodes
   Stationary circles with fingers in front of and behind the ear, followed by stationary circles along the deep lateral cervical lymph nodes (sagittal plane)

8. Effleurage (as in step 1)

Posterior Thorax

The treatment area is outlined by the lower horizontal watershed (caudal limitation), the upper horizontal watershed (cranial limitation), and the sagittal watershed (medial limitation) (Fig. 5–7).

Selected indications: Pretreatment for unilateral secondary upper extremity lymphedema (this sequence is applied on the healthy quadrant); postsurgical and post-traumatic swellings; general increase in lymph circulation, or to achieve a common soothing effect by decreasing sympathetic activity

Pretreatment: lateral neck (abbreviated; see lateral neck sequence, steps 1–3)

Patient in prone position, therapist contralateral to the healthy quadrant:

1. Manipulation of the axillary lymph nodes
   Stationary circles bimanually with flat hands between the latissimus dorsi and

pectoral muscles (sagittal plane), with the working direction toward the apex of the axilla (subclavian trunk)

2. Effleurage, two or three times in several pathways, starting at the posterior sagittal watershed in the direction of the axillary lymph nodes (following the pathway of the collectors)

3. Manipulation of the lateral thorax
Stationary circles alternating and dynamic from the horizontal watershed toward the axillary lymph nodes (sagittal plane). This sequence follows the thoracic portion of the inguinal axillary (IA) anastomosis.

4. Manipulation of the posterior thorax (Fig. 5–8)
Rotary techniques in several tracks starting at the sagittal watershed in the direction of the axillary lymph nodes (following the pathway of the collectors). This technique should cover the entire treatment area as outlined previously (Fig. 5–7).

5. Manipulation of the posterior and lateral thorax
Combination of alternating rotary techniques (upper and lower hands) starting at the sagittal watershed (lower hand is parallel to and just above the lower horizontal watershed). The rotary techniques travel alternating toward the lateral direction until the thoracic portion of the IA anastomosis is reached. Dynamic stationary circles follow this technique as outlined in step 3.

6. Manipulation of the posterior axillo-axillary (PAA) anastomosis
Bimanual stationary circles, with the working phase directed toward the axillary lymph nodes. The hands are aligned parallel with the sagittal watershed (frontal plane).

7. Manipulation of the paravertebral lymph nodes and vessels (if necessary)
Stationary circles paravertebrally with the finger pads (working deep)

8. Manipulation of intercostal lymph vessels
Stationary circles, with the finger pads working from lateral placements to medial placements, using wavelike movements, with pressure working deep (perforating precollectors)

9. Effleurage (as in step 1)

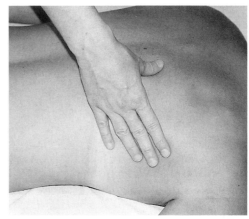

Figure 5–8 Rotary technique on the posterior thorax.

Lumbar Area

The treatment area is outlined by the lower horizontal watershed (cranial limitation), the horizontal gluteal fold (caudal limitation), and the sagittal watershed (medial limitation) (Fig. 5–9).

Selected indications: Pretreatment for unilateral secondary and primary lower extremity lymphedema (this sequence is applied on the healthy quadrant); phlebolymphostatic edema; lipedema and lipolymphedema; postsurgical and post-traumatic swellings; general increase in lymph circulation, or to achieve a common soothing effect by decreasing sympathetic activity

Pretreatment: lateral neck (abbreviated; see lateral neck sequence, steps 1–3), abdomen, inguinal lymph nodes

Patient in prone position, therapist contralateral to the healthy quadrant:

1. Effleurage, two or three times in several pathways, starting at the posterior sagittal watershed toward the inguinal lymph nodes (remaining in the lumbar quadrant)

2. Manipulation of the lumbar area
Alternating rotary techniques from the sagittal watershed toward the hip (ASIS). The upper hand is parallel to and just below the lower horizontal watershed; the lower hand follows the collectors of the posterior interinguinal (PII) anastomosis.

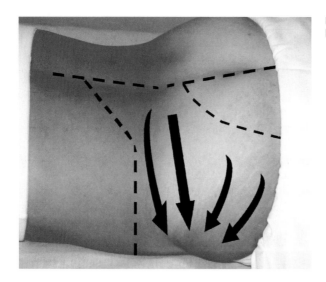

Figure 5–9 Drainage areas for the lumbar area.

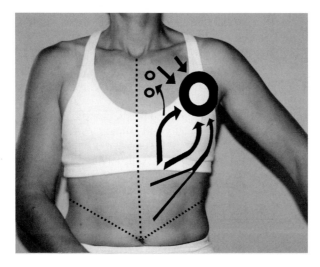

Figure 5–10 Drainage areas for the anterior thorax.

3. Manipulation of the PII anastomosis
   Bimanual stationary circles simultaneously on the PII anastomosis, with working direction toward the inguinal lymph nodes. Both hands are parallel to the sagittal watershed (frontal plane).

4. Manipulation of the paravertebral lymph nodes and vessels (if necessary)
   Stationary circles paravertebrally with the finger pads (working deep)

5. Effleurage (as in step 1)

Anterior Thorax

The treatment area is outlined by the lower horizontal watershed (caudal limitation), the upper horizontal watershed (cranial limitation), and the sagittal watershed (medial limitation) (Fig. 5–10).

Selected indications: Pretreatment for unilateral secondary and primary upper extremity lymphedema (this sequence is applied on the healthy quadrant); postsurgical and post-traumatic swellings; general increase in lymph circulation, or to achieve a common soothing effect by decreasing sympathetic activity

Pretreatment: lateral neck (abbreviated; see lateral neck sequence, steps 1–3)

Patient in supine position, therapist contralateral to the healthy quadrant:
1. Manipulation of the axillary lymph nodes
   Bimanual stationary circles, with flat hands between the latissimus dorsi and pectoral muscles (sagittal plane), with the working direction toward the apex of the axilla (subclavian trunk)
2. Effleurage, two or three times in several pathways (following the collectors), starting at the anterior sagittal watershed in the direction of the axillary lymph nodes (not over the nipple)
3. Manipulation of the lymph vessels in the healthy mammary gland
   This technique is performed with a combination of alternating and dynamic pump and rotary techniques. The lower hand starts with dynamic pump techniques in three placements in the direction of the axillary lymph nodes: the first placement is on the mammary fold, the second placement in the glandular tissue, and the third placement below the nipple.
   The upper hand uses rotary techniques starting at the anterior sagittal watershed, following a line below the upper horizontal watershed in three hand placements toward the axillary lymph nodes.
4. Manipulation of the lateral thorax
   Dynamic and alternating stationary circles from the lower horizontal watershed toward the axillary lymph nodes (sagittal plane). This sequence follows the thoracic portion of the IA anastomosis.
5. Manipulation of the anterior and lateral thorax
   Combination of alternating rotary techniques (upper and lower hands) starting at the anterior sagittal watershed (lower hand is parallel to and just above the lower horizontal watershed). The rotary techniques travel alternating in the lateral direction until the thoracic portion of the IA anastomosis is reached. The technique is then followed by dynamic stationary circles, which follow the IA anastomosis toward the axillary lymph nodes (as outlined in step 4).

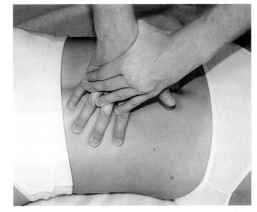

Figure 5–11 Intercostal technique on the anterior thorax.

6. Manipulation of the anterior axillo-axillary (AAA) anastomosis
   Bimanual stationary circles, with the working phase directed toward the axillary lymph nodes. The hands are aligned parallel with the anterior sagittal watershed (frontal plane).
7. Manipulation of the parasternal lymph nodes and vessels (if necessary)
   Stationary circles parasternally with finger pads (working deep)
8. Manipulation of intercostal lymph vessels (Fig. 5–11)
   Stationary circles with 3 or 4 finger pads working from lateral placements to medial placements, using wavelike movements with pressure working deep (perforating precollectors)
9. Effleurage (as in step 2)

Abdomen (Superficial and Deep Manipulations)

Refer to the list of local contraindications for the abdominal area in Chapter 4, Contraindications for Manual Lymph Drainage. Abdominal techniques should not be applied if they cause pain or discomfort, or directly following meals. Patients should empty their bladder before treatment starts.

Abdominal sequences can be separated into superficial and deep techniques. The skillful manipulation of the intra-abdominal areas, especially when combined with diaphragmatic

141

breathing, results in increased lymph transport within the thoracic duct and larger lymphatic trunks. A decongestive effect on organ structures located within the abdominal and pelvic cavities, as well as on lymphatic drainage areas located more distally (the lower extremities), is additionally realized when performing abdominal techniques.

Selected indications: part of the treatment sequence for lower extremity lymphedema (primary and secondary) as well as lymphedema involving the external genitalia; chronic venous insufficiency stages II and III (phlebolymphostatic edema); lipedema and lipolymphedema; part of the treatment sequence for primary lymphedema of the genitalia; part of the treatment sequence for upper extremity lymphedema (particularly with removal or radiation of both axillary lymph node groups); part of the treatment for cyclic idiopathic edema; general increase in lymph circulation

Superficial abdominal treatment (modified)

Pretreatment: lateral neck (abbreviated; see lateral neck sequence, steps 1–3)

Patient in supine position, with the legs and the head elevated and the arms resting on the patient's side; therapist on patient's right side (next to pelvis):

1. Effleurage
   Two or three times starting at the pubic bone, following the rectus abdominis muscle to the xiphoid process, then along the thoracic cage and the iliac crest back to the pubic bone
   Two or three times following the ascending, transverse, and descending part of the colon

2. Manipulation of the colon
   Descending colon: The right hand is placed on the descending colon, with the fingertips on the thoracic cage and the fingers pointing up toward the midclavicular point. This is a two-handed technique; the bottom hand (right hand) is in contact with the skin and remains passive; pressure is applied with the left hand, which rests on top of the right hand. Working phase: Moderate (but soft) pressure is applied down into the abdomen (deep), then along and in the direc-

tion of the descending colon (caudal), ending in a partial supination directed toward the cisterna chyli. The hand relaxes in the resting phase, and the tissue elasticity carries the hand back to the beginning position. This sequence is repeated two or three times.
Ascending colon: The therapist is on the patient's right side (next to the thorax, facing the direction of the patient's feet). The right hand is placed on the ascending colon, with the fingertips near the inguinal ligament and the fingers pointing downward toward the pubic bone. The right hand, which is in contact with the skin, remains passive; pressure is applied with the left hand, which rests on top of the right hand. Working phase: Moderate (but soft) pressure is applied down into the abdomen (deep), then along and in the direction of the ascending colon (cranial), ending in a partial supination directed toward the cisterna chyli. The hand relaxes in the resting phase, and the tissue elasticity carries the hand back to the beginning position. This sequence is repeated two or three times.

3. Effleurage (as in step 1)

Deep abdominal treatment (modified)

With this technique, the caudal part of the thoracic duct, the cisterna chyli, the larger lymphatic trunks, the pelvic and lumbar lymph nodes, and the organ structures with their lymphatic system are stimulated. Deep abdominal sequences are applied on five different hand placements on the abdominal area and are combined with the patient's diaphragmatic breathing (Fig. 5–12). To avoid hyperventilation, the therapist performs only one sequence per placement. Ideally, the placements on the thoracic cage and in the center of the abdomen are repeated during the full sequence, resulting in a total of nine manipulations (depending on the patient's reaction). During each manipulation, the therapist's hand follows the patient's exhalation into the abdominal area and offers moderate (but soft) resistance to the initial subsequent inhalation phase. The therapist then releases the resistance and stays in skin contact until the end of the inhalation phase. The hand is moved to the next placement on the abdomen during the pause be-

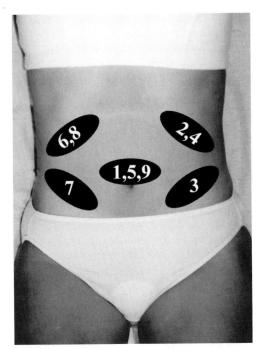

Figure 5–12 Hand placements for the deep abdominal technique.

tween inhalation and the next exhalation phase. To avoid discomfort, the hand, which is in contact with the patient's skin, remains soft and passive. Pressure is applied with the top hand, which rests on top of the working hand.

Pretreatment: lateral neck (abbreviated; see lateral neck sequence, steps 1–3)

Patient in supine postion, with the legs and the head elevated and the arms resting on the patient's side; therapist on the patient's side, with the hand placements as follows:

1. Center of the abdomen, over the umbilicus (this placement should be avoided if pulsating aorta is felt with the soft and passive hand)
2. Below and parallel with the thoracic cage on the contralateral side
3. Above and parallel with the inguinal ligament on the contralateral side
4. Repeat step 2.
5. Repeat step 1.
6. Below and parallel with the thoracic cage on the ipsilateral side

7. Above and parallel with the inguinal ligament on the ipsilateral side
8. Repeat step 6.
9. Repeat step 1.

Upper Extremity

Selected indications: postsurgical and post-traumatic swellings (including edema caused by immobility due to partial or complete paralysis); reflex sympathetic dystrophy; rheumatoid arthritis; lipedema; general increase in lymph circulation, or to achieve a common soothing effect by decreasing sympathetic activity

Pretreatment: lateral neck (abbreviated; see lateral neck sequence, steps 1–3 and 6–shoulder collectors)

Patient in supine position; therapist on the patient's side ipsilateral to the involved quadrant (in sequence 1–3, the therapist stands next to the patient's head):

1. Manipulation of the axillary lymph nodes
   Stationary circles on the axillary lymph nodes in two hand placements; the hand closer to the patient's head is working, the other hand holds the arm in proper elevated position.
2. Effleurage, two or three times covering the entire arm
3. Manipulation of the medial aspect of the upper arm
   Stationary circles with the hand closer to the patient's head, beginning on the medial epicondyle. Several hand placements are applied to cover the medial upper arm, with the working phase direction toward the axillary lymph nodes. The other hand holds the patient's arm in a comfortable and elevated position.
4. Manipulation of the tissues covering the anterior and posterior portion of the deltoid muscle
   Stationary circles bimanually and alternating on the anterior and posterior portion of the deltoid muscle; the working phase is directed toward the axillary lymph nodes.
   Note: In the treatment of upper extremity lymphedema, the working phase of this sequence is directed toward the AAA and PAA anastomoses (Fig. 5–13).

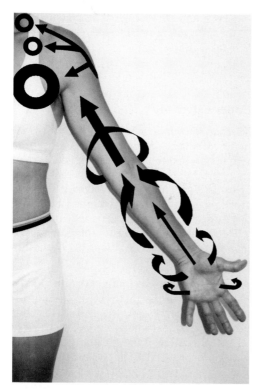

Figure 5–13 Drainage areas for the upper extremity.

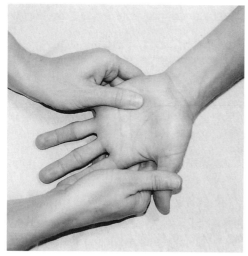

Figure 5–14 Thumb circles on the palm (ulnar bundle).

5. Manipulation of the lateral aspect of the upper arm
Pump technique, with the hand closer to the patient's head on the lateral upper arm

in several placements from the lateral epicondyle toward the acromion. The other hand holds the patient's arm in a comfortable and elevated position.
Combination of pump technique and stationary circle (alternating hands) on the lateral aspect of the upper arm, beginning at the lateral epicondyle in several hand placements toward the olecranon

6. Manipulation of the antecubital fossa
Thumb circles (one hand or alternating) covering the antecubital fossa from ~2 inches below to ~2 inches above. Several pathways are applied to cover the antecubital fossa from distal to proximal. This area can also be treated using stationary circles with the palmar surfaces of the fingers.

7. Manipulation of the forearm
Scoop techniques with one hand on the anterior and posterior aspect of the forearm between the wrist and the elbow. To manipulate both aspects with the same hand, the patient's forearm is rotated in pronation and supination, respectively. The other hand holds the patient's arm at the wrist in a comfortable and elevated position.
Combination of pump technique and stationary circles between the wrist and the elbow to cover the patient's anterior and posterior aspects of the forearm
The patient's forearm is rotated in pronation and supination, respectively, to cover both surfaces.

8. Manipulation of the dorsum of the hand and wrist
Thumb circles (one thumb or alternating) over dorsum of the hand and posterior wrist, starting on the metacarpophalangeal joints, ending at the styloid processes

9. Manipulation of the palmar aspect of the hand and the anterior wrist (Fig. 5–14)
Thumb circles (one thumb or alternating) in the palm, following the ulnar and radial bundle from the center of the palm toward the ulnar and radial edges of the hand (following the path of the collectors)

10. Manipulation of the fingers
Combination of thumb/finger circles on each individual finger from the distal to the proximal ends

11. Rework

Appropriate techniques are used (depending on the patient's condition) covering specific parts of the limb or the entire extremity to increase lymph angiomotoricity

12. Final effleurage (as in 2)

Lower Extremity

Selected indications: postsurgical (joint replacement, etc.) and post-traumatic swellings (including edema caused by immobility due to partial or complete paralysis); chronic venous insufficiency stages II and III (phlebolymphostatic edema); lipedema; part of the treatment sequence for primary lymphedema of the genitalia; part of the treatment for cyclic idiopathic edema; general increase in lymph circulation, or to achieve a common soothing effect by decreasing sympathetic activity

Pretreatment: lateral neck (abbreviated; see lateral neck sequence, steps 1–3), abdomen

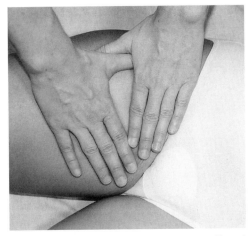

Figure 5–15 Stationary circles on the inguinal lymph nodes (second hand placement).

Anterior leg

Patient in supine position, with the leg slightly abducted and externally rotated; therapist on the patient's involved side:

1. Manipulation of the inguinal lymph nodes
   Stationary circles with both hands at the same time, with the working phase directed toward the inguinal ligament; three hand placements in the medial femoral triangle (Fig. 5–15)
   First hand placement: the upper hand lies parallel to the inguinal ligament (the fifth metacarpophalangeal joint is aligned with the patient's ASIS), the lower hand is positioned diagonally to the upper hand (with the fingertips touching the inguinal ligament).
   Second hand placement: the same hand positions are applied on the medial thigh (medial aspect of the femoral triangle).
   Third placement: both hands lie parallel on the medial aspect of the thigh (sagittal plane) to address the lymph nodes located in the distal apex of the medial femoral triangle.

2. Effleurage, two or three times covering the entire leg

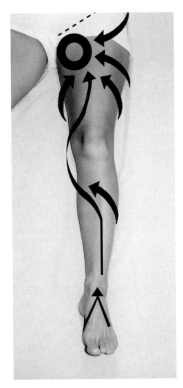

Figure 5–16 Drainage areas for the anterior lower extremity.

3. Manipulation of the anterior thigh
   Alternating pump techniques following the rectus femoris muscle between the base of the patella and the ASIS

4. Manipulation of the anterior and lateral thigh

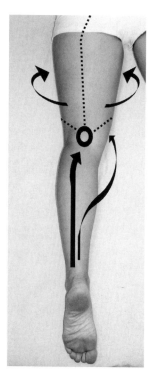

Figure 5–17
Drainage areas for the posterior lower extremity.

Combinations of pump techniques and stationary circles with alternating hands, beginning at the knee to proximal. The lateral pathway follows the iliotibial tract; the anterior pathway follows the rectus femoris muscle.

5. Manipulation of the medial thigh
Stationary circles alternating and dynamic at the medial thigh, beginning at the medial aspect of the knee to the groin (sagittal plane)

6. Manipulation of the knee
Pump technique in several hand placements (three or four) covering the anterior knee
Stationary circles (dynamic and simultaneously) on the medial and lateral knee, covering the knee from distal to proximal
Stationary circles in several hand placements covering the popliteal fossa from distal to proximal
Stationary circles (bimanual and simultaneous) below the medial aspect of knee ("bottle neck" area)

7. Manipulation of the lower leg
Scoop technique alternating at the calf between the malleoli and the popliteal fossa

(patient's knee is flexed). Either hand can be used by the therapist.
Pump technique on the anterior aspect of the lower leg, scoop technique on the calf (alternating and dynamic), between the malleoli and the knee

8. Manipulation on the foot
Stationary circles (simultaneous and dynamic) between the malleoli and the Achilles tendon in several hand placements
Thumb circles (one thumb or alternating) covering the dorsum of the foot and the ankle. Thumb circles may start on the toes or the metatarsophalangeal joints.

9. Rework
Appropriate techniques are used (depending on the patient's condition), covering specific parts of the limb, or the entire extremity to increase lymph angiomotoricity.

10. Final effleurage (as in step 2)

Posterior leg

The treatment of the posterior leg with the patient in the prone position is recommended in those cases where the decongestion of the limb does not advance as expected ("stubborn legs") with the treatment in supine, or if the swelling is more distally emphasized (e.g., larger swelling on the lower leg). The techniques on the posterior leg are similar to the sequences for the anterior leg (Figs. 5–16, 5–17). Manipulation of the inguinal lymph nodes in the supine position precedes the treatment of the posterior leg (Fig. 5–15).

Patient in prone position, with the leg slightly abducted; therapist on the patient's same side:

1. Effleurage, two or three times covering the entire leg

2. Manipulation of the posterior thigh
Alternating pump techniques between the popliteal fossa and the horizontal gluteal fold (frontal plane)

3. Manipulation of the medial thigh
Stationary circles alternating and dynamic at the medial thigh, beginning at the medial aspect of the knee to the groin (sagittal plane)

4. Manipulation of the posterior and lateral thigh

Combinations of pump techniques and stationary circles with alternating hands, beginning at the popliteal fossa to proximal. The lateral pathway follows the iliotibial tract; the posterior pathway follows the posterior thigh musculature in a frontal plane.

5. Manipulation of the knee

Stationary circles or pump techniques covering the popliteal fossa from distal to proximal (three or four hand placements)

Stationary circles (bimanual and simultaneous) below the medial aspect of knee ("bottle neck" area)

6. Manipulation of the lower leg

Alternating pump techniques in several hand placements covering the calf musculature between the heel and the popliteal fossa

Combination of pump techniques and stationary circles covering the calf musculature between the heel and the popliteal fossa in several hand placements

Thumb circles (one thumb or alternating) between the malleoli and the Achilles tendon. To include joint and muscle pump functions, this technique can be combined with passive ankle movements.

7. Rework

Appropriate techniques are used (depending on the patient's condition) covering specific parts of the limb, or the entire extremity to increase lymph angiomotoricity.

8. Final effleurage (as in step 1)

◆ Treatment Sequences

In the treatment of lymphedema, in particular in those cases where lymph node groups are removed and/or radiated, some of the sequences outlined above in Application of Basic MLD Techniques on Different Parts of the Body, are modified. These modifications are noted in the appropriate sections in the text.

In many cases of extremity lymphedema, the ipsilateral truncal quadrant (this may include the external genitalia) is also congested.

Truncal involvement may be visible or palpable (skinfolds), but they may also be difficult to identify, particularly if obesity is a factor.

It is therefore recommended to generally assume truncal involvement in extremity lymphedema, in which case the decongestion of the involved trunk has priority over the treatment of the swollen extremity (see also Chapter 4, The Two-Phase Approach in Lymphedema Management), and the truncal preparation is more complex. The following treatment sequences are based on this assumption.

Once the adjacent truncal quadrant is successfully decongested (this is generally the case if volume reduction in the involved extremity is noted), the treatment of the lymphedematous extremity becomes the priority, and the truncal preparation may be abbreviated.

Unilateral Secondary Upper Extremity Lymphedema

This condition is most often the result of mastectomy or lumpectomy with the removal and/or radiation of the axillary lymph nodes in breast cancer surgery.

The following sequence should be used until the truncal quadrant is decongested (Fig. 5–18).

Patient in supine position:

1. Abbreviated manipulation of the lateral neck lymph nodes, including the shoulder collectors (observe contraindications)

2. Anterior thorax on the contralateral side (omit intercostal and parasternal techniques)

3. Activation and utilization of the AAA anastomosis to move lymph fluid from the affected to the unaffected side

4. Manipulation of the inguinal lymph nodes on the ipsilateral, affected side

Therapist moves to other side of table:

5. Activation and utilization of the AI anastomosis on the affected side

6. Manipulation of lymph fluid from the congested upper quadrant in the direction of the inguinal lymph nodes on the same side, utilizing the AI anastomosis. Rotary

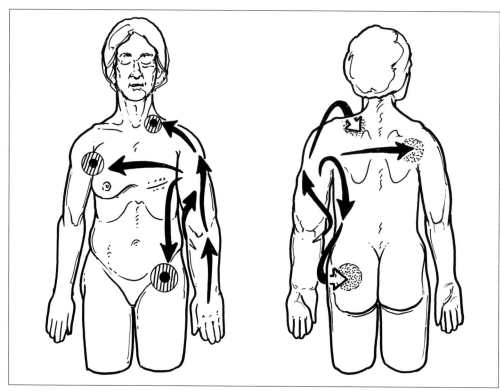

Figure 5–18 Drainage directions for unilateral lymphedema on the upper extremity.

techniques and stationary circles should be used.

7. Intercostal and parasternal techniques on the affected trunk quadrant to utilize deep drainage pathways

Patient on the side (or prone position), with the affected extremity on top:

8. Rework of the AI anastomosis and shoulder collectors

Patient in prone position (or on the side):

9. Posterior thorax on the unaffected side (omit intercostal and paravertebral techniques)

10. Activation and utilization of the PAA anastomosis to move lymph fluid from the affected to the unaffected side. Stationary circles should be used.

Therapist moves to other side of table:

11. Manipulation of lymph fluid from the congested posterior upper quadrant in the direction of the inguinal lymph nodes on the same side, utilizing the AI anastomo-sis. Rotary techniques and stationary circles should be used.

12. Intercostal and paravertebral techniques on the affected trunk quadrant to utilize deep drainage pathways

Patient on the side (or prone position), with the affected extremity on top:

13. Rework of PAA anastomosis, AI anastomosis, and shoulder collectors

Patient in supine position:

14. Rework of AAA anastomosis, axillary lymph nodes on the contralateral side, and inguinal lymph nodes on the ipsilateral side

15. Application of compression bandages on the involved extremity
    The following sequence should be used if the truncal quadrant is decongested and the treatment of the upper extremity is the primary focus:

Patient in supine position. Abbreviated trunk preparation (pretreatment):

1. Abbreviated manipulation of the lateral neck lymph nodes, including the shoulder collectors (observe contraindications)
2. Manipulation of the axillary lymph nodes on the contralateral side
3. Activation and utilization of the AAA anastomosis to stimulate lymph flow from the affected to the unaffected side
4. Manipulation of the inguinal lymph nodes on the ipsilateral (affected) side
   Therapist moves to other side of table:
5. Activation and utilization of the AI anastomosis on the affected side to stimulate lymph flow toward the drainage area

Patient on the side (or prone position), with the affected extremity on top:
6. Rework of AI anastomosis and shoulder collectors
7. Activation and utilization of the PAA anastomosis to stimulate lymph flow from the affected to the unaffected side

Treatment of the upper extremity:

> If the extremity is considerably swollen, it is not recommended to treat the entire extremity during one setting. The treatment should proceed in steps; for example, only the upper arm (or parts of it) may be treated, which prevents overload of the healthy lymphatics in the drainage areas.

8. Manipulation of the lateral upper arm between the lateral epicondyle and the acromion, using basic techniques ("bulk flow" techniques)
9. Rework of shoulder collectors, AI and PAA anastomosis

Patient in supine position:
10. Rework of AAA anastomosis
11. Manipulation of the lateral upper arm between the lateral epicondyle and the acromion. Modified effleurage as well as pump techniques and combination of pump and stationary circles should be used (see sequence 4–5, upper arm)
    This sequence should be followed up with rework techniques across the watershed into pretreated drainage areas.
12. Manipulation of the medial aspect of the upper arm toward the lateral aspect, using

stationary circles (dynamic technique). This technique should be followed up with rework techniques of drainage areas as in step 11. The entire length of the upper arm is treated in this manner.

13. Vasa vasorum technique in the area of the cephalic vein (Fig. 4–9)
14. Manipulation of elbow, forearm, and hand as outlined in the basic sequence techniques
15. If necessary, edema or fibrosis techniques should be incorporated at this point.
16. Rework of upper extremity, AAA anastomosis, axillary lymph nodes on contralateral side, inguinal lymph nodes on ipsilateral side, and shoulder collectors

Patient on the side (or prone position), with the affected extremity on top:
17. Rework of the PAA and AI anastomoses (on the same side)
18. Application of compression bandages on involved extremity

Bilateral Secondary Upper Extremity Lymphedema

This condition is most often the result of mastectomy or lumpectomy with the removal and/or radiation of the axillary lymph nodes in breast cancer surgery. Ideally, bandages should be applied on both upper extremities. If this is not possible, compression bandages should be applied to the more involved extremity.

The following sequence should be used until the truncal quadrant(s) is/are decongested (Fig. 5–19).

Patient in supine position:
1. Abbreviated manipulation of the lateral neck lymph nodes, including the shoulder collectors (observe contraindications)
2. Abdominal treatment: superficial and deep (modified) techniques as outlined in the basic sequences (observe contraindications). If abdominal techniques are contraindicated, diaphragmatic breathing should be used to substitute.
3. Manipulation of the inguinal lymph nodes on both sides
4. Activation and utilization of the AI anastomoses on both sides to promote lymph

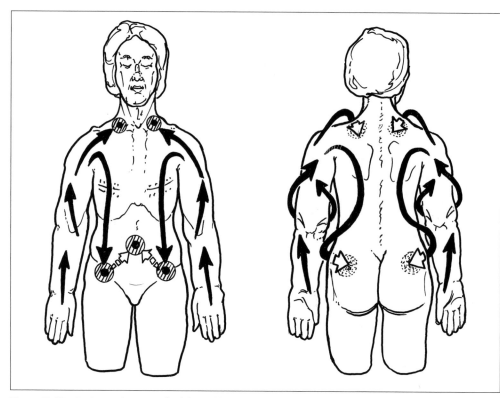

Figure 5–19   Drainage directions for bilateral lymphedema on the upper extremities.

flow from the congested quadrants to the drainage areas

5. Manipulation of lymph fluid from the congested upper quadrants in the direction of the inguinal lymph nodes, utilizing the AI anastomoses. Rotary techniques and stationary circles should be used.

6. Intercostal and parasternal techniques on both affected trunk quadrants to utilize deep drainage pathways

Patient in prone position (or on side):

7. Rework of both AI anastomoses

8. Manipulation of lymph fluid from the congested posterior upper quadrants in the direction of the inguinal lymph nodes, utilizing the AI anastomoses. Dynamic rotary techniques and stationary circles should be used.

9. Intercostal and paravertebral techniques on both affected trunk quadrants to utilize deep drainage pathways

Patient in supine position:

10. Rework of AI anastomoses on both sides, deep abdominal technique (modified), inguinal lymph nodes on both sides, and shoulder collectors

11. Application of compression bandages on both, or the more involved extremity

The following sequence should be used if the truncal quadrant(s) is/are decongested and the treatment of the upper extremities becomes the primary focus.

It is not recommended to treat both extremities in the same session. The more involved extremity should be treated first until decongested, then fitted with a compression sleeve. If the extremity is considerably swollen, it should be treated in steps; for example, only the upper arm (or parts of it) may be treated, which prevents overload of the healthy lymphatics in the drainage areas.

Therapy proceeds with the other arm, once the more involved extremity is decongested.

Patient in supine position:

1. Abbreviated manipulation of the lateral neck lymph nodes, including the shoulder collectors (observe contraindications)

2. Deep abdominal technique (modified) as outlined in the basic sequence (observe contraindications). If abdominal techniques are contraindicated, diaphragmatic breathing should be used to substitute.

3. Manipulation of the inguinal lymph nodes on both sides

4. Activation and utilization of the AI anastomoses on both sides to promote lymph flow across the watersheds into the drainage areas

Patient on the side (or prone position), with the more involved extremity on top:

5. Rework of AI anastomosis on the more involved side, and the shoulder collectors

6. Manipulation of the lateral upper arm between the lateral epicondyle and the acromion, using basic techniques ("bulk flow" techniques)

7. Rework of shoulder collectors and AI anastomosis on more involved side

Patient in supine position:

8. Manipulation of the lateral upper arm (more involved extremity) between the lateral epicondyle and the acromion. Modified effleurage as well as pump techniques and combination of pump and stationary circles should be used (see sequence 4–5, upper arm). This sequence should be followed up with rework techniques across the watershed into pretreated drainage areas.

9. Manipulation of the medial aspect of the upper arm toward the lateral aspect, using stationary circles (dynamic technique). This technique should be followed up with rework techniques of drainage areas. The entire length of the upper arm is treated in this manner.

10. Vasa vasorum technique in the area of the cephalic vein

11. Manipulation of elbow, forearm, and hand as outlined in the basic sequence techniques

12. If necessary, edema or fibrosis techniques should be incorporated at this point.

13. Rework of upper extremity, inguinal lymph nodes on both sides, AI anastomoses on both sides, shoulder collectors, and deep abdominal technique (modified)

14. Application of compression bandages on both, or the more involved extremity

Unilateral Secondary Lower Extremity Lymphedema

This condition is most often the result of the removal and/or radiation of the inguinal and/or pelvic lymph nodes in cancer surgery (prostate, bladder, female reproductive organs, melanoma). Secondary lower extremity lymphedema may also occur as a result of trauma and may be combined with swelling of the lower truncal quadrant on the same side, and/or the external genitalia.

The following sequence should be used until the truncal quadrant is decongested (Fig. 5–20).

Patient in supine position:

1. Abbreviated manipulation of the lateral neck lymph nodes (observe contraindications)

2. Manipulation of the axillary lymph nodes on the ipsilateral side

3. Activation and utilization of the IA anastomosis to move lymph fluid from the swollen lower quadrant toward the drainage area

4. Manipulation of the inguinal lymph nodes on the contralateral side

5. Activation and utilization of the AII anastomosis to move lymph fluid from the swollen lower quadrant toward the drainage area on the opposite side

6. Abdominal treatment: superficial and deep (modified) techniques as outlined in the basic sequences (observe contraindications). If abdominal techniques are contraindicated, diaphragmatic breathing should be substituted.

Patient on the side (or prone position), with the affected extremity on top:

7. Rework of the IA anastomosis on the affected side

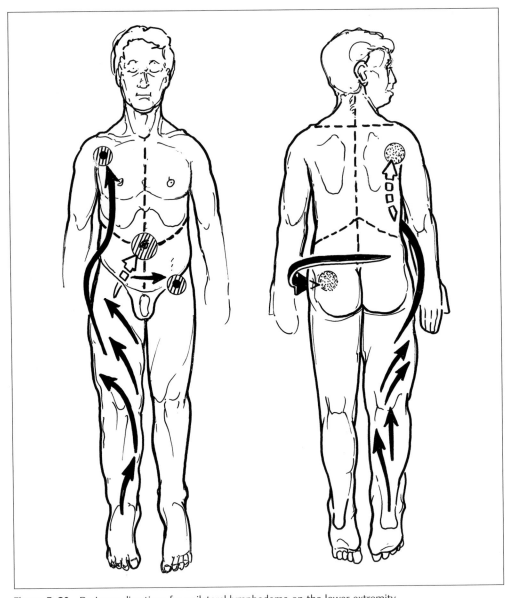

Figure 5–20 Drainage directions for unilateral lymphedema on the lower extremity.

Patient in prone position (or on side):

8. Manipulation of the lumbar area on the unaffected side (omit step 4)

9. Activation and utilization of the PII anastomosis to move lymph fluid from the swollen lower quadrant toward the drainage area on the opposite side

10. Paravertebral techniques on the affected lumbar area to promote deep lymphatic pathways

11. Rework of the PII anastomosis

Patient in supine position:

12. Rework of AII anastomosis, IA anastomosis on the affected side, inguinal lymph nodes

on contralateral and axillary lymph nodes on ipsilateral sides, and deep abdominal techniques (modified)

13. Application of compression bandages on the affected extremity
The following sequence should be used if the truncal quadrant is decongested and the treatment of the lymphedematous leg is the primary focus.

Patient in supine position. Abbreviated trunk preparation (pretreatment):

1. Abbreviated manipulation of the lateral neck lymph nodes (observe contraindications)

2. Manipulation of the axillary lymph nodes on the ipsilateral side

3. Activation and utilization of the IA anastomosis to promote lymph flow across the watershed toward the drainage area

4. Manipulation of the inguinal lymph nodes on the contralateral side

5. Activation and utilization of the AII anastomosis to promote lymph flow across the watershed toward the drainage area on the opposite side

6. Deep abdominal technique (modified) as outlined in the basic sequences (observe contraindications). If abdominal techniques are contraindicated, diaphragmatic breathing should be substituted.

Patient on the side (or prone position), with the affected extremity on top:

7. Rework of the IA anastomosis on the affected side

8. Activation and utilization of the PII anastomosis to promote lymph flow across the watershed toward the drainage area on the opposite side

9. Manipulation of the lateral thigh between the lateral knee and the iliac crest, using basic techniques ("bulk flow" techniques)

10. Rework of the PII and IA anastomoses (on the affected side)

Patient in supine position:

11. Rework of the AII anastomosis
Treatment of the lower extremity:

> If the extremity is considerably swollen, it is not recommended to treat the entire extremity in one session. The treatment should proceed in steps; for example, only the thigh (or parts of it) may be treated, which prevents overload of the healthy lymphatics in the drainage areas.

12. Manipulation of the lateral thigh between the knee and the iliac crest. Modified effleurage as well as pump techniques, combination of pump and stationary circles, and rotary techniques should be used.
This sequence should be followed up with rework techniques across the watersheds into pretreated drainage areas.

13. Manipulation of the medial aspect of the thigh toward the lateral aspect, using stationary circles (dynamic technique). This technique should be repeated over the entire length of the thigh and followed up with rework techniques toward the drainage areas.

14. Vasa vasorum technique in the area of the femoral vein

15. Manipulation of knee, lower leg, and foot as outlined in the basic sequence techniques

16. If necessary, edema or fibrosis techniques should be incorporated at this point. It may also be necessary to turn the patient in the prone position for the treatment of the posterior leg.

17. Rework of lower extremity, AII anastomosis, IA anastomosis on the affected side, axillary lymph nodes on ipsilateral side, inguinal lymph nodes on contralateral side, and deep abdominal techniques (modified)

Patient on the side (or prone position), with the affected extremity on top:

18. Rework of the PII anastomosis

19. Application of compression bandages on the affected extremity

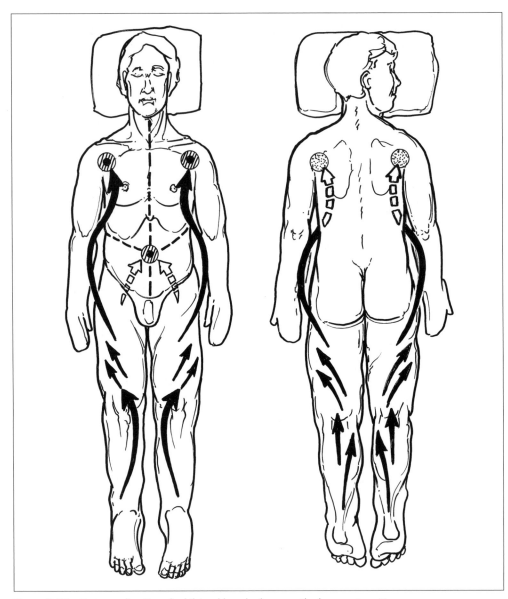

Figure 5–21 Drainage directions for bilateral lymphedema on the lower extremities.

Bilateral Secondary Lower Extremity Lymphedema

This condition is most often the result of the removal and/or radiation of the inguinal and/or pelvic lymph nodes in cancer surgery (prostate, bladder, female reproductive organs, melanoma). Secondary lower extremity lymphedema may also occur as a result of trauma and may be combined with swelling of the lower truncal quadrant on the same side, and/or the external genitalia. Ideally, bandages should be applied on both lower extremities. If this is not possible, compression bandages should be applied to the more involved extremity.

The following sequence should be used until the truncal quadrant(s) is/are decongested (Fig. 5–21).

Patient in supine position:

1. Abbreviated manipulation of the lateral neck lymph nodes (observe contraindications)

2. Manipulation of the axillary lymph nodes on both sides

3. Activation and utilization of the IA anastomoses on both sides to promote lymph flow from the congested quadrants to the drainage areas

4. Abdominal treatment: superficial and deep (modified) techniques as outlined in the basic sequences (observe contraindications). If abdominal techniques are contraindicated, diaphragmatic breathing should be substituted.

Patient in prone position (or on side):

5. Rework of IA anastomoses on both sides

6. Decongestion of the swollen lower truncal quadrants on both sides toward the axillary lymph nodes, using modified lumbar techniques: modified effleurage; rotary techniques starting at the sagittal watershed to the side, followed by stationary circles (dynamic technique) toward the axilla using the IA anastomosis; paravertebral techniques to utilize deep drainage pathways

Patient in supine position:

7. Rework of IA anastomoses and axillary lymph nodes on both sides

8. Rework abdominal area: superficial and deep (modified) techniques

9. Application of compression bandages on both or the more involved extremity

The following sequence should be used if the truncal quadrant(s) is/are decongested and the treatment of the lower extremities becomes the primary focus.

> It is not recommended to treat both extremities in the same session. The more involved extremity should be treated first until decongested. If the extremity is considerably swollen, it should be treated in steps; for example, only the thigh (or parts of it) may be treated, which prevents overload of the healthy lymphatics in the drainage areas.

Therapy proceeds with the other leg, once the more involved extremity is decongested. Generally, a pantyhose-style compression garment is ideal for this condition once both extremities are decongested. To preserve the results in the leg that was treated first, compression bandages should be applied. If this is not possible, the patient should be fitted with a thigh-high compression garment (preferably a relatively inexpensive standard-size garment) while the other extremity receives treatment, then be fitted with a pantyhose-style garment.

Patient in supine position. Abbreviated trunk preparation (pretreatment):

1. Abbreviated manipulation of the lateral neck lymph nodes (observe contraindications)

2. Manipulation of the axillary lymph nodes on both sides

3. Activation and utilization of the IA anastomoses on both sides to promote lymph flow across the watersheds into the drainage areas

4. Abdominal treatment: superficial and deep (modified) techniques as outlined in the basic sequences (observe contraindications). If abdominal techniques are contraindicated, diaphragmatic breathing should be substituted.

Patient on the side (or prone position), with the more involved extremity on top:

5. Rework of the IA anastomosis on the more involved side

6. Manipulation of the lateral thigh between the lateral knee and the iliac crest, using basic techniques ("bulk flow" techniques)

Patient in supine position:

7. Rework of IA anastomoses on both sides

Treatment of the lower extremity:

8. Manipulation of the lateral thigh between the knee and the iliac crest. Modified effleurage as well as pump techniques, combination of pump and stationary circles, and rotary techniques should be used.
   This sequence should be followed up with rework techniques across the watersheds into pretreated drainage areas.

9. Manipulation of the medial aspect of the thigh toward the lateral aspect, using stationary circles (dynamic technique). This technique should be repeated over the entire length of the thigh and followed-up with rework techniques toward the drainage areas.

10. Vasa vasorum technique in the area of the femoral vein

11. Manipulation of knee, lower leg, and foot as outlined in the basic sequence techniques

12. If necessary, edema or fibrosis techniques should be incorporated at this point. It may also be necessary to turn the patient in the prone position for the treatment of the posterior leg.

13. Rework of lower extremity, IA anastomoses on both sides, axillary lymph nodes on both sides and abdominal techniques

14. Application of compression bandages on both, or the more involved extremity

Unilateral Primary Lower Extremity Lymphedema

This condition is the result developmental abnormalities (see Chapter 3, Primary Lymphedema) of the lymphatic system, which are either congenital or hereditary. Primary lower extremity lymphedema may be combined with swelling of the adjacent truncal quadrant and/or the external genitalia.

Congenital malformations of the lymphatic system may also be present in the contralateral leg. If the volume of the unaffected leg increases, or if any changes in tissue consistency are noted during the treatment, the use of interinguinal anastomoses (AII and PII) should be discontinued.

Treatment sequences for this condition are very similar to the treatment of secondary lymphedema of the lower extremity. The inguinal lymph nodes in primary lymphedema are still present and should be stimulated. The goal of intervention, however, is to relieve these lymph nodes; lymph fluid is therefore rerouted around the inguinal lymph nodes toward sufficient drainage areas located in the adjacent trunk territories.

The following sequence should be used until the truncal quadrant is decongested (Fig. 5–20).

Patient in supine position:
1. Abbreviated manipulation of the lateral neck lymph nodes (observe contraindications)

2. Manipulation of the axillary lymph nodes on the ipsilateral side

3. Activation and utilization of the IA anastomosis to move lymph fluid from the swollen lower quadrant toward the drainage area

4. Manipulation of the inguinal lymph nodes on the contralateral side

5. Activation and utilization of the AII anastomosis to move lymph fluid from the swollen lower quadrant toward the drainage area on the opposite side

6. Abdominal treatment: superficial and deep (modified) techniques as outlined in the basic sequences (observe contraindications). If abdominal techniques are contraindicated, diaphragmatic breathing should be substituted.

Therapist moves to the other side of the treatment table:
7. Manipulation of the inguinal lymph nodes on the affected side

Patient in prone position (or on side):
8. Manipulation of the lumbar area on the unaffected side (omit manipulation of the inguinal lymph nodes)

9. Activation and utilization of the PII anastomosis to move lymph fluid from the swollen lower quadrant toward the drainage area on the opposite side

10. Paravertebral techniques on the affected lumbar area to promote deep lymphatic pathways

11. Rework of the PII anastomosis

Patient in supine position:
12. Rework of AII anastomosis, IA anastomosis on the affected side, axillary lymph nodes on the ipsilateral side, inguinal lymph nodes on both sides, and deep abdominal techniques (modified)

13. Application of compression bandages on the affected extremity

The following sequence should be used if the truncal quadrant is decongested and the treatment of the lymphedematous leg is the primary focus.

Patient in supine position. Abbreviated trunk preparation (pretreatment):
1. Abbreviated manipulation of the lateral neck lymph nodes (observe contraindications)

2. Manipulation of the axillary lymph nodes on the ipsilateral side

3. Activation and utilization of the IA anastomosis to promote lymph flow across the watershed toward the drainage area

4. Manipulation of the inguinal lymph nodes on the contralateral side

5. Activation and utilization of the AII anastomosis to promote lymph flow across the watershed toward the drainage area on the opposite side

6. Deep abdominal technique (modified) as outlined in the basic sequences (observe contraindications). If abdominal techniques are contraindicated, diaphragmatic breathing should be substituted.

Patient on the side (or prone position), with the affected extremity on top:

7. Rework of the IA anastomosis on the affected side

8. Activation and utilization of the PII anastomosis to promote lymph flow across the watershed toward the drainage area on the opposite side

9. Manipulation of the lateral thigh between the lateral knee and the iliac crest, using basic techniques ("bulk flow" techniques)

10. Rework of the PII and inguinal-axillary anastomoses (on the affected side)

Patient in supine position:

11. Rework of the AII anastomosis
Treatment of the lower extremity:

> If the extremity is considerably swollen, it is not recommended to treat the entire extremity in one session. The treatment should proceed in steps; for example, only the thigh (or parts of it) may be treated, which prevents overload of the healthy lymphatics in the drainage areas. If the swelling is more distally pronounced (as is often the case in primary lymphedema), more time should be spent to treat the areas below the knee.

12. Manipulation of the inguinal lymph nodes on the affected leg
As discussed earlier, inguinal lymph nodes in primary lymphedema are used as additional drainage areas. Lymph fluid from more distal sections of the leg should not be manipulated toward the inguinal nodes but rerouted around them as in the treatment of secondary lymphedema.

13. Manipulation of the lateral thigh between the knee and the iliac crest. Modified effleurage as well as pump techniques, combination of pump and stationary circles, and rotary techniques should be used. This sequence should be followed up with rework techniques across the watersheds into pretreated drainage areas.

14. Manipulation of the medial aspect of the thigh toward the lateral aspect, using stationary circles (dynamic technique). This technique should be repeated over the entire length of the thigh and followed up with rework techniques toward the drainage areas.

15. Vasa vasorum technique in the area of the femoral vein

16. Manipulation of knee, lower leg, and foot as outlined in the basic sequence techniques

17. If necessary, edema or fibrosis techniques should be incorporated at this point. It may also be necessary to turn the patient in prone position for the treatment of the posterior leg.

18. Rework of lower extremity, including the inguinal lymph nodes; rework of the anterior AII anastomosis, IA anastomosis on the affected side, axillary lymph nodes on ipsilateral side, inguinal lymph nodes on the contralateral side, and deep abdominal techniques (modified)

Patient on the side (or prone position), with the affected extremity on top:

19. Rework of the PII anastomosis

20. Application of compression bandages on the affected extremity

Bilateral Primary Lower Extremity Lymphedema

This condition is the result of developmental abnormalities (see Chapter 3, Primary Lymphedema) of the lymphatic system, which are either congenital or hereditary. Primary lower extremity lymphedema may be combined with swelling of the adjacent truncal quadrant and/or the external genitalia.

Treatment sequences for this condition are very similar to the treatment of bilateral secondary lymphedema of the lower extremities. The inguinal lymph nodes in primary lymphedema are still present and should be stimulated. The goal of intervention, however, is to relieve these lymph nodes; lymph fluid is therefore rerouted around the inguinal lymph nodes toward sufficient drainage areas located in the upper truncal territories (axillary lymph nodes).

The following sequence should be used until the truncal quadrant(s) is/are decongested (Fig. 5–21).

Patient in supine position:
1. Abbreviated manipulation of the lateral neck lymph nodes (observe contraindications)
2. Manipulation of the axillary lymph nodes on both sides
3. Manipulation of the inguinal lymph nodes on both sides
4. Activation and utilization of the IA anastomoses on both sides to promote lymph flow from the congested quadrants to the drainage areas
5. Abdominal treatment: superficial and deep (modified) techniques as outlined in the basic sequences (observe contraindications). If abdominal techniques are contraindicated, diaphragmatic breathing should be substituted.

Patient in prone position (or on side):
6. Rework of IA anastomoses on both sides
7. Decongestion of the swollen lower truncal quadrants on both sides toward the axillary lymph nodes, using modified lumbar techniques: modified effleurage; rotary techniques starting at the sagittal watershed to the side, followed by stationary circles (dynamic technique) toward the axilla using the IA anastomosis; paravertebral techniques to utilize deep drainage pathways

Patient in supine position:
8. Rework of IA anastomoses and axillary lymph nodes on both sides
9. Rework abdominal area: superficial and deep (modified) techniques
10. Application of compression bandages on both or the more involved extremity

The following sequence should be used if the truncal quadrant(s) is/are decongested and the treatment of the lower extremities becomes the primary focus.

It is not recommended to treat both extremities in the same session. The more involved extremity should be treated first until decongested. If the extremity is considerably swollen, it should be treated in steps; for example, only the thigh (or parts of it) may be treated, which prevents overload of the healthy lymphatics in the drainage areas.

Therapy proceeds with the other leg, once the more involved extremity is decongested. Generally, a pantyhose-style compression garment is ideal for this condition, once both extremities are decongested. To preserve the results in the leg that was treated first, compression bandages should be applied. If this is not possible, the patient should be fitted with a thigh-high compression garment (preferably a relatively inexpensive standard-size garment) while the other extremity receives treatment, then be fitted with a pantyhose-style garment.

Patient in supine position. Abbreviated trunk preparation (pretreatment):
1. Abbreviated manipulation of the lateral neck lymph nodes (observe contraindications)
2. Manipulation of the axillary lymph nodes on both sides
3. Activation and utilization of the IA anastomoses on both sides to promote lymph flow across the watersheds into the drainage areas
4. Manipulation of the inguinal lymph nodes on both sides

   As discussed earlier, inguinal lymph nodes in primary lymphedema are used as additional drainage areas. Lymph fluid from more distal sections of the leg should not be manipulated toward the inguinal nodes, but rerouted around them, as in the treatment of secondary lymphedema (see secondary lower extremity lymphedema)
5. Abdominal treatment: superficial and deep (modified) techniques as outlined in the basic sequences (observe contraindications). If abdominal techniques are

contraindicated, diaphragmatic breathing should be substituted.

Patient on the side (or prone position), with the more involved extremity on top:

6. Rework of the IA anastomosis on the more involved side

7. Manipulation of the lateral thigh between the lateral knee and the iliac crest, using basic techniques ("bulk flow" techniques)

Patient in supine position:

8. Rework of IA anastomoses on both sides

Treatment of the lower extremity:

9. Rework the inguinal lymph nodes on the more involved leg

10. Manipulation of the lateral thigh between the knee and the iliac crest. Modified effleurage as well as pump techniques, combination of pump and stationary circles, and rotary techniques should be used.

This sequence should be followed up with rework techniques across the watersheds into pretreated drainage areas.

11. Manipulation of the medial aspect of the thigh toward the lateral aspect, using stationary circles (dynamic technique). This technique should be repeated over the entire length of the thigh and followed up with rework techniques toward the drainage areas.

12. Vasa vasorum technique in the area of the femoral vein

13. Manipulation of knee, lower leg, and foot as outlined in the basic sequence techniques

14. If necessary, edema or fibrosis techniques should be incorporated at this point. It may also be necessary to turn the patient in prone position for the treatment of the posterior leg.

15. Rework of lower extremity, including the inguinal lymph nodes; rework of the IA anastomoses on both sides, axillary lymph nodes on both sides, inguinal lymph nodes on the less swollen leg, and abdominal techniques

16. Application of compression bandages on both, or the more involved extremity

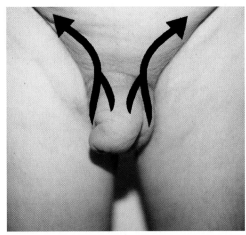

Figure 5–22 Genital lymphedema with involvement of the penis in an uncircumcised patient. Arrows indicate drainage directions.

Genital Lymphedema

Genital lymphedema is a challenging condition that very often causes real and long-lasting physical, emotional, and social problems for the affected patients. This condition can affect both males and females but is more common in males due to the greater tissue elasticity of the scrotum and penis, combined with the effects of gravity (Fig. 5–22).

Reliable numbers on the incidence of genital swelling are unavailable because this condition often remains undiagnosed; genital edema is generally not a topic of conversation, such as swelling of an extremity following surgery.

Genital lymphedema is usually irreversible without treatment, and once it develops, it tends to become more fibrotic and increases in size. It can be effectively controlled and maintained with complete decongestive therapy (CDT). In some cases, genital swelling may occur acutely following surgery or trauma and may resolve completely by itself.

In most cases genital lymphedema is combined with lower extremity lymphedema.

Classification

Genital swelling can be classified as malignant, benign, primary, and secondary.

Malignant conditions

Advanced pelvic and/or abdominal malignancies may block or reduce the lymphatic and venous return from the genital area.

The onset of genital swelling without apparent reason, the presence of a clear vaginal discharge, or lymphorrhea, may be a symptom of an active malignant process and needs to be thoroughly examined by a physician.

Primary conditions

Primary genital swelling is usually the result of congenital malformations (dysplasia) of lymph vessels and/or lymph nodes in the region. As with all primary forms, the swelling may be present at birth (rare) or develop later in life with or without obvious cause. Minor surgical interventions, such as a circumcision, may trigger the onset of pediatric genital swelling if congenital malformations of the lymphatic system are present.

Isolated swelling of the genital region is not common. In many cases other parts of the body are involved in the swelling as well, such as the lower quadrant(s) and/or one or both of the lower extremities.

It was also reported that obese patients with lower extremity lymphedema have an increased risk of developing genital swelling due to greater pressure on the lymphatic system in the groin from the enlarged abdomen.

Secondary conditions

Trauma or surgical interventions in combination with the removal and/or radiation of lymph vessels and/or lymph nodes (especially pelvic lymph nodes) to remove gynecological, testicular, penile, urological, abdominal, intestinal, or prostatic cancers are a common cause.

The incidence of genital swelling tends to increase with the combination of surgery and radiation, and if the patient has a history of recurrent episodes of cellulitis.

The swelling may occur immediately post surgery or years later as with other forms of lymphedema. Reports suggest that genital swelling in combination with lower extremity lymphedema occurs in about 10% of patients.

The incidence of genital swelling in females has been estimated to occur in 10 to 20% of patients following surgery.

In males, the incidence of genital edema following oncological surgery (prostatectomy, bladder cancer) and/or radiation seems to be considerably higher.

Filariasis is another common cause of genital swelling in endemic regions (See Chapter 3 Pathology, and Fig. 3–4 A/B).

A very common reason for the onset of genital swelling is the use of pneumatic compression pumps for the treatment of lower extremity lymphedema. Boris, Weindorf and Lasinski published a paper in the March 1998 edition of Lymphology Magazine and concluded that the use of external pneumatic compression pumps in the treatment of lower extremity lymphedema produces an unacceptable high incidence of genital edema (please refer to Chapter 3, Lymphedema—Therapeutic Approach).

Clinical Picture

Various combinations of genital anatomy swelling may occur. In males, isolated penile swelling is rare. Combined penile and scrotal swelling is a more common presentation. The scrotum may swell to such an extent that ambulation becomes difficult. The lower quadrants and/or lower extremities often accompany genital swelling. Additional involvement of the pubic area frequently causes the penis to retract into the scrotum.

In females, the labia minora and the labia majora may be included in the swelling. These areas could project several inches out of the vagina. Clear labial/vaginal discharge (lymphorrhea), the appearances of papillomas or warty growths are often symptoms indicating genital involvement, especially if the patient had pelvic or gynecological procedures. Vaginal discharge for other reasons often has a curdish, white, thick discharge.

Genital swelling frequently causes problems in urination and sexual activity, depending on the extent of the involvement.

Evaluation

Other conditions, such as active malignancies, renal, liver, cardiac or venous problems can cause genital edema. A thorough evaluation with a clear diagnostic picture is necessary before MLD/CDT can be initiated.

History

- What kind of surgery (if any) was performed and how many lymph nodes were excised?
- Were there any cellulitis attacks in the past? Where did they start?
- Pain? Some patients describe bursting sensation or an ache around the genital area (pain generally recedes with treatment). Males often complain about painful erections.
- Were/are there any problems with bowel or bladder function following surgery or radiation?
- Are appropriate hygienic measures possible?
- Is the patient circumcised?

Inspection

- Any moist areas, lymphatic cysts, lymphatic fistulas (Fig. 5–23), lymphorrhea (patients often use sanitary or incontinence pads)
- Extent of the swelling? Penis/scrotum; external/internal labiae; pubic area; lower quadrant and/or lower extremity (unilateral/bilateral)
- Scars?
- Skin folds in the genital region?
- Papillomas, warts?
- Bacterial or mycotic infections? (Patients with discharge from the area often complain about malodor; lymph itself has no odor, but is very high in protein content, which presents an excellent breeding ground for bacteria, causing malodor.)

Palpation

- Tissue quality—fibrosis, scars
- Tissue quality in other involved areas
- Can the foreskin be pulled back in uncircumcised male patients?

Treatment

As discussed earlier, genital swelling is often associated with lower extremity lymphedema.

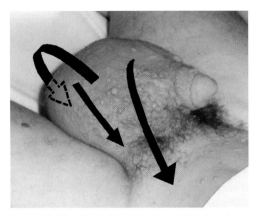

Figure 5–23 Genital lymphedema with lymphatic cysts and fistulas. Arrows indicate drainage directions.

The treatment of the genital swelling may be included in the treatment sequence or it may be performed as a stand-alone treatment.

If lower extremity swelling (or trunkal edema) is present, the treatment of the genital swelling should precede the sequence for leg lymphedema.

Lymphatic cysts and/or fistulas, lymphorrhea, bacterial and mycotic infections are common complicating factors found in combination with this condition. Meticulous hygiene is therefore imperative. If fistulas are present, the area must be cleaned and disinfected with proper agents, and the treatment should be performed wearing sterile gloves.

To maximize the therapeutic effect, genital bandaging may be performed prior to the application of hands-on techniques for the pretreatment of the drainage areas. Following the treatment sequence, the bandages are removed and the MLD techniques in the swollen genital area are performed. The therapist then proceeds with the application of the final compression bandage. The application of compression bandages on the genital area is discussed later in this chapter.

Patient in supine position:

1. Abbreviated manipulation of the lateral neck lymph nodes (observe contraindications)
2. Manipulation of the axillary lymph nodes on both sides
3. Activation and utilization of the IA anastomoses on both sides to promote lymph flow

across the watershed into the drainage areas

4. If inguinal lymph nodes are present, manipulation of the inguinal lymph nodes on both sides

5. Abdominal treatment: superficial and deep (modified) techniques as outlined in the basic sequences (observe contraindications). If abdominal techniques are contraindicated, diaphragmatic breathing should be substituted.

If the lower truncal quadrants are congested, the patient is turned in the prone position at this point, an the lumbar areas are decongested in the following manner. Decongestion of the swollen lower truncal quadrants on both sides toward the axillary lymph nodes, using modified lumbar techniques; modified effleurage; rotary techniques starting at the sagittal watershed to the side, followed by stationary circles (dynamic techniques) toward the axilla using the IA anastomosis; paravertebral techniques to utilize deep drainage pathways. The patient is then turned back in the supine position.

6. Treatment of the scrotum: stationary circles on both sides of the scrotum to manipulate the lymph fluid toward the pubic area, and from here toward the axillary lymph nodes on the respective side, utilizing the IA anastomoses.

7 Application of bandages (see Lower Extremity Bandaging later in this chapter)

Phlebolymphostatic Edema

This condition is a result of a venous insufficiency (for pathology, refer to Chapter 3, Chronic Venous and Lymphovenous Insufficiency). The deficient venous valves in chronic venous insufficiency (CVI) fail to prevent retrograde flow of venous blood during muscle pump activity, which in turn directly affects the lymphatic system.

Over time, and if CVI is left without treatment, damage to the lymphatic system, combined with reduction in transport capacity is unavoidable. The presence of lymphedema in stage II and III of CVI necessitates the application of the complete spectrum of complete decongestive therapy. If venous ulcerations are present, appropriate wound dressings and skin care products, prescribed by the physician, are applied before CDT starts (refer to Chapter 3, Complete Decongestive Therapy). The wound remains covered during the treatment, and MLD techniques are directed away from and around the ulcer bed. Treatment in and around the wound area is performed wearing sterile gloves. Decongestion of the extremity greatly increases the tendency of venous stasis ulcerations to heal.

The treatment protocol for lymphedema associated with CVI corresponds with the protocol for primary lymphedema; fibrosis and edema techniques are contraindicated.

> Should any signs or symptoms of thrombophlebitis in deep veins or symptoms of pulmonary embolism develop (see Chapter 3, Thrombophlebitis in Deep Veins), the patient must see a doctor immediately, and any treatment must be interrupted until the condition is cleared up.

Patient in supine position. Abbreviated trunk preparation (pretreatment):

1. Abbreviated manipulation of the lateral neck lymph nodes (observe contraindications)

2. Manipulation of the axillary lymph nodes on the ipsilateral side

3. Activation and utilization of the IA anastomosis to promote lymph flow across the watershed toward the drainage area

4. Manipulation of the inguinal lymph nodes on the contralateral side

5. Activation and utilization of the AII anastomosis to promote lymph flow across the watershed toward the drainage area on the opposite side

6. Deep abdominal technique (modified) as outlined in the basic sequences (observe contraindications). If abdominal techniques are contraindicated, diaphragmatic breathing should be used to substitute.

Patient on the side (or prone position), with the affected extremity on top:

7. Rework of the IA anastomosis on the affected side

8. Activation and utilization of the PII anastomosis to promote lymph flow across the watershed toward the drainage area on the opposite side

9. Manipulation of the lateral thigh between the lateral knee and the iliac crest, using basic techniques ("bulk flow" techniques)

10. Rework of the PII and IA anastomosis (on the affected side)

Patient in supine position:

11. Rework of the AII anastomosis
Treatment of the lower extremity (experience shows that the swelling in phlebolymphostatic edema is generally pronounced more distally; in these cases, more time should be spent treating the tissues distal to the knee joint):

12. Manipulation of the inguinal lymph nodes on the affected leg

13. Manipulation of the lateral thigh between the knee and the iliac crest. Modified effleurage as well as pump techniques, combination of pump and stationary circles, and rotary techniques should be used.

This sequence should be followed up with rework techniques across the watersheds into pretreated drainage areas.

14. Manipulation of the medial aspect of the thigh toward the lateral aspect, using stationary circles (dynamic technique). This technique should be repeated over the entire length of the thigh and followed up with rework techniques toward the drainage areas.

15. Manipulation of knee, lower leg, and foot as outlined in the basic sequence techniques

16. To maximize the decongestive effect, it is often beneficial to turn the patient in the prone position at this point for the treatment of the posterior lower leg.

17. Rework of lower extremity, including the inguinal lymph nodes. Rework of the AII anastomosis, IA anastomosis on the affected side, axillary lymph nodes on the ipsilateral side, inguinal lymph nodes on the contralateral side, and deep abdominal techniques (modified)

Patient on the side (or prone position), with the affected extremity on top:

18. Rework of the PII anastomosis

19. Application of compression bandages on the affected extremity. In many cases of phlebolymphostatic insufficiency, compression bandages need to be applied only up to the knee; this depends on the severity of the swelling and is determined by the physician.

Lipolymphedema

Lipolymphedema generally involves both lower extremities, and the treatment protocol of this condition corresponds with that for primary lymphedema. The lymphedematous component responds well and relatively fast to CDT; the lipedema itself responds more slowly, sometimes not at all. Lighter pressures in manual and compression bandage techniques during the initial treatment sessions may be necessary because lipedema and lipolymphedema are often associated with hypersensitivity and pain, which typically diminish after several treatments. Patients often require more padding under the compression bandages, particularly in the anterior tibial area. In some cases, it may be necessary not to apply a bandage at all during the first few treatments. Edema and fibrosis techniques are contraindicated in the treatment of this condition.

The following sequence should be used until the truncal quadrant(s) is/are decongested.

Patient in supine position:

1. Abbreviated manipulation of the lateral neck lymph nodes (observe contraindications)

2. Manipulation of the axillary lymph nodes on both sides

3. Manipulation of the inguinal lymph nodes on both sides

4. Activation and utilization of the IA anastomoses on both sides to promote lymph flow from the congested quadrants to the drainage areas

5. Abdominal treatment: superficial and deep (modified) techniques as outlined in the basic sequences (observe contraindications). If abdominal techniques are contraindicated, diaphragmatic breathing should be substituted.

Patient in prone position (or on side):

6. Rework of IA anastomoses on both sides

7. Decongestion of the swollen lower truncal quadrants on both sides toward the axillary lymph nodes, using modified lumbar

techniques: modified effleurage; rotary techniques starting at the sagittal watershed to the side, followed by stationary circles toward the axilla using the IA anastomosis (IA); paravertebral techniques to utilize deep drainage pathways

Patient in supine position:

8. Rework of IA anastomoses and axillary lymph nodes on both sides

9. Rework abdominal area: superficial and deep (modified) techniques

10. Application of compression bandages on both, or the more involved extremity

The following sequence should be used if the truncal quadrant(s) is/are decongested and the treatment of the lower extremities becomes the primary focus.

> It is not recommended to treat both extremities in the same session. The more involved extremity should be treated first until decongested. If the extremity is considerably swollen, it should be treated in steps; for example, only the thigh (or parts of it) may be treated, which prevents overload of the healthy lymphatics in the drainage areas.

Therapy proceeds with the less involved leg, once the more involved extremity is decongested. Generally, a pantyhose-style compression garment is ideal for this condition, once both extremities are decongested. To preserve the results in the leg that was treated first, compression bandages should be applied. If this is not possible, the patient should be fitted with a thigh-high compression garment (preferably a relatively inexpensive standard-size garment) while the other extremity receives treatment, then be fitted with a pantyhose-style garment.

Patient in supine position. Abbreviated trunk preparation (pretreatment):

1. Abbreviated manipulation of the lateral neck lymph nodes (observe contraindications)

2. Manipulation of the axillary lymph nodes on both sides

3. Activation and utilization of the IA anastomoses on both sides to promote lymph flow across the watersheds into the drainage areas.

4. Manipulation of the inguinal lymph nodes on both sides

5. Deep abdominal techniques (modified) as outlined in the basic sequences (observe contraindications). If abdominal techniques are contraindicated, diaphragmatic breathing should be substituted.

Patient on the side (or prone position), with the more involved extremity on top:

6. Rework of the IA anastomosis (IA) on the more involved side

7. Manipulation of the lateral thigh between the lateral knee and the iliac crest, using basic techniques ("bulk flow" techniques)

Patient in supine position:

8. Rework of IA anastomoses on both sides

Treatment of the lower extremity:

9. Rework the inguinal lymph nodes on the more involved leg

10. Manipulation of the lateral thigh between the knee and the iliac crest. Modified effleurage as well as pump techniques, combination of pump and stationary circles, and rotary techniques should be used.
This sequence should be followed up with rework techniques across the watersheds into pretreated drainage areas.

11. Manipulation of the medial aspect of the thigh toward the lateral aspect, using stationary circles. This technique should be repeated over the entire length of the thigh and followed up with rework techniques toward the drainage areas.

12. Vasa vasorum technique in the area of the femoral vein

13. Manipulation of knee, lower leg, and foot as outlined in the basic sequence techniques

14. Rework of lower extremity, including the inguinal lymph nodes

If necessary, patient in prone position:

15. Manipulation of the posterior knee and lower leg as outlined in the basic sequence techniques

Patient in supine position:

16. Rework of the IA anastomoses (IA) on both sides, axillary lymph nodes on both sides, inguinal lymph nodes on the less swollen leg, and abdominal techniques

17. Application of compression bandages on both, or the more involved extremity

Lymphedema of the Head and Neck

This condition is often the result of cancer treatment for malignancies in the neck (larynx, pharynx, thyroid gland, tonsils) or the head region (bottom of the mouth, tongue, lips, salivary glands). Cancers in the head and neck region commonly metastasize to cervical lymph nodes.

The term *neck dissection* refers to a surgical procedure in which the fibrofatty contents of the neck are removed for the treatment of cervical lymphatic metastases. Depending on the malignancy and the severity of the condition, a radical, modified radical, or selective neck dissection may be performed. These procedures are often combined with radiation therapy.

Radical neck dissection: En bloc clearance of all fibrofatty tissue from one or both sides of the neck, including the lymph nodes, the spinal accessory nerve, the internal jugular vein, and the sternocleidomastoid muscle.

Modified radical neck dissection: This procedure involves the removal of the same lymph node groups as the radical neck dissection, but requires preservation of one or more of the three non-lymphatic structures (spinal accessory nerve, the internal jugular vein, and the sternocleidomastoid muscle).

Selective neck dissection: This term refers to a type of neck dissection in which certain lymph node groups in the neck are preserved, while others are removed. Included in this category are supraomohyoid neck dissection, lateral neck dissection, anterior compartment neck dissection, and posterolateral neck dissection.

Depending on the extent of the surgical procedure, additional damage to the facial nerves, diaphragm, brachial plexus, and vocal chords may be observed.

The swelling, which is usually more pronounced in the morning, may involve the neck, submandibular area, cheek, nose, and eyelids. Forehead and scalp are generally not involved. The therapeutic benefit can often be considerably enhanced by facial exercises, chewing (gum), and meticulous oral hygiene. The patient should be fitted with a compression garment for the face and neck. These garments are available in different styles and can be ordered in either standard or custom-made sizes. Compression masks should be worn at night.

Drainage areas in post–neck dissection conditions are the cranial portions of the upper quadrants (anterior and posterior) and the axillary lymph node groups.

Patient sitting (or in supine position) (Fig. 5–24):

1. Manipulation of the axillary lymph node groups on both sides with stationary circles

2. Manipulation of the lymph vessels on the upper part of the anterior thorax with stationary circles (dynamic technique) or rotary techniques (along the pectoralis muscle). These vessels represent a connection between the edematous and the drainage areas

3. Manipulation of the lymph vessels on the upper part of the posterior thorax with stationary circles (dynamic technique) or rotary techniques (along the descending trapezius muscle). These vessels represent a connection between the edematous and the drainage areas. For this technique, the patient may be in the prone position.

4. Manipulation of the lymph vessels on the posterior neck and scalp with stationary circles. The working phase is directed toward the drainage areas on the thorax. For this technique, the patient may be in the prone position.

Treatment of the face: This area is treated with stationary circles, which may be performed with either the entire surface of the palmar fingers or with the (individual) finger pads. Thumb circles may also be used. The primary focus is to soften the fibrotic tissues and to redirect the edematous fluid toward the posterior neck and the drainage areas located on the trunk. Ideally, the patient should be in the supine position with an elevated upper thorax, neck, and head. Early in the intervention phase, the patient should be taught simple stationary circles with one or more finger pads to soften up the fibrotic areas in the neck

5. Stationary circles or thumb circles starting at the angle of the jaw toward the posterior neck in multiple placements

6. Rework the posterior neck toward the thorax.

7. Stationary circles or thumb circles starting at the temple toward the posterior head and neck in multiple placements

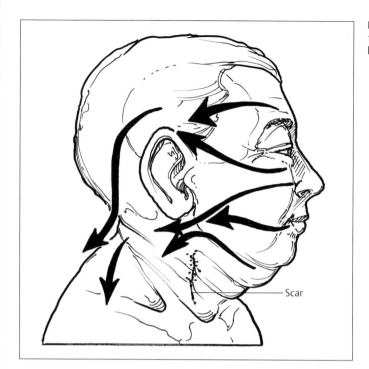

Figure 5–24 Drainage directions for lymphedema of the head and neck.

Scar

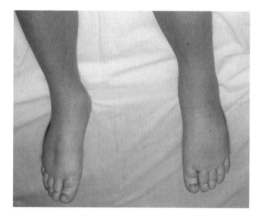

Figure 5–25 Pediatric lymphedema (note pitting edema, nail fungus, and positive Stemmer sign).

8. Rework the posterior neck toward the thorax.

9. The remaining face is treated with stationary circles or thumb circles starting at the sagittal watershed, with the working phase directed toward the posterior scalp and neck in several placements. The previously cleared pathways above and below the ears are used to move lymph fluid toward the drainage areas.

10. Rework the posterior neck toward the thorax.

11. Rework the lymph vessels on the upper portions of the anterior and posterior thorax and the axillary lymph nodes on both sides.

Pediatric Lymphedema

In the majority of cases, pediatric lymphedema is caused by congenital malformations of the lymphatic system and may be present at birth or later in life. It can be divided into two groups, based on the age of onset. Primary lymphedema, which is present at birth and associated with a family history, is termed *Milroy's disease*. This form of pediatric lymphedema is described as typically involving the lower extremities (Fig. 5–25), but the arms, hands, and face may be involved. It also may be associated with malformations of the lymphatics in the intestinal system. The term *Meige's disease* (lymphedema praecox) is often used to describe primary lymphedema that occurs after birth, but before the age of 35; the age of onset is generally in adolescence. Both types can affect both sexes; however, the majority of cases occurs in females.

Various other conditions may be associated with pediatric lymphedema and include

Amniotic band syndrome: this congenital disorder is caused by intrauterine constriction rings or bands that cause tissue depressions or strangulation marks on the digits, extremities, and sometimes the thorax, neck, and abdomen. These constriction rings are caused by strands of amniotic tissues adherent to the embryo or fetus and often cause the onset of swelling.

Turner's syndrome: this genetic disorder involves girls and is characterized by the absence of an X chromosome. Turner's syndrome is associated with multiple malformations, such as deformed fingernails, anomalies of the ears and palate, skeletal deformities, dwarfism, and dysplasia of the ovaries and kidneys. Lymphedema may present in the extremities, head, trunk, and other areas.

Noonan's syndrome: this condition resembles Turner's syndrome; however, Noonan's syndrome involves males and females, and no chromosomal abnormality is present.

Klippel-Trénaunay-Weber syndrome: this disorder is sporadic in appearance, with unknown cause, and includes vascular, skeletal, and soft tissue malformations. Skeletal malformations include asymmetric enlargement of bones (and the soft tissues); the vascular abnormalities involve varicose veins, arteriovenous fistulas, hemangiomas, and lymphatic malformations. There are also often nevi (pigmented moles) present on the skin.

The most important aspect in the treatment of pediatric lymphedema is the education and training of the parents. It is necessary for the parents to invest time and effort to learn basic hands-on MLD skills and bandaging techniques from a lymphedema therapist in the clinic. Parents cannot learn these techniques from a book; interaction between the parent and the therapist in the clinic setting is necessary to provide for feedback, question-and-answer sessions, and so on. Early on in the treatment, the parent(s) should be actively involved in the treatment process. The treatment sequences and bandaging techniques can be observed during the therapy session and repeated at home. Well-educated parents are capable of providing good-quality care for their child.

Pediatric lymphedema may benefit greatly from a course of CDT initiated as early as possible. Following an intensive course consisting of daily treatments, routine check-ups with the lymphedema therapist ensure continuous feedback regarding the parents' treatment skills and bandaging technique. Normal limb size may be achieved and maintained, and the typical secondary tissue changes associated with lymphedema may be greatly reduced or eliminated. The general approaches concerning MLD and compression therapy used in adult patients, as well as the duration of the individual treatment session, have to be modified significantly, especially in lymphedematous children of up to 3 years of age. It is also important to realize that treatment progress generally is slower in pediatric lymphedema.

Manual Lymph Drainage

Because the tissues in pediatric cases are delicate, great care should be taken to avoid discomfort or injury. Depending on the age and size of the child, soft stationary circles and pump techniques may be used; these soft skin manipulations are generally well received by the child. Abdominal techniques are absolutely contraindicated.

Children generally are very active and will not lie still for the entire length of the treatment session. It is therefore recommended that parents bring distractions, such as a favorite toy, game, or book, and the treatment room should be equipped with a television set, preferably to include a video player. If therapy is not possible on a treatment table, the session may be performed on the floor, or the parent may hold the child in his or her lap during treatment.

Compression Therapy

The application of compression bandage materials requires great care and may not be possible in infants. In standing or walking children, gravity represents an additional factor that may exacerbate the swelling, and compression therapy becomes necessary. In very young children, feedback regarding pressure and comfort is not provided; therefore, the therapist and parents need to embrace a very careful approach when it comes to bandaging. Materials and techniques used in compression bandaging (see later in this chapter) depend on the child's age and developmental situation. Bandages must not interfere with normal growth and should not greatly compromise the patient's ability to toddle and walk. In older children, normal activities and play should not be considerably restricted. In general, 4 cm and 6 cm wide short-stretch bandages are used, toes are not wrapped, and 1-inch gauze bandages are recommended to bandage the fingers, if appropriate. The delicate tissues require extra-soft padding, which can be achieved with nonwoven padding bandages (Artiflex, Cellona), soft foam, or foam containing a fleece lining (Velfoam), or a combination of these materials. It is necessary to check the bandage several times during the day for possible slipping or tourniquet effects; in most cases, the bandages have to be renewed multiple times a day during the intensive phase. Compression garments are not recommended for children younger than 1 year of age. When compression garments are needed, custom garments are used. Close interaction with the referring pediatrician is necessary to determine the appropriate compression level. In general, 20 to 30 mm/Hg of compression should not be exceeded in children < 4 years of age.

Home Care

In addition to wearing the compression garment during the day, in many cases it is necessary to apply a mild bandage during the nighttime. It is recommended that MLD treatments be administered at least once a day. In infants and young children, parents may find that the best time to provide treatment is when the child is asleep. Older children should be taught appropriate self-care techniques as they mature.

The use of compression garments during the day generally does not affect normal activities, such as sports and play, as long as they fit properly. The therapist or the physician should check the compression garment(s) every 4 to 6 months for general condition, proper compression, and size. More frequent assessments may be required for children experiencing growth spurts.

◆ Application of Compression Bandages

Successful treatment of lymphedema requires the use of a vast assortment of compression materials, which are applied using specialized bandage techniques. Only trained individuals with a thorough knowledge of lymphedema and its implications should apply compression bandages to patients with lymphedema.

General goals in compression bandaging are the following:

◆ To create a palpable compression gradient from the distal to the proximal end of the extremity.

◆ To create a functional, effective, comfortable, and durable compression environment.

Functional: Joint and muscle movements should be only minimally restricted; joints are bandaged in a functional position.

Effective: The pressure values should be high enough to achieve the goals outlined in Chapter 4, Effects of Compression Therapy, but not limit arterial blood supply or cause tourniquet effects, discomfort, or pain.

Comfortable: The skin and other structures (tendons, bony prominences, areas of small circumference) are protected with specialized padding.

Durable: Bandage materials should be applied to minimize slippage. This is important because the patient wears the compression bandages while decongestive exercises are performed.

◆ To create a structure for the external short-stretch bandages to adhere to

Lymphedematous extremities are often abnormally shaped, and deepened skinfolds are present in the vicinity of joints. These uneven circumferences and lobuli are padded to create a more physiologic structure for the compression bandages.

Required Materials

The use of various compression materials is essential to reduce limb volume safely and effectively. The following is a list of materials that are commonly used in skin care and compres-

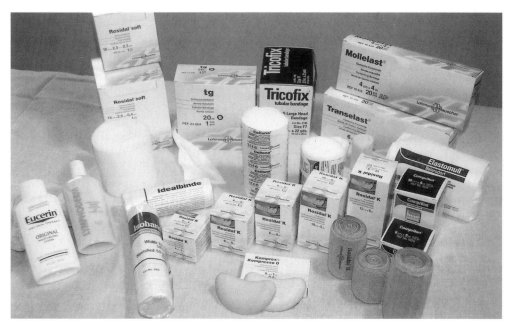

Figure 5–26 Materials used in lymphedema management.

sion bandaging for lymphedema and related conditions. To avoid allergic reactions, all materials used should be free of latex. The main manufacturers for compression materials in the United States are Lohmann & Rauscher and BSN-Jobst. The materials listed can be obtained from specialty distributors (Fig. 5–26).

Lotions: Patients are instructed in proper cleansing and moisturizing techniques to maintain the health and integrity of the skin. Suitable neutral or low-pH ointments and lotions commonly used in lymphedema are Lymphoderm and Eucerin.

Stockinettes: These tubular bandages are made from cotton and are used as an underlay to protect the skin from the padding materials and the bandages from lotions and perspiration. An assortment of different sizes to accommodate smaller extremities (children) as well as extremely large lymphedematous extremities are available from both manufacturers. Brand names are TG or K (Lohmann & Rauscher) and Tricofix (BSN-Jobst).

Stockinettes are packed in rolls of ~22 yards, which is generally sufficient for the duration of the decongestive phase of the treatment. A portion of this roll is cut before each bandage application to fit the length of the patient's extremity and should be replaced with every treatment.

Gauze bandages: Made from elastic cotton material, gauze bandages are applied on fingers and toes and also are used to bandage male genitalia. Gauze is available as cohesive bandages, which are often used with male genitalia. Gauze bandages may be applied to keep foam pieces (padding) in place. They are available in different widths and colors (white and beige). Brand names are Mollelast or Transelast (Lohmann & Rauscher) and Elastomull (BSN-Jobst). Gauze bandages should be used for one application only and replaced with every treatment.

Padding materials: Padding ensures an even distribution of pressure supplied by the short-stretch bandages and avoids tourniquet effects around the circumference of the extremity. These materials are applied on top of the stockinette and under the short-stretch bandages. Different materials can be used for the purpose of padding, such as nonwoven synthetic bandages or foam.

Synthetic padding bandages: These can be used over the entire length of the limb (except phalanges) and to pad deep skinfolds and

169

creases. Synthetic padding is available in different widths; brand names are Cellona (Lohmann & Rauscher) and Artiflex (BSN-Jobst). Nonwoven synthetic padding should not be washed and should be replaced when dirty (usually once a week)

Soft foam: Foam materials provide sufficient padding and prevent bandages from sliding. Soft foam is available as foam rolls or sheets. Foam rolls (Rosidal Soft from Lohmann & Rauscher) provide extra-soft padding and are more durable than synthetic padding bandages and soft foam sheets. The interlocking surface area of foam rolls makes the compression bandages slip-resistant. Foam rolls can be used in place of, or in addition to, nonwoven synthetic padding bandages and 0.25-inch-thick foam sheets. Foam rolls are washable and available in different widths and thicknesses.

Sheets of soft foam (generally 3 feet × 6 feet, with a recommended density of ~1.6 lbs per cubic foot) may be cut by the clinician into individual sizes and patterns to provide extra-soft and uniform pressure distribution. Custom-cut foam pieces may be used in abnormally shaped extremities and lobuli to provide a more even surface area for the compression bandages to adhere to. They are held in the proper position with gauze bandages. Foam materials with 0.25- to 0.5-inch thickness are typically used. Quarter-inch foam is less bulky, has minimal rebound effect, and spreads the pressure more evenly than nonwoven synthetic padding bandages. Half-inch-thick foam is more bulky, more durable, has a moderate rebound effect, and distributes the pressure very evenly. Foam sheets cannot be washed and are typically used throughout the decongestive phase.

High-density foam: This material is used to increase the radius of an extremity in certain areas, such as the palmar surface of the hand and the area between the malleoli and the Achilles tendon. As discussed in Chapter 4, Laplace's Law, the surface pressure of a bandage increases if the radius decreases. It is therefore necessary to pad areas of concavity to achieve an increase in radius, thus preventing extremes. High-density foam has fibrinolytic qualities and is applied in areas of lymphostatic fibrosis, with the goal to soften fibrotic sections in the tissue. Foam rubber pieces are available as rolls, sheets, and precut pieces (oval and kidney

shapes). The edges of foam rubber pieces used in compression bandaging should be beveled to avoid pressure marks on the skin; the edges of precut pieces are beveled by the manufacturer. To protect the patient's skin as well as the foam rubber pieces from lotion and perspiration, the pieces should be covered in stockinette. High-density foam rubber is available under the brand name Komprex (Lohmann & Rauscher). Komprex rubber foam is typically used throughout the decongestive phase.

Chip bags: Chip bags are used to soften "stubborn" areas of lymphostatic fibrosis in appropriate cases. Bags may be fabricated by the clinician using small pieces of foam cubes (~0.25–0.75 inch) that are placed in a stockinette. The open ends of the stockinette are sealed with tape. Contents of the chip bags may be composed of cubes made from soft foam (mildest effects), high-density foam (most aggressive effects), or a mixture of both (not too aggressive). The fibrinolytic qualities of the foam are enhanced by a "micromassaging" effect to the tissues produced by the foam cubes. It is important to understand that chip bags work well, but more aggressively than foam pieces by themselves. Upon removal of the chip bags following a period of wearing the compression bandages, deep indentations on the tissue surface may be observed. Chip bags should not be incorporated in the compression bandage on a daily basis. The use of chip bags is up to the clinician's discretion, but they cannot be used with patients on anticoagulant medication, hemophilic patients, over varicose veins, and if they cause discomfort or pain.

Short-stretch bandages: The pressure qualities of the cotton bandages (working pressure and resting pressure) are described in Chapter 4, Compression Bandages. Several layers of these textile-elastic bandages have to be applied to achieve the desired pressure values and effects on the swollen extremity. Short-stretch bandages are available in different widths (4, 6, 8, 10, and 12 cm); brand names are Rosidal (Lohmann & Rauscher) and Comprilan (BSN-Jobst). The length of short-stretch bandages is ~5.5 yards; 10 and 12 cm wide bandages are also available in lengths of ~11 yards. These double-length bandages simplify the application of compression bandages on the thigh, as well as the application of self-bandages by the patient. Short-stretch bandages should be cleaned when dirty (usually once a week) and when there is a noticeable decrease in elasticity. Washing guidelines are discussed below.

Wide-width short-stretch bandages: These bandages are available in widths of 15 and 20 cm and are applied primarily on the thorax and abdominal areas. Wider bandages are also applied over the narrower short-stretch bandages on the thigh to increase stability or to hold larger foam pieces in place. Brand names are Idealbinde (Lohmann & Rauscher) and Isoband (BSN-Jobst).

Tape (~1 inch wide) should be used to affix the bandage material and not clips or pins. Sharp bandaging clips or pins may cut into the patient's skin and provide an avenue for infection.

Washing Guidelines for Compression Bandages

Short- and medium-stretch bandages can be cleaned in the washing machine in lukewarm water. To avoid tangling and knotting of the bandages during the washing process, they should be placed in a pillowcase or laundry bag. Mild liquid detergents may be used, such as Ivory and Dreft (powder detergents or Woolite should not be used). Bandages can be dried on air setting or delicate setting in the dryer. The bandages may lose their elasticity after several applications; washing restores the memory of the braided cotton fibers needed for the working pressure.

During the evaluation, the clinician determines the quantity of materials needed for the application of the compression bandages during the decongestive phase of the therapy. To ensure successful intervention, adequate supplies have to be on hand before treatment starts. The treatment center either keeps a sufficient quantity of compression materials in stock, or the patients themselves are responsible to order the materials needed from a distributor before the initial treatment. Approximate stock quantities for lymphedema treatment centers are listed in Chapter 6 (6.2)

The life of short- and medium-stretch bandages can be considerably extended by using two sets, one to wear and one to wash (the manufacturers recommend to replace the bandages every 3 months if used daily).

Upper Extremity Bandaging

Recommended materials to apply a compression bandage on the upper extremity during the decongestive phase of CDT (phase 1) are listed below. The quantities listed below represent two sets of compression bandages:

- 1 Bottle of skin lotion
- 1 Box of stockinette (tubular bandage) in the appropriate size
- 1–2 boxes (20 individual rolls in a box) of gauze bandages (4 or 6 cm width)
- 4–6 synthetic nonwoven padding bandages (10 cm) or 2 Rosidal Soft foam bandages (10 cm)
- 2 short-stretch bandages (6 cm), or 2 short-stretch bandages (4 cm, for smaller hands)
- 2 short-stretch bandages (8 cm)
- 4–6 short-stretch bandages (10 cm)
- 2 short-stretch bandages (12 cm)
  Tape to secure the bandages
- If necessary: 1 sheet of soft foam (about 0.25–9nch thickness)
- If necessary: 1 sheet of Komprex or 1 roll of soft foam rubber

Application

Generally, bandages are applied with an even pre-stretch of ~30 to 40% and an overlap of ~50 to 70%. The patient should be in the sitting position.

Skin care: Wash and bathe the skin, then apply the appropriate lotion thoroughly.

Stockinette: The tubular bandage should be cut to a length that allows for an overlap of ~5 inches on the proximal end of the extremity. This overlap is used to extend over and cover the complete compression bandage on the proximal border to protect it from axillar perspiration. A hole is cut for the thumb on the distal end (Fig. 5–27).

Finger bandages: The patient's fingers are spread slightly, and the hand is in pronation. A bolster should be placed under the elbow to support the patient's arm.

Start the first gauze bandage with a loose anchor turn around the wrist (Fig. 5–28), then proceed over the dorsum of the hand to the little finger (or the thumb). The fingers should

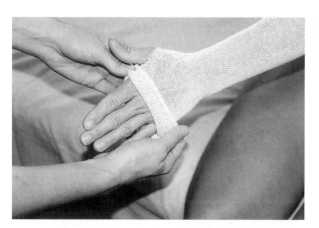

Figure 5–27 Application of stockinette.

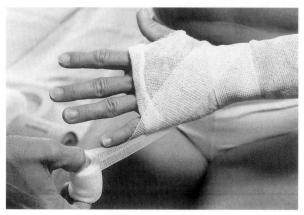

Figure 5–28 Application of gauze bandages on the fingers.

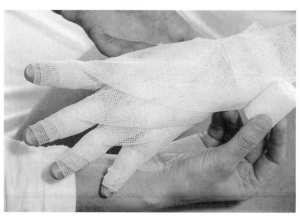

Figure 5–29 Application of gauze bandages on the fingers; fingertips remain unbandaged.

be bandaged with light pressure from the distal to the proximal ends with ~50% overlap. The fingertips are not covered. Leave the finger over the dorsum of the hand toward the wrist, apply a half turn (complete anchoring turns should be always avoided) around the wrist, and proceed to bandage the remaining fingers in the same fashion (Fig. 5–29). The borders of the gauze bandage should not slide or roll in on the distal and proximal ends of the fingers. One and a half to two gauze bandages are typically necessary to bandage all fingers. Any unused part of the second gauze bandage should be wrapped spirally (not circular) around the forearm.

Upon completion, the fingertips should be checked for proper circulation. The bandages

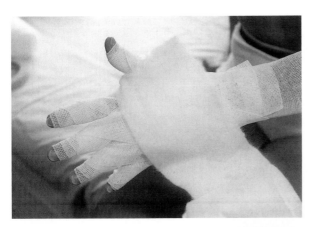

Figure 5–30 Application of padding materials on the hand.

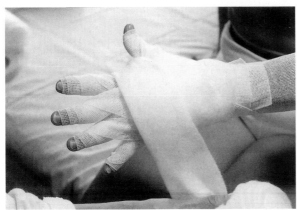

Figure 5–31 Application of padding materials on the hand.

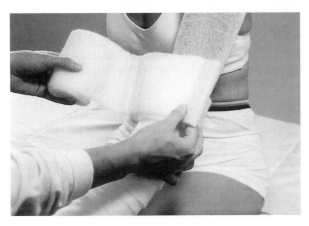

Figure 5–32 Application of extra padding materials on the antecubital fossa.

should not slide over the knuckles when the patient makes a fist, and no skin area over the fingers should be visible.

Padding materials: Nonwoven synthetic padding (Artiflex, Rosidal) or soft foam rolls (Rosidal Soft) are used to pad the hand and arm. A hole is cut for the thumb (Fig. 5–30); the pad-

ding bandage is secured around the wrist with a circular turn. The hand is then padded down to the knuckles using two to four circular turns, with the padding bandage folded in half (Fig. 5–31). The padding bandage then proceeds in the proximal direction to cover the forearm and upper arm. The cubital fossa is protected with extra layers of padding (Fig. 5–32). Two rolls of

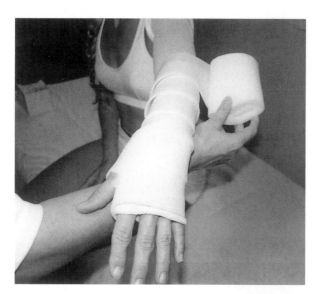

Figure 5–33 Application of padding materials (soft foam roll) on the arm.

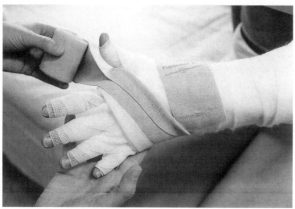

Figure 5–34 Application of 6 cm bandage on the hand.

padding bandages typically are used for an upper extremity (Fig. 5–33).

◆ **Short-stretch bandages:.** Starting a 6 cm wide bandage with a loose anchor turn around the wrist, the hand is bandaged to include the knuckles, with the patient spreading the fingers slightly (Fig. 5–34). To avoid irritation in the web space between the thumb and the index finger, the bandage should be folded over about one third of its width (depending on the size of the hand), without twisting the bandage (Fig. 5–35). The bandage is anchored between each turn around the hand with half turns on the wrist (thenar area). To avoid bulking, the fold on the hand should alternate between the proximal and distal border of the

bandage with each turn (Fig. 5–36). The double bandage layer resulting from folding the bandage provides increased pressure on the distal portion of the hand, where the swelling is usually more pronounced. Any remaining bandage material is used on the forearm (Fig. 5–37).

The successive bandages are applied in opposite directions to each other. This provides for a more functional and durable bandage. The next bandage (8 cm) starts on the wrist, with a loose anchor (Fig. 5–38) in the opposite direction of the first bandage, and proceeds to cover the forearm and the elbow area (depending on the size of the extremity). Typically, the bandages are applied with ~30 to 40% stretch and 50 to 70% overlap in a circular manner. While bandaging the forearm, the

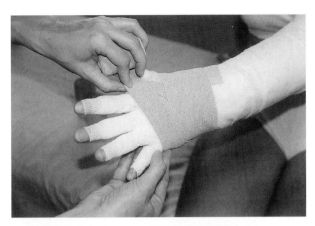

Figure 5–35 Folding of the 6 cm bandage on the dorsum of the hand.

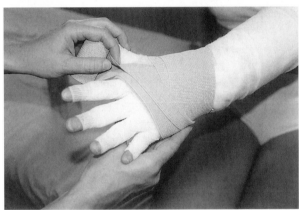

Figure 5–36 Alternating folds to avoid excessive pressure.

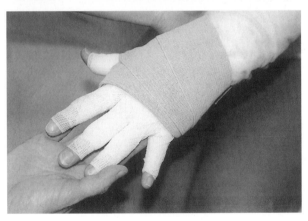

Figure 5–37 Finished bandage on the hand.

patient should make a fist and push the arm against the therapist's abdominal area (Fig. 5–39). This technique provides for a functional bandage on the forearm and prevents tourniquet effects during the use of the forearm musculature while wearing the bandage. The next two bandages (either two 10 cm or one 10 cm and one 12 cm) are applied in opposite directions to each other. To provide a smooth gradient from distal to proximal, the individual bandages are started in areas of soft pressure (Fig. 5–40). The therapist continues to check the gradient of the compression bandage during the entire process of

175

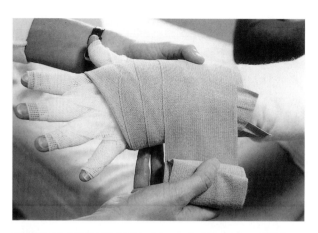

Figure 5-38 Application of the 8 cm bandage on the hand and forearm.

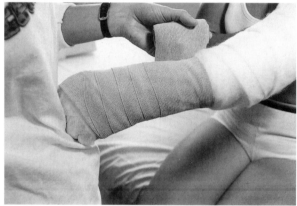

Figure 5-39 Application of the 8 cm bandage on the forearm.

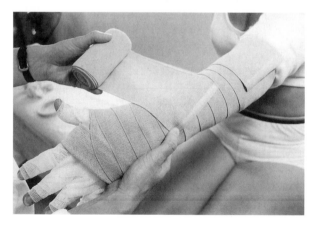

Figure 5-40 The 10 cm bandage starts on the area of lowest pressure.

application. Feedback from the patient is necessary and helpful. It is important that the bandage ends in the axillary fold to prevent accumulation of fluid between the armpit and the proximal end of the bandage (Fig. 5–41). Compression bandages are secured with tape, and the proximal overlap of the stockinette is folded over the external bandage.

Special padding: If additional padding is required, soft foam sheets may be cut to fit the patient's hand and forearm and/or upper arm (Fig. 5–42). Soft foam may be used in combination with nonwoven synthetic padding bandages (especially in areas where foam pieces overlap, e.g., joints). Foam pieces are held in place with gauze bandages (Figs. 5–43, 5–44).

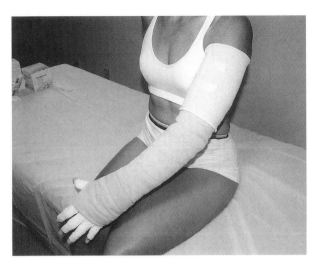

Figure 5–41 Complete bandage on the upper extremity.

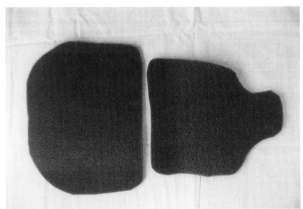

Figure 5–42 Soft foam padding for hand and forearm (right) and upper arm (left).

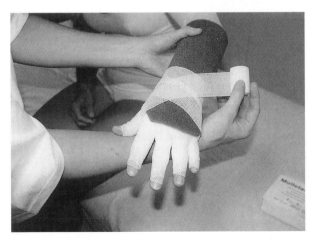

Figure 5–43 Soft foam padding is held in place with gauze bandages.

To increase the radius in the sides of the hand, kidney-shaped pieces of soft foam or high-density foam (Komprex) may be used in the palm of the hand (Fig. 5–45). In appropriate cases, pieces of custom-cut high-density foam or chip bags may be used to soften areas of lymphostatic fibrosis.

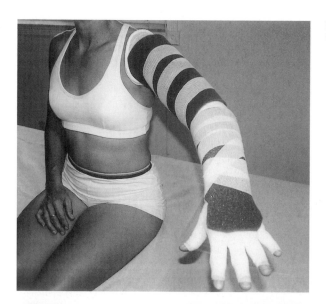

Figure 5–44 Soft foam padding on the upper extremity.

Figure 5–45 High-density foam (Komprex) on the palm.

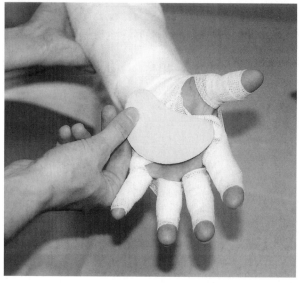

High-density foam must never be applied in layers. If used circumferentially on parts of the extremity, it should be applied using the "sandwich" technique (not in one piece around the extremity).

Lower Extremity Bandaging

Following is a list of recommended materials to apply a compression bandage on the lower extremity during the decongestive phase of

CDT (phase 1). The quantities listed represent two sets of compression bandages:

- ◆ 1 bottle of skin lotion
- ◆ 1 box of stockinette (tubular bandage) in the appropriate size
- ◆ 1–2 boxes of gauze bandages (4 cm width)
- ◆ 2 high-density foam pieces (kidney-shaped)
- ◆ 6 synthetic nonwoven padding bandages (10 cm) or 2–3 Rosidal Soft foam bandages (10 cm)

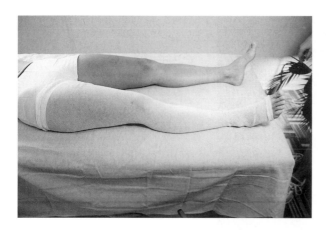

Figure 5–46 Application of stockinette.

- 4–6 synthetic nonwoven padding bandages (15 cm) or 2–3 Rosidal Soft foam bandages (15 cm)
- 2 short-stretch bandages (6 cm)
- 2 short-stretch bandages (8 cm)
- 6–8 short-stretch bandages (10 cm)
- 8–12 short-stretch bandages (12 cm)
- 4 wide-width short-stretch bandages (15 or 20 cm, depending on the patient's size)
- Tape to secure the bandages
- If necessary: 1 sheet of soft foam ~3 feet x 6 feet (about 0.5-inch thickness)
- If necessary: 2 sheets of Komprex or 2 rolls of soft foam rubber

Application

Generally, bandages are applied with an even pre-stretch of ~30 to 40% and an overlap of ~50 to 70%. To bandage the foot and the lower leg, the patient should be in the supine position and should stand on the floor during the application of the compression bandages from the knee up to the groin.

Skin care: Wash and bathe the skin, then apply the appropriate lotion thoroughly.

Stockinette: The tubular bandage should be cut to a length that allows for an overlap of ~5 inches on the proximal end of the extremity. This overlap is used to extend over and cover the complete compression bandage on the proximal border (Fig. 5–46).

Toe bandages: Start the first gauze bandage with a loose anchor turn around the dorsum of the foot (in the metatarsophalangeal joint area), then proceed to bandage the big toe (Fig. 5–47). Enter the toe over the dorsum, apply two or three circular turns, and leave the toe again over the dorsum; avoid sliding or rolling of the bandages in the web space area. The tips of the toes remain unbandaged. Proceed to bandage the remaining toes (except the fifth toe, which generally is not involved in the swelling) in the same manner (Fig. 5–48). One 4 cm gauze bandage (usually folded to half width) is generally sufficient to cover the toes. Any unused part of the gauze bandage should be wrapped spirally (not circular) around the foot. Upon completion, the tips of the toes should be checked for proper circulation.

Padding materials: Nonwoven synthetic padding (3 rolls) or soft foam rolls (2 rolls of Rosidal Soft) are applied on the foot and lower leg (Figs. 5–49, 5–50). Komprex foam kidneys are secured between the medial and lateral malleolus and the Achilles tendon with the padding bandages (Fig. 5–51). Synthetic padding bandages may be doubled over the shin area to provide additional protection.

Short-stretch bandages: Using a 6 or 8 cm wide bandage (depending on the size of the foot), do a loose anchor turn around the metatarsus (Fig. 5–52). The foot is bandaged down to the web spaces with three or four circular turns in the metatarsophalangeal joint area. The bandage should roll from lateral to medial (toward the big toe) and is applied without tension on the foot. The same bandage proceeds to cover the heel, using the "heel lock" technique, which provides addi-

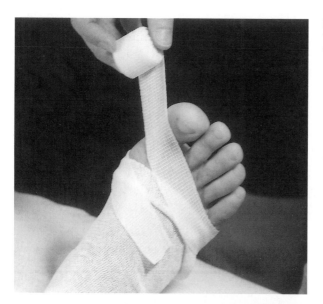

Figure 5–47 Gauze bandages start with a loose anchoring turn around the dorsum of the foot.

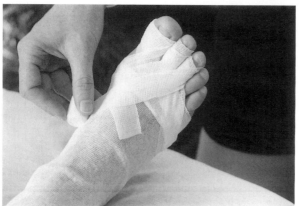

Figure 5–48 Application of gauze bandages on the toes.

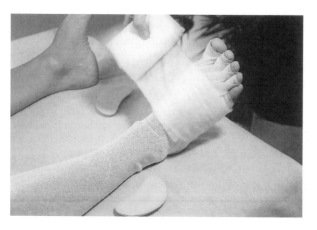

Figure 5–49 Application of padding materials on the foot.

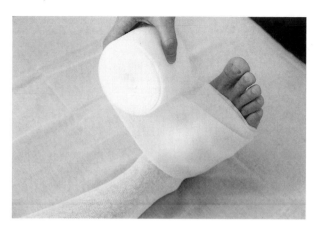

Figure 5–50 Application of padding materials (soft foam roll) on the foot.

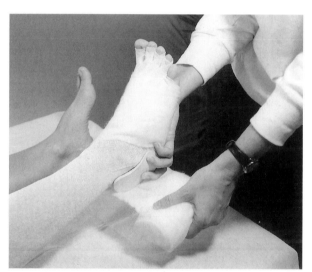

Figure 5–51 High-density foam (Komprex) pieces behind the ankles are held in place by padding bandages.

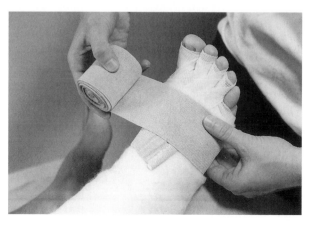

Figure 5–52 Loose anchor turn around the metatarsus with the first short-stretch bandage.

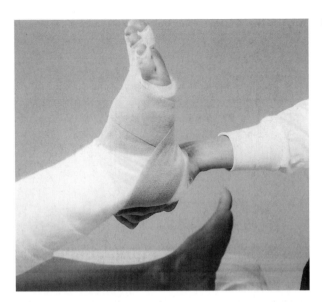

Figure 5–53 "Heel lock" technique around the lateral ankle.

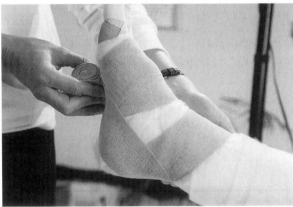

Figure 5–54 "Heel lock" technique around the medial ankle.

tional support for the ankle and keeps the bandage from sliding (Figs. 5–53, 5–54). During the application of compression bandages on the heel, the ankle is in ~70 to 90 degrees of dorsiflexion. The bandage is guided from the plantar surface toward the Achilles tendon, covering the area between the heel and the lateral malleolus, from here around the ankle to the area between the medial malleolus and the heel, and again down to the plantar surface of the foot (Fig. 5–55). Proceed with a circular turn without tension around the foot, and repeat the heel lock technique until the bandage is used up; secure with tape. The next bandage (8 or 10 cm) starts above the ankle with a loose anchor in the opposite direction of the previous bandage (applying compression bandages in the opposite direction to each other prevents bandaging the foot in eversion or inversion; i.e., it provides for a functional bandage and adds durability). The goal is to cover the heel and the foot with the second bandage in a circular technique (Figs. 5–56, 5–57). The lower leg is bandaged with 10 or 12 cm wide bandages (typically 2–4 rolls). To provide a smooth gradient from distal to proximal, the individual bandages are started in areas of soft pressure (Fig. 5–58). The therapist continues to check the gradient of the compression bandage during the entire process of application. Feedback from the patient is necessary and helpful. Secure the last bandage on the lower leg with tape (Fig. 5–59).

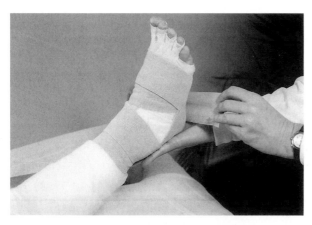

Figure 5–55 Complete application of the first short-stretch bandage on the foot.

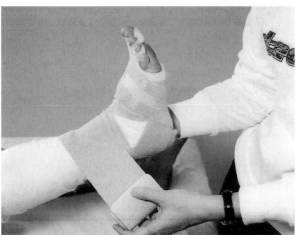

Figure 5–56 Start of the second short-stretch bandage with a loose anchor around the ankle.

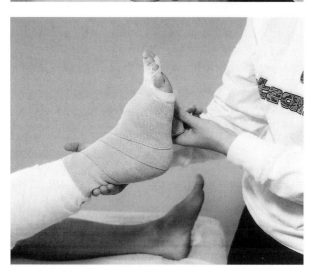

Figure 5–57 The heel and foot are covered with the second short-stretch bandage.

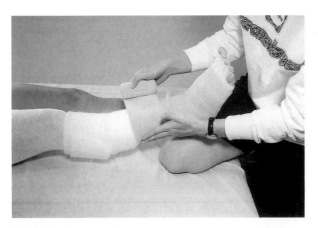

Figure 5–58 Bandaging of the lower leg.

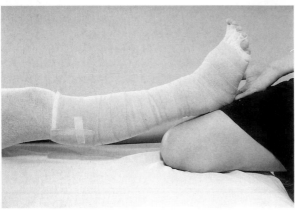

Figure 5–59 Finished bandage on the lower leg and foot.

The remaining compression bandage is applied with the patient in standing. The patient should shift the body weight to the extremity being bandaged, with the knee slightly bent. Padding materials using nonwoven synthetic padding or soft foam rolls are applied on the knee and thigh. When using synthetic padding bandages, the layers may be doubled in the popliteal fossa to provide additional protection. The knee and thigh should be bandaged using 12 cm wide short-stretch bandages (typically 4–6 rolls). The first bandage starts with a loose anchor turn below the knee, proceeding to cover the knee using the figure-eight technique (Figs. 5–60, 5–61). The remaining thigh is bandaged in a circular manner up to the groin area; the last bandage (or each individual bandage) is secured with tape (Fig. 5–62). An additional 15 or 20 cm wide medium-stretch bandage may be applied on the thigh to add stability.

Hip attachments: If the lower truncal quadrants are involved in the swelling, or to prevent the compression bandages on the leg from sliding, the hip may be bandaged using one or two rolls (depending on the size of the patient) of 20 cm wide short stretch bandages. (Note: Hip attachments are applied directly on the skin; the patient wears the underwear on top of the bandages.) Start the first bandage with a loose turn around the proximal thigh to secure (Fig. 5–63), then proceed to cover the trunk, guiding the bandage from the lateral thigh to the opposite iliac crest (to prevent sliding, at least one third of the width of the bandage should be cranial to the iliac crest). From here, apply a complete circular turn around the trunk, and proceed with the bandage over the buttocks back down to the thigh (Fig. 5–64). Proceed with the same technique until the lower trunk is thoroughly covered. Circular turns on the proximal thigh should be

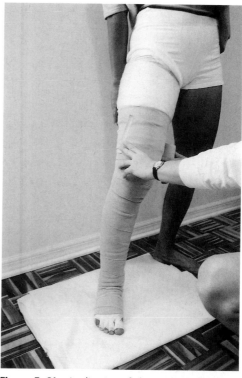

Figure 5–60 Application of short-stretch bandages on the knee using the figure eight technique.

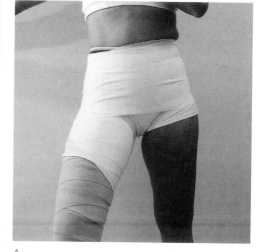

Figure 5–61 Application of short-stretch bandages on the thigh starting with a loose anchor turn.

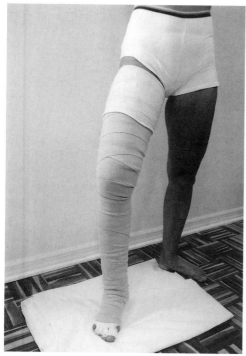

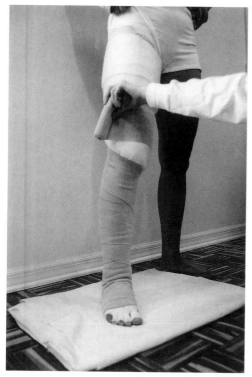

△
Figure 5–63 Hip attachment using wide short-stretch bandages (15–20 cm).

◁ **Figure 5–62** Finished bandage on the lower extremity.

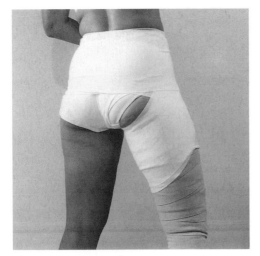

Figure 5–64 Hip attachment, posterior view.

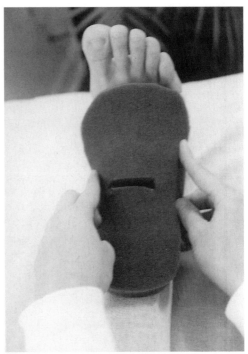

Figure 5–65 Special padding on the foot using soft foam.

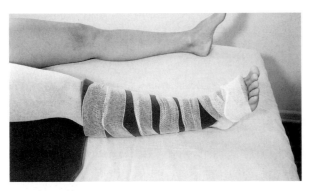

Figure 5–66 Special padding on the foot and lower leg using soft foam.

Figure 5–67 Soft foam padding is held in place by gauze bandages.

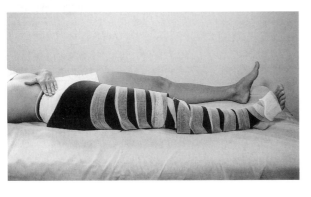

avoided to prevent tourniquet effects. Upon completion, the bandage is checked again for correct pressure gradient. If two rolls of bandages are needed for the hip attachment, the ends may be sewn together to simplify the application.

Special padding: If additional padding is required, or to prevent the compression bandage from sliding, soft foam sheets may be cut to fit the patient's foot, lower leg, and thigh (Fig. 5–65). Soft foam may be used in combination with nonwoven synthetic padding bandages (especially in areas where foam pieces overlap, e.g., joints). Foam pieces are held in place with gauze bandages (Figs. 5–66, 5–67). In appropriate cases, pieces of custom-cut high-density foam or chip bags (Fig. 5–68) may be used to soften areas of lymphostatic fibrosis.

Note: High-density foam must never be applied in layers. If used circumferentially on parts of the extremity, it should be applied using the "sandwich" technique (not in one piece around the extremity).

Genital Bandaging

Female patients: Soft foam pieces or pieces of high-density foam rubber are custom cut in the shape of sanitary pads. These pads are placed directly on the skin, which makes it necessary to place the pads in several layers of stockinette, which should be renewed daily. To maximize the therapeutic benefit, compression pantyhose should be worn. Compressive garments for the lower trunk with thigh attachments (biker-shorts style) may be used if the lower extremities are uninvolved.

Male patients: The soft tissues of the penis and scrotum are usually involved in the swelling. The bandages on the scrotum may become loose during the day, and renewal may be necessary. Therefore, patients should be taught early in the treatment phase how to apply compression bandages on the genital tissues. During the decongestive phase, the scrotal compression bandages may be held in place by wearing biker shorts, athletic support (jockstraps), or briefs (instead of shorts). In the self-management phase, slipping of the bandages is usually prevented by compression pantyhose if genital lymphedema is combined with lower extremity swelling. Compressive

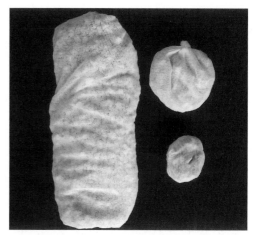

Figure 5–68   Chip bags.

garments for the lower trunk with thigh attachments (biker-shorts style) may be used if the lower extremities are uninvolved. In most cases, genital bandaging has to be applied lifelong to avoid reaccumulation of fluid.

Recommended materials to apply a compression bandage on the penis and scrotum:
1 pair of surgical gloves
1 bottle of skin lotion
Stockinette (tubular bandage) in the appropriate size to cover the scrotum
Gauze bandages (4 or 6 cm width) for the application on penis and scrotum
Fastening options for the bandage on the scrotum: Because slippage is a common problem, the bandages can be held in place by using cohesive gauze bandages (4 or 6 cm width) or special foam materials (Velfoam). Velfoam is covered with a hook-sensitive material on one side (Fig. 5–69).

If lymphatic cysts and/or fistulas are present (Fig. 5–23), appropriate skin cleansing products (as prescribed by the physician) and sterile gauze should be incorporated.

Application

Proper hygiene is of utmost importance. Appropriate products, as prescribed by the physician, should be used.

Application on the penis: The penis is bandaged with circular turns using one or two rolls of gauze bandages (Figs. 5–70, 5–71). In

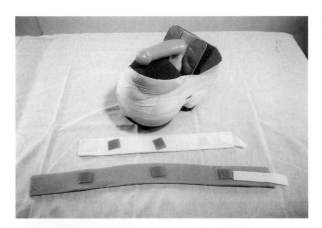

Figure 5–69 Fastening system to hold scrotum bandage in place.

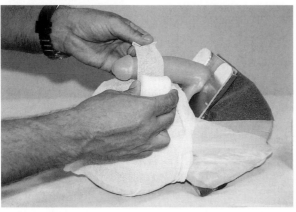

Figure 5–70 Application of gauze bandage on the penis starting behind the glans penis.

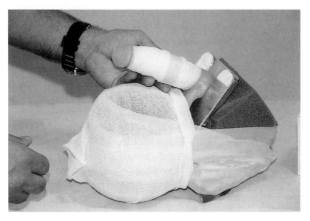

Figure 5–71 The finished gauze bandage on the penis is affixed with tape.

uncircumcised patients, the bandages should be applied with the foreskin pulled back and the first bandage starting proximal to the glans penis. If the foreskin cannot be pulled back, a separate bandage should be used to bandage the foreskin. This bandage is renewed every time the patient urinates. Soft foam pieces (wrapped in stockinette) may be used if unpadded gauze bandages cause discomfort.

Scrotal bandage: A stockinette of appropriate size and length is used to cover the scrotum (Fig. 5–72). To provide a secure base for the gauze bandages to adhere to, a Velfoam piece

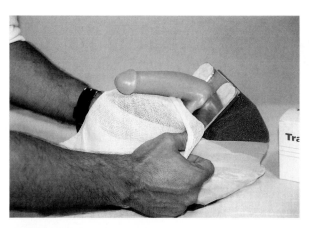

Figure 5–72 Application of stock-inette on the scrotum.

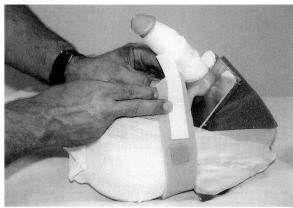

Figure 5–73 Application of the fastening system around the base of the scrotum.

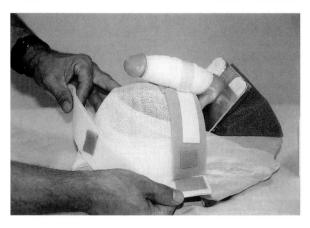

Figure 5–74 Application of the fastening system around the circumference of the scrotum.

(2 inches wide) is cut to the appropriate length and placed around the base of the scrotum (Fig. 5–73). Velcro is used to secure the foam and on several areas on the foam to provide a hook system for the gauze bandages. An additional Velfoam piece is then applied to the circumference of the scrotum and secured with Velcro to the foam on the base of the scrotum (Fig. 5–74). These foam pieces provide a sufficient base for the gauze bandages; upon decongestion of the scrotum, the foam pieces are shortened as necessary. Velcro spots affixed to the foam pieces prevent the gauze bandages from sliding (Fig. 5–75). The scrotum is then

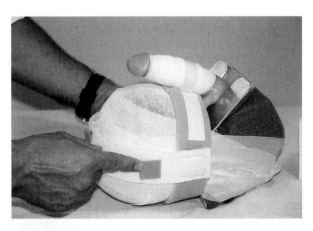

Figure 5–75 Velcro pieces attached to the fastening system prevents sliding of gauze bandages.

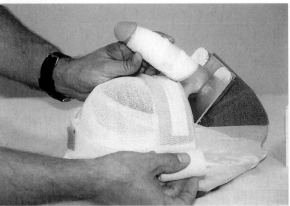

Figure 5–76 Application of gauze bandages on the scrotum.

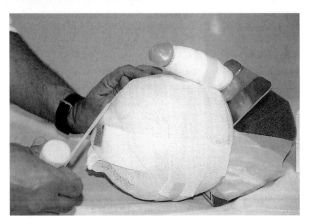

Figure 5–77 Velcro pieces prevent slippage of the gauze bandages.

wrapped with gauze bandages, which are secured with tape (Figs. 5–76, 5–77, 5–78). Instead of foam pieces, cohesive gauze bandages may be used to prevent sliding.

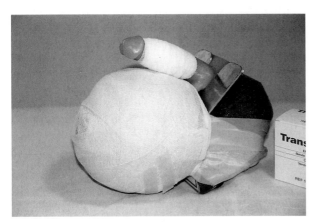

Figure 5–78 Finished bandage on penis and scrotum.

◆ Measurements for Compression Garments

To ensure preservation and improvement of the therapeutic success achieved in phase 1 of the treatment, it is imperative that a compression garment is chosen that meets the patient's individual needs. To select the correct style (ready-made or custom-made), compression level, length, and, if necessary, fastening systems, the patient's age, physical abilities (and limitations), lifestyle, type of lymphedema, and any other conditions must be taken into consideration.

Most manufacturers provide compression garments in a variety of sizes. Custom garments should be ordered if the extremity is either too large or too small for standard size garments or if a single compression garment with a compression level of more than 50 mmHg is necessary. The length of a compression garment is indicated by a system of letters used by the manufacturers. These letters represent the measuring points on both ends of the garment; an arm sleeve that covers the extremity from the wrist (measuring point C) to the axilla (measuring point G), for example, is called a C-G sleeve. An open-toe stocking covering the lower extremity from the foot (point A) to the groin (point G) would be referred to as an A-G stocking.

Only trained individuals with a thorough understanding of lymphedema and its implications should take measurements. Ill-fitted and ineffective compression garments not only produce poor results but also can be dangerous to the patient.

To increase effectiveness, it would be beneficial to have an assistant present at the time of measurements to complete the data on the measuring forms.

Measurements should be taken at the end of the intensive phase of CDT (phase 1), when the extremity is at its most reduced state. Ideally, the measurements should be taken early in the morning, at the end of a treatment, or after the compression bandages have been removed.

Materials needed to take measurements include a measuring board obtained from the manufacturers. These boards simplify the measuring process and increase accuracy. Other materials needed are a metric system measuring tape (measurements should be taken in centimeters), a nontoxic skin marker, a pen, and a measuring form (order form).

Measuring for Stockings and Pantyhose

Circumferential as well as length measurements are required. The skin of the patient should be marked with a nontoxic, nonpermanent marker on each circumferential measuring point (these markings also determine the length measurements). The length measurements are taken on the inside of the leg from each circumferential point to the sole of the foot (Fig. 5–79).

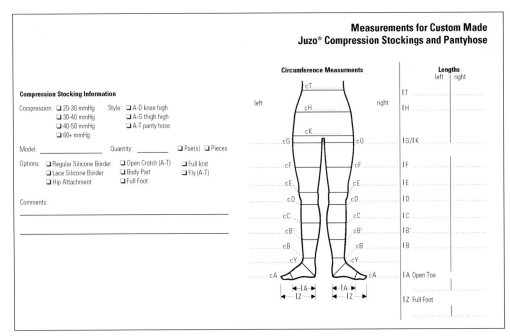

Figure 5–79 Measurement form for compression stockings and pantyhose (with permission from JUZO, Inc.).

If the lymphedematous leg is unusually shaped, the positions of the circumferential measurement points, as well as the length measurements, should be taken first on the nonaffected extremity. This technique helps to identify the position of the measuring points on the affected extremity.

Required Measurements for Custom-Made Knee-High Stockings (A-D)

Circumferential measuring points (indicate the position of all measuring points with nontoxic, nonpermanent marker):

◆ Point cA: around the metatarsal heads, horizontally around the base of the fifth metatarsal base

◆ Point cY: around the instep and the heel at a 45-degree angle, taken with the ankle in maximum dorsiflexion

◆ Point cB: around the smallest circumference above the malleoli

◆ Point cB1: around the lower leg at the transition between the Achilles tendon and the calf musculature (plantar flexion in the ankle helps to find this measuring point)

◆ Point cC: around the largest circumference of the calf

◆ Point cD: smallest circumference of the knee, in the area of the fibular head.

Length measurements:

For open-toe stockings, take the length measurement from point cA to the heel (l-A); if a closed toe stocking is required, the length measurement from the longest toe to the heel is taken (l-Z). The length measurements from the sole of the foot (even with the floor or the measuring board) to the circumferential measurements points cB to cD are taken with the ankle in 90 degrees of dorsiflexion.

Required Measurements for Standard-Size Knee-High Stockings (A-D)

◆ Circumferential measuring points: points cB and cC

◆ Length measurements: from the floor to circumferential measuring point cD (determines the length of the stocking)

Required Measurements for Custom-Made Thigh-High Stockings (A-G)

Circumferential measuring points in addition to the ones taken for A-D stockings (indicate the position of all measuring points with non-toxic, nonpermanent marker):

◆ Point cE: around the popliteal fossa and the patella with the leg slightly bent
◆ Point cF: around the middle of the thigh
◆ Point cG: horizontally around the proximal end of the thigh with the patient standing.

Length measurements: taken on the inside of the leg between the floor and each circumferential measuring point

Required Measurements for Standard-Size Thigh-High Stockings (A-G)

Circumferential measuring points: points cB, cC, and cG
    Length measurements: from the floor to circumferential measuring point cG, on the inside of the leg

Required Measurements for Custom-Made Pantyhose (A-T)

Circumferential measuring points in addition to the ones taken for A-G stockings (indicate the position of all measuring points with non-toxic, nonpermanent marker):
    All measurements are taken with the patient standing.

◆ Point cK: taken at the same height as measuring point cG, but includes the circumference of both thighs and buttocks
◆ Point cH: around the greatest circumference of the hips
◆ Point cT: around the waist, just above the iliac crest

Depending on the condition, the abdominal part of the compression pantyhose may be ordered with full, partial, or neutral compression. Adjustable and highly elastic abdominal parts are available (pregnancy, postsurgical conditions). Front openings may be ordered for male patients.
    Length measurements between the floor and up to circumferential point cG are taken on

the inside of the leg. Length measurements between the floor to points cH and cT are taken on the outside.

Required Measurements for Standard Size Pantyhose (A-T)

◆ Circumferential measuring points: points cB, cC, cG, and cH
◆ Length measurements: from the floor to circumferential measuring point cG

Depending on the condition, the abdominal part of the compression pantyhose may be ordered with full, partial, or neutral compression. Adjustable and highly elastic abdominal parts are available (pregnancy, postsurgical conditions). Front openings may be ordered for male patients.

Measuring for Arm Sleeves

Circumferential as well as length measurements are required. The skin of the patient should be marked with a nontoxic, nonpermanent marker on each circumferential measuring point. The length measurements are taken on the anterior arm from the wrist (point c) to each circumferential measuring point (Fig. 5–80).

Required Measurements for Custom-Made Arm Sleeves (C-G)

Circumferential measuring points (indicate the position of all measuring points with nontoxic, nonpermanent marker):

◆ Point c: around the smallest circumference of the wrist, on the transition from the hand to the forearm
◆ Point c1: this measurement is necessary for arm sleeves worn in combination with compression gauntlets. The measurement is taken around the forearm, 6 cm (may vary; see Measuring for Hand and Finger Compression Garments later in this chapter) proximal to circumferential measuring point c.
◆ Point d: around the forearm, at the midpoint between point c and the elbow
◆ Point e: around the elbow, in the cubital fossa, with the arm slightly bent

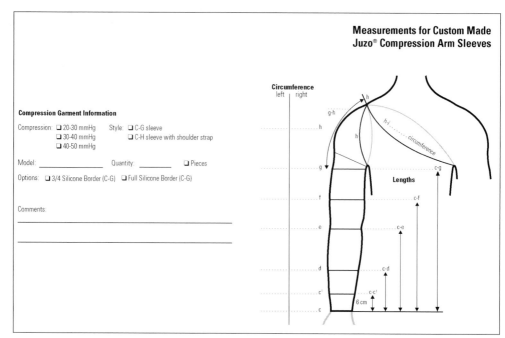

Figure 5–80 Measurement form for compression arm sleeves (with permission from JUZO, Inc.).

- ◆ Point f: around the middle of the upper arm
- ◆ Point g: around the proximal end of the upper arm, in the axillary fold

If a shoulder cover and strap is required:

- ◆ Point h: vertically around the axilla and the shoulder
- ◆ Point h–i: this measurement is necessary to require the length of the shoulder strap. It is taken circumferentially from measuring point h across the thorax to the opposite axilla.

Length measurements are taken from the circumferential measuring point c along the anterior arm (the arm is in supination) to each circumferential measuring point.

For arm sleeves with a shoulder cover and strap, an additional length measurement is required:

- ◆ g–h: this length is taken on the outside of the shoulder between circumferential measuring points g and h.

Required Measurements for Standard-Size Arm Sleeves (C-G)

- ◆ Circumferential measuring points: points c, e, and g
- ◆ Length measurements: from circumferential measuring point c to circumferential measuring point g along the anterior arm (forearm in supination)

Measuring for Hand and Finger Compression Garments

See Figure 5–81 for example of measurement form for hand and finger compression garments.

Required Measurements for Compression Gauntlets with Finger Stubs or Closed Fingers

Circumferential measuring points (indicate the position of all measuring points with nontoxic, nonpermanent marker) (the fingers should be slightly spread for points a and b):

- ◆ Point a: around the metacarpus (bases of the second and fifth metacarpal bones)

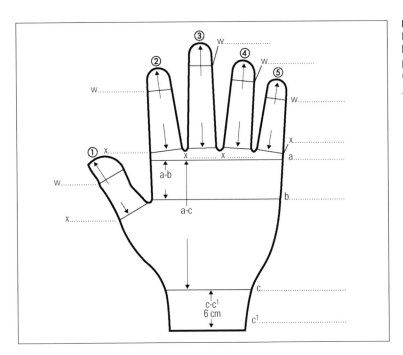

Figure 5–81
Measurement form for hand and finger compression garments (with permission from JUZO, Inc.).

- Point b: around the metacarpus, at the web space between the thumb and the index finger (parallel to point a)
- Point c: around the smallest circumference of the wrist, on the transition from the hand to the forearm
- Point c1: around the forearm, 6 cm (see also length measurement c–c1) proximal to circumferential measuring point c
- Point w: around the distal end of each finger and the thumb, at the point where the end of the finger portion is desired (finger stubs should not end in the joint/crease area of the finger)
- Point x: around the proximal end of each finger and the thumb. Point x can be easily identified using the crease on the palmar surface of the finger bases

Length measurements:

a–b: distance between circumferential measuring points a and b. Take measurement with open palm.

c–c1: distance between circumferential measurements c and c1. This measurement determines the length of the wrist extension. If an extension shorter than 6 cm is desired, cir-cumferential measurement c1 should be taken at the appropriate point.

w–x: the length of each finger is measured between the circumferential measuring points w and x.

For a gauntlet with closed fingers, the length of the fingers between circumferential measuring points x and the fingertips are taken.

Required Measurements for Compression Gauntlets with Thumb Stub (no Finger Swelling)

Circumferential measuring points (indicate the position of all measuring points with nontoxic, nonpermanent marker):

- Point a: around the metacarpus (bases of the second and fifth metacarpal bones). The fingers should be slightly spread for this measurement.
- Point c: around the smallest circumference of the wrist, on the transition from the hand to the forearm

No length measurements are necessary for standard-size compression gauntlets.

Compression Neck and Chin Straps and Face Masks

Pressure garments for the face are available as neck and chin straps and as partial or full-face masks. Full-face masks may be ordered with or without openings for the eyes, nose, or mouth.

Depending on the severity and chronicity of the swelling, compression garments for the face may be ordered in knitted materials or other synthetic fabric.

Custom-made face masks in knitted materials generally provide firmer and more durable compression, but they often have a long turn-around time and are costly to produce. Face masks made of other materials (often used in burn care and post–facial surgery) are manufactured in the more cost-effective "cut and sewn" technique. These garments are available in standard sizes, but they tend to be less durable.

See Figure 5–82 for example of measurement form for neck and chin compression garments.

Compression Garments for the Upper Thorax and Breast

Compression bras (Fig. 5–83)*:* these garments typically are used if swelling in the mammary gland is an issue.

Advantages: Velcro closure in the back allows for adjustments; fashionable; available in

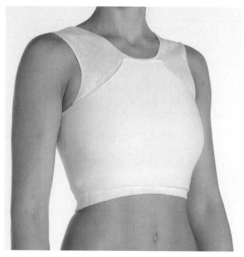

Figure 5–83 Compression bra (with permission from JUZO, Inc.).

a variety of standard sizes; only one circumferential measurement on the chest (below the breast) required; relatively inexpensive.

Disadvantages: Closure in the back may be difficult to reach; does not provide sufficient support in truncal swelling; the low cut in the axillary area may allow fluid to accumulate.

Compression vests (Fig. 5–84): These custom-made garments are available in different compression levels (20–30 and 30–40 mmHg) and are appropriate for patients with a tendency to swell in the upper quadrant(s). Compression vests may be ordered as slip-ons or with optional closure systems (Velcro, zipper), which may be located in the front or back. Vests can be ordered with attached compression arm sleeves.

Required Measurements for Compression Vests

Circumferential measuring points (indicate the position of all measuring points with nontoxic, nonpermanent marker):

◆ Point h: vertically around the axilla and the shoulder. The arm should not be elevated during this measurement.

◆ Point m: around the waist (just below the last rib)

◆ Point n: around the chest, under the axilla

Length measurements:

◆ s–s: this measurement determines the neck opening. It is taken on the front of the neck between the desired points of the neck opening on the shoulder height (point s represents the height of the shoulders).

◆ qu–r: this measurement determines the lower portion of the neck opening and is taken between the desired points of the opening.

◆ r–s: determines the height of the opening between the shoulder height (point s) and the lower portion of the neck opening (point r)

◆ m–s: determines the length between the waist measurement (point m) and the shoulder height (point s)

◆ m–n: the distance between the circumferential measurements on the waist (point m) and the chest (point n)

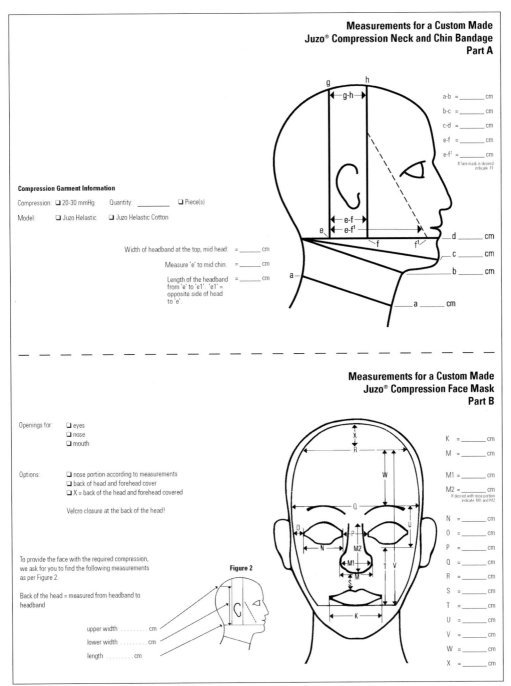

**Measurements for a Custom Made
Juzo® Compression Neck and Chin Bandage
Part A**

g   h

g-h

a-b = _____ cm

b-c = _____ cm

c-d = _____ cm

e-f = _____ cm

e-f¹ = _____ cm
If face mask is desired
indicate F1

Compression Garment Information

Compression: ❏ 20-30 mmHg   Quantity: _____   ❏ Piece(s)

Model: ❏ Juzo Helastic   ❏ Juzo Helastic Cotton

Width of headband at the top, mid head: = _____ cm

Measure 'e' to mid chin: = _____ cm

Length of the headband = _____ cm
from 'e' to 'e1'. 'e1' =
opposite side of head
to 'e'.

e-f
e-f¹

e   f   f¹

d   _____ cm

c   _____ cm

b   _____ cm

a—

a   _____ cm

**Measurements for a Custom Made
Juzo® Compression Face Mask
Part B**

Openings for: ❏ eyes
                 ❏ nose
                 ❏ mouth

Options: ❏ nose portion according to measurements
            ❏ back of head and forehead cover
            ❏ X = back of the head and forehead covered

Velcro closure at the back of the head!

To provide the face with the required compression,
we ask for you to find the following measurements
as per Figure 2.

Back of the head = measured from headband to
headband

upper width . . . . cm

lower width . . . . cm

length . . . . cm

Figure 2

K = _____ cm

M = _____ cm

M1 = _____ cm

M2 = _____ cm
If desired with nose portion
indicate M1 and M2

N = _____ cm

O = _____ cm

P = _____ cm

Q = _____ cm

R = _____ cm

S = _____ cm

T = _____ cm

U = _____ cm

V = _____ cm

W = _____ cm

X = _____ cm

Figure 5–82 Measurement form for neck and chin compression garments and compression face masks (with permission from JUZO, Inc.).

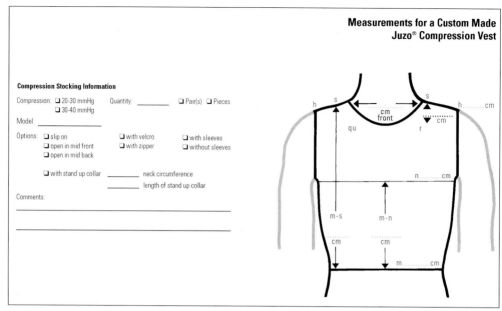

Measurements for a Custom Made Juzo® Compression Vest

Compression Stocking Information

Compression: ❏ 20-30 mmHg   Quantity: _____   ❏ Pair(s) ❏ Pieces
                    ❏ 30-40 mmHg

Model: _____

Options: ❏ slip on   ❏ with velcro   ❏ with sleeves
             ❏ open in mid front   ❏ with zipper   ❏ without sleeves
             ❏ open in mid back

             ❏ with stand up collar _____ neck circumference
                                          _____ length of stand up collar

Comments: _____

_____

Figure 5–84   Measurement form for compression vest (with permission from JUZO, Inc.).

◆ Patient Education

Providing patients with appropriate information and education facilitates long-term success of lymphedema management. A dialogue between the patient and the lymphedema therapist covering all relevant aspects of lymphedema management should be initiated early on in the intensive phase of the treatment. Sufficient knowledge of the patient regarding his or her condition is the key to compliance. Patients need to know what causes lymphedema to understand fully why self-management is a necessary component of CDT (easy to understand terms should be used; a sample patient information form is given in Chapter 6, Information on Lymphedema). Patients should be informed about the possible consequences if self-care for lymphedema is neglected. Knowledge about the risks involved in certain activities (air travel, extremes in temperature, etc.) helps to avoid the recurrence of symptoms.

At the end of the intensive phase, the patient should have the necessary skills to perform self-bandaging and self-MLD techniques safely and effectively and to execute a customized program of decongestive exercises. A thorough understanding in preventive measures (see Do's and Don'ts for Upper Extremity Lymphedema and Do's and Don'ts for Lower Extremity Lymphedema later in this chapter) as well as high- and medium-risk activities for lymphedema should be achieved at the time the patient transitions into phase 2 of the treatment.

Self-Bandaging

During the intensive phase of the therapy (phase 1), the compression bandages applied by the therapist may slide somewhat over the treatment-free weekend days. Sliding is usually limited to the upper arm or thigh. The patient should be able to reapply the bandages in these areas to avoid reaccumulation of fluid and/or tourniquet effects caused by bunching up of the compression bandages. It is therefore necessary to involve the patient in the bandaging process as soon and as much as possible. At the end of the first week of treatment, the patient should be able to apply padding and compression bandages on the proximal parts of the extremity without major difficulty.

To maintain and improve the success achieved in the first phase of treatment and to further reduce and soften areas of fibrotic tissue, most patients have to continue to wear bandages at night. Even patients who do not experience an increase in extremity volume during the nighttime and who do not have any areas of fibrotic tissue may experience fluctuation in limb volume at times (lifestyle, during menstrual period, weight gain, climate, etc.). It is therefore imperative for long-term success that every patient learns appropriate self-bandaging techniques while under the care of an experienced and properly trained lymphedema therapist.

To support patient compliance, it is essential to keep the self-bandaging techniques as simple as possible. It cannot be expected that a patient will be able to use the same techniques as the lymphedema therapist. The use of high-density foam without the supervision of the clinician is not advisable. Bandages in the self-management phase are primarily worn at nighttime, when the patient sits or lies down. Much less bandage pressure is needed to achieve the beneficial effects of compression therapy. The quantity of materials is therefore much lower than during the intensive phase of therapy, during which the compression bandages are worn 22 to 23 hours a day.

Upper Extremity

The following is a list of the recommended materials for applying a compression bandage during the night on the upper extremity (self-management phase). The quantities represent two sets of compression bandages, which are recommended for hygienic reasons (one to wear and one to wash):

- 1 bottle of skin lotion
- 1 box of stockinette (tubular bandage) in the appropriate size
- 1–2 boxes (20 individual rolls in a box) of gauze bandages (4 or 6 cm width)
- 2–4 synthetic nonwoven padding bandages (10 cm) or 2 Rosidal Soft foam bandages (10 cm)
- 2 short-stretch bandages (4 or 6 cm)
- 2–4 short-stretch bandages (10 or 12 cm)
- Tape to secure the bandages

◆ **Application.** Bandages generally are applied with an even prestretch of ~30 to 40% and an overlap of ~50 to 70%. The patient should apply the bandages while sitting at a table.

All materials should be arranged in the order in which they are applied; two or three strips of tape per compression bandage (~5 inches long) should be prepared. Padding bandages are not taped.

Skin care: Appropriate skin care products are applied thoroughly, without causing redness of the skin.

Stockinette: The tubular bandage should be cut to a length that allows for an overlap of ~5 inches on the proximal end of the extremity. This overlap is used to extend over and cover the complete compression bandage on the proximal border to protect it from axillar perspiration. A hole is cut for the thumb on the distal end.

Finger bandages: Fingers are slightly spread, and the palm of the hand faces down. A bolster should be placed under the elbow to support the weight of the arm.

Start the gauze bandage with a loose anchor turn around the wrist, then proceed over the back of the hand to the little finger (or the thumb). The fingers should be bandaged with light pressure from the nail bed up with ~50% overlap (Fig. 5–85). The fingertips are not covered. Leave the finger with the gauze bandage toward the back of the hand and proceed to the wrist; apply a half turn (complete anchoring turns should be avoided) around the wrist, and continue to bandage the remaining fingers in the same fashion. The borders of the gauze bandage should not slide or roll in on the distal and proximal ends of the fingers. One gauze bandage is generally used to bandage all fingers. Any unused part of the second gauze bandage should be wrapped spirally (not circular) around the forearm. The finger bandage should never start or end at a finger. Upon completion, the fingertips should be checked for proper circulation.

Padding materials: Nonwoven synthetic padding or soft foam rolls (Rosidal Soft) are used to pad the hand and arm. A hole is cut for the thumb; the padding bandage is secured around the wrist with a circular turn. The hand

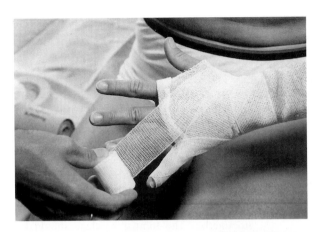

Figure 5–85 Application of gauze bandages on the fingers.

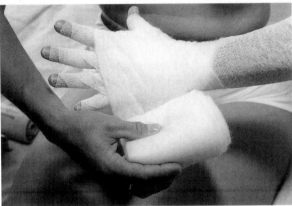

Figure 5–86 Application of synthetic padding bandages on the hand, including the knuckles.

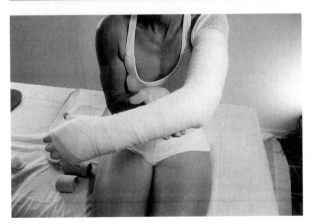

Figure 5–87 Padding of the arm using synthetic padding bandages.

is then padded down to the knuckles using two to four circular turns (Fig. 5–86). The padding bandage proceeds to cover the forearm and upper arm. Two rolls of padding bandages are used to cover the hand and arm (Fig. 5–87). Do not use tape to secure the padding materials.

Short-stretch bandages: Starting a 6 cm (or 4 cm) wide bandage with a loose anchor turn around the wrist, the hand is bandaged to include the knuckles with slightly spread fingers (Fig. 5–88). The bandage is anchored between each turn around the hand with half turns on

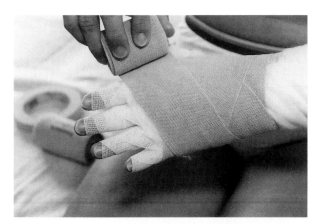

Figure 5–88 Application of short-stretch bandages on the hand and wrist.

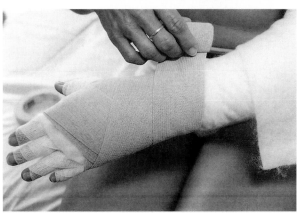

Figure 5–89 The remaining short-stretch bandage is used to apply compression on the forearm.

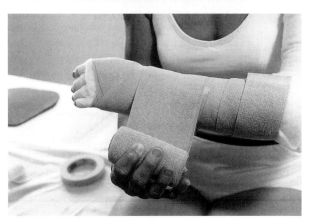

Figure 5–90 Application of the second short-stretch bandage starting at the wrist.

the wrist. Any remaining bandage material is used on the forearm (Fig. 5–89). The end of the bandage is secured with two strips of tape. The subsequent bandage (10 or 12 cm) is applied in the opposite direction of the first bandage. This provides for a more functional and durable bandage. The bandage starts on the wrist with a loose anchor and proceeds to cover the forearm, elbow area, and upper arm with circular turns and ~50% overlap (Fig. 5–90). A third bandage may be used if necessary. It is important that the last bandage ends in the axillary

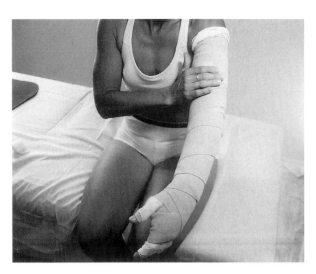

Figure 5–91 Finished compression bandage on the upper extremity.

fold to prevent accumulation of fluid between the armpit and the end of the bandage (Fig. 5–91).

The end of the bandage is secured with two or three strips of tape, and the overlap of the stockinette is folded over the bandage.

Lower Extremity

Following is a list of the recommended materials for applying a compression bandage on the lower extremity during the self-management phase of CDT (phase 2). The quantities represent two sets of compression bandages, which are recommended for hygienic reasons (one to wear and one to wash):

- 1 bottle of skin lotion
- 1 box of stockinette (tubular bandage) in the appropriate size
- If toe bandages are necessary:1–2 boxes of gauze bandages (4 cm width)
- 2 high-density foam pieces (kidney-shaped)
- 3–5 synthetic nonwoven padding bandages (10 cm) or 2 Rosidal Soft foam bandages (10 cm)
- 2–4 synthetic nonwoven padding bandages (15 cm) or 2 Rosidal Soft foam bandages (15 cm)
- 4–6 short-stretch bandages (10 cm) or 2 double-length (11 yards) 10 cm rolls

- 4–6 short-stretch bandages (12 cm) or 2 double-length (11 yards) 12 cm rolls
- Tape to secure the bandages
- If necessary: additional foam pieces provided by the therapist

◆ **Application.** Bandages generally are applied with an even prestretch of ~30 to 40% and an overlap of ~50 to 70%. All materials should be arranged in the order in which they are applied; two or three strips of tape per compression bandage (~5 inches long) should be prepared. Padding bandages are not taped.

To bandage the foot and the lower leg, the patient should be sitting, with the foot of the affected leg resting on another chair or on the knee of the other leg. Bandages from the knee up to the groin are applied while standing.

Skin care: Appropriate skin care products are applied thoroughly, without causing redness on the skin.

Stockinette: The tubular bandage should be cut to a length that allows for an overlap of ~5 inches on the proximal end of the extremity. This overlap is used to extend over and cover the complete compression bandage on the proximal border (Fig. 5–92).

Toe bandages (if necessary): Start the first gauze bandage with a loose anchor turn around the foot, then proceed to bandage the big toe. Enter the toe from the dorsum of the

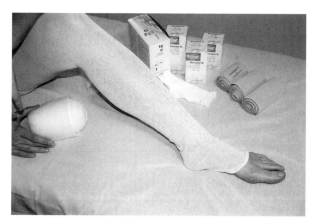

Figure 5-92 Application of stockinette on the leg.

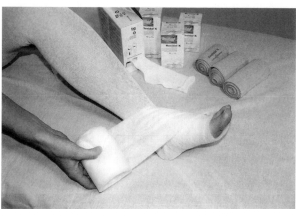

Figure 5-93 Application of synthetic padding bandages on the foot, ankle, and lower leg.

foot, apply two or three circular turns, and leave the toe again over the dorsum of the foot. Avoid sliding or rolling of the bandages in the web space area. The tips of the toes remain unbandaged. Proceed to bandage the remaining toes (except the fifth toe, which generally is not involved in the swelling) in the same manner. One 4 cm bandage (usually folded to half width) is generally sufficient to cover the toes. Any unused part of the gauze bandage should be wrapped spirally (not circular) around the foot. Upon completion, the tips of the toes should be checked for proper circulation.

Padding materials: Two or three rolls of nonwoven synthetic padding, or one or two rolls of soft foam (Rosidal Soft) are applied on the foot and lower leg (Fig. 5-93). Komprex foam kidneys are secured between the medial and lateral anklebone and the Achilles tendon with

the padding bandages. Synthetic padding bandages may be doubled over the shin area to provide additional protection.

Short-stretch bandages: Starting a 10 cm wide bandage with a loose anchor turn around the foot, the foot is bandaged down to the web spaces with three or four circular turns (Fig. 5-94). The same bandage proceeds to cover the heel in a crisscross fashion. During the application of compression bandages on the heel, the ankle is in ~70 to 90 degrees of flexion (Figs. 5-95, 5-96). Secure the bandage with tape. The next bandage (10 cm) starts above the ankle with a loose anchor in the opposite direction of the previous bandage (applying compression bandages in the opposite direction to each other prevents bandaging the foot in a nonfunctional position; i.e., it provides for a functional bandage and adds durability). The goal is to cover the lower leg up to the knee

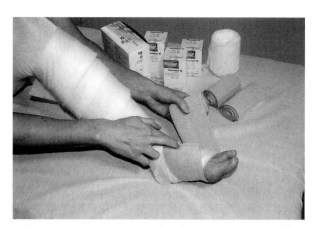

Figure 5–94 Start of the first short-stretch bandage with a loose anchor around the foot.

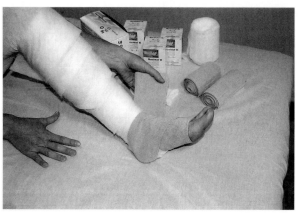

Figure 5–95 The ankle is in 70 to 90 degrees of flexion while applying bandages around the heel.

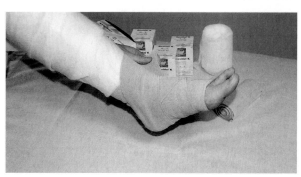

Figure 5–96 Short-stretch bandages around the ankle are applied in a criss-cross fashion.

using circular turns (Figs. 5–97, 5–98). Secure the bandage on the lower leg with tape. If a double-length bandage is used, the foot as well as the lower leg may be bandaged using the same roll.

The remaining compression bandage is applied while standing up, and the body weight should be shifted to the extremity being bandaged, with the knee slightly bent. Pad-

ding materials using nonwoven synthetic padding or soft foam rolls are applied on the knee and thigh (Fig. 5–99). When using synthetic padding bandages, the layers may be doubled in the back of the knee to provide additional protection. The knee and thigh should be bandaged using two or three rolls of 12 cm wide short-stretch bandages (or one double-length roll). The first bandage starts with a

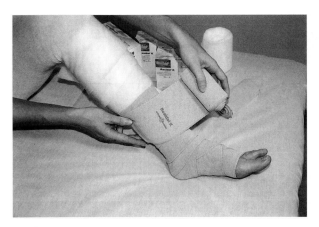

Figure 5–97 The second short-stretch bandage starts with a loose anchor around the ankle.

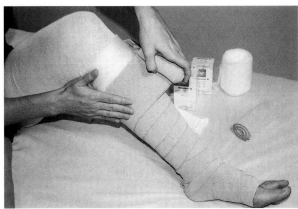

Figure 5–98 Application of short-stretch bandages on the lower leg.

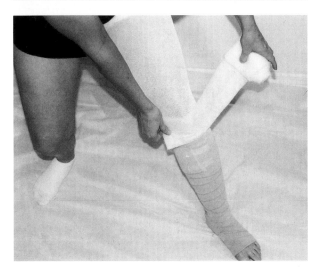

Figure 5–99 Application of synthetic padding bandages on the knee and thigh.

loose anchor turn below the knee, proceeding to cover the knee and parts of the thigh using circular techniques (Fig. 5–100). The remaining thigh is bandaged with the next bandage roll. Secure the bandage with tape, and fold the overlap of the stockinette over the bandage (Fig. 5–101).

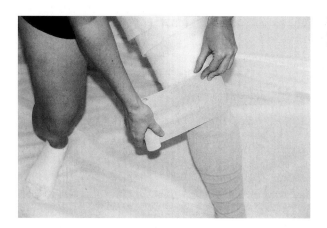

Figure 5–100 Application of short-stretch bandages on the knee and thigh.

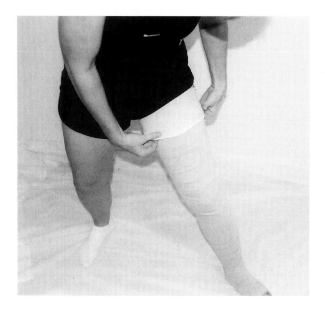

Figure 5–101 Finished compression bandage on the leg.

Decongestive Exercises

The following exercises serve as guidelines for an exercise program that can be performed by the patient without major difficulties during the decongestive and self-management phases of therapy. The exercise protocol may be changed to accommodate the patient's limitations. Generally, the exercise program should not be too difficult or too lengthy to perform, and the movements must not cause discom-

fort, pain, or soreness in the musculature. The affected extremity should be elevated as often as possible during the day.

Ideally, the exercises are performed 10 to 15 minutes following the MLD session, and the patient should rest with the limb elevated for ~10 to 15 minutes after the exercises.

Stretching exercises (yoga), swimming, water aerobics, and walking are beneficial additions to the decongestive exercise program. Higher impact activities (e.g., step aerobics) may exacerbate lymphedema and should be avoided. A summary of high- and medium-risk activities for patients with upper and lower extremity lymphedema are listed in Do's and Don'ts for Upper Extremity Lymphedema and Do's and Don'ts for Lower Extremity Lymphedema in this chapter.

Upper Extremity

◆ Exercises should be performed wearing compression bandages or compression sleeves (except when exercises are performed in the water).

◆ Tight or restrictive clothing (tight underwear or bra, heavy breast prosthesis) should not be worn while performing the exercises.

◆ Exercises should be performed twice daily for ~10 to 15 minutes. The duration of the program should be increased slowly over a comfortable period of time.

◆ Movements should be performed in a slow and controlled manner, and the musculature should be relaxed between each individual exercise. The relaxation phase should last at least as long as the time spent during the exercise.

Exercises should be performed sitting on stool or a chair without leaning back. Many of the exercises, however, may be performed while lying on the floor. Proper breathing techniques should be used throughout the session.

◆ Abdominal Breathing (3 repetitions)

1. Place both hands on your belly.
2. Inhale deeply through your nose into your belly (feel how you breathe against your hands).
3. Exhale through your mouth.

Perform breathing exercises as often as possible during the day.

◆ Neck Exercises (2–3 repetitions each)

1. Turn your head slowly and look to the right as far as possible; return to normal position; repeat on the left side.
2. Bend your head to the right and try to touch the shoulder with your ear (do not shrug

your shoulder). Return to the starting position and repeat for left side.

◆ Shoulder Exercises

Shoulder Rolls (3–5 repetitions each)

1. Rotate shoulders alternately on the right and left side.
2. Perform shoulder rolls, forward and backward, using both shoulders.

Shoulder Shrug (3–5 repetitions each)

1. Shrug both shoulders and inhale. Exhale while relaxing your shoulders.

◆ Arm Exercises (3–5 repetitions each)

Fingers

1. Place palms and fingers together.
2. Move little fingers away from each other and back together.
3. Move ring fingers away from each other and back together.

Continue with each finger.

Alternate Position

1. Hold palms out in front of the body with the palms facing up.
2. Move thumb and index finger together, so the finger pads touch each other; return to open hand.
3. Move thumb and ring finger together, so the finger pads touch each other; return to open hand.

Continue with each finger.

Hand

Alternate between hands; the relaxed hand rests on the leg.

1. Make a fist and hold for ~3 seconds.
2. Open the fist and relax the hand for ~3 seconds.
3. Make a fist and rotate the wrist clockwise and counterclockwise.
4. Make a fist and touch it to the opposite shoulder.

Arm and Hands

Picking Oranges

1. Stretch out arm and lean forward.
2. Make a fist and return hand to leg.

Climb up the Ladder

Alternate between arms and continue for ~30 to 40 seconds.

1. Hold arms above head.
2. Grasp rungs of imaginary ladder and "climb" as high as possible (remain seated).

Swimming

Use breaststrokes as far as possible to the front, move arms to the side, then to the knees and to the front again.

Hand to Opposite Knee

Alternate between arms.

1. Place the palm of one hand on the opposite knee and push down with your hand, then upward with your knee.
2. Hold for 5 seconds.

◆ **Exercises with a Broomstick (3–5 repetitions each).**

Climbing Up and Down the Stick

1. Hold the stick vertically between your knees with your hands.
2. Take the stick at the bottom with one hand and "climb" up and down the stick with alternating hands.

Weight Lifting

1. Hold the stick with both hands horizontally, with the palms up.
2. Lift the stick up and toward your head, then return to the original position.

Wringing the Stick

1. Hold the stick with both hands horizontally, with the palms down and about 1 foot apart.
2. Attempt to wring the stick, moving one hand forward and the other back.
3. Hold for ~3 to 5 seconds and wring in the other direction.

Canoeing

1. Hold the stick with both hands horizontally, with the palms down and about 1 foot apart.

2. Start to "paddle" to either side with nice, big strokes.

Pendulum

1. Hold the stick vertically in front of you on one end.
2. Move the stick slowly from one side to the other like a pendulum.
3. Change hands and repeat.

◆ **Exercises with a Soft Ball (3–5 repetitions each).**

Biceps Curl

1. Hold the ball with one hand, palm up.
2. Curl the ball to your shoulder, then return to the starting position.
3. Alternate hands (the relaxed hand rests on the thigh).

Sponge Squeeze

1. Hold ball with both hands in your lap and squeeze as hard as you can.
2. Hold the squeeze for ~10 seconds.

Roll the Dough

1. Place the ball on one thigh and roll the ball with your whole hand (fingers and palm) to the knee. Return to the lap, and alternate the hands.

Soft Ball Circles

1. Hold the ball in one hand, with the arm extended.
2. Guide the ball with two or three big circles around your body by switching the ball between the hands.
3. Alternate directions.
4. Lift one thigh and guide the ball under the thigh to the other hand; alternate between the hands and legs.

Lower Extremity

◆ Exercises should be performed while wearing compression bandages or compression garments (except when exercises are performed in the water).
◆ Tight or restrictive clothing should not be worn while performing the exercises.

- Exercises should be performed twice daily for ~10 to 15 minutes. The duration of the program should be increased slowly over a comfortable period of time.
- Movements should be performed in a slow and controlled manner, and the musculature should be relaxed between each individual exercise. The relaxation phase should last at least as long as the time spent during the exercise.

Exercises should be performed while lying supine on the floor, preferably on a cushioned mat or other surface that maintains some firmness. Proper breathing techniques should be used throughout the session. To avoid back strain, a small pillow may be placed under the knees.

◆ Abdominal Breathing (3 repetitions)

1. Place both hands on your belly.
2. Inhale deeply through your nose into your belly (feel how you breathe against your hands).
3. Exhale through your mouth.

Perform breathing exercises as often as possible during the day.

◆ Foot and Leg Exercises (3–5 repetitions each)

Toe Clenches   (either alternating or with both feet at the same time)

1. Curl your toes and squeeze for about 3 seconds.
2. Relax the toes for 3 seconds.

Spread the Toes   (either alternating or with both feet at the same time)

1. Spread the toes as far as possible and hold for about 3 seconds.
2. Relax the toes for about 3 seconds.

Ankle Curls   (either alternating or with both feet at the same time)

1. Flex the foot as far as possible at the ankle, with the toes pointing away from the body (back of the knee remains on the floor).
2. Hold for about 3 seconds.

3. Flex the foot as far as possible at the ankle, with the toes pointing to the shin.
4. Relax for about 3 seconds.

Ankle Rotation   (either alternating or with both feet at the same time)

1. Rotate foot at the ankle, both clockwise and counterclockwise.

Riding the Bike   (for about 1 minute)

1. While lying on your back, move your legs in the air as if you are riding a bicycle.
(If you use a stationary bike, keep it on a low setting to avoid soreness or strain.)

Heel Sliding

1. Move the heel of your foot as close as possible to your buttocks.
2. Return to the starting position, and alternate the legs.

Hand and Knee Touch

1. Lift one knee and push the palm of the opposite hand against the knee. Hold for about 3 seconds.
2. Relax for about 3 seconds, then alternate sides.

Butt Lift

1. Bend the knees and place your feet flat on the floor.
2. Raise your buttocks off the floor and hold for about 3 seconds.
3. Bring the buttocks back to the floor and relax for about 3 seconds.

◆ Exercises for the Lower Back (3–5 repetitions each)

Knee Hugs   (keep your head on the floor)

1. Bend one knee and hug the knee with both arms.
2. Bring the knee with your arms as close as possible to your chest.
3. Hold for about 3 seconds.
4. Bring the foot back to the floor.
5. Alternate legs.

Back Stretch 1   (keep your head and shoulders on the floor and stabilize your body with both palms pressing down on the floor)

1. Bend both knees and move them as close to the chest as possible.

2. Hold for about 3 seconds.

3. Bring the feet back to the floor and relax for about 3 seconds.

Back Stretch 2 (keep your head and shoulders on the floor and stabilize your body with both palms pressing down on the floor)

1. Bend both knees with the foot flat on the floor.

2. Move both knees to the right side as close to the floor as possible, and hold for 3 seconds.

3. Move the knees back to the middle position and relax for about 3 seconds.

4. Alternate sides.

◆ **Exercises with a Soft Ball (3–5 repetitions each)**

Squeeze

1. Hold the ball between your knees and squeeze together for about 3 seconds; relax for about 3 seconds.

2. Place the ball under your thigh and squeeze to the floor for about 3 seconds; relax for about 3 seconds.

3. Alternate legs.

Circles

1. Bend one knee, and lead the ball behind the thigh and back to the front using both hands.

2. Alternate legs.

Walking

Walking is a great exercise for lymphedema of the lower extremities. If you use a stair exerciser or treadmill, keep it on a low setting to avoid soreness or strain.

Remember to walk with a normal gait. Do not drag the affected leg, and avoid limping.

Self-MLD

Simple and easy-to-perform MLD techniques are an integral part of the self-management program. In this stage, the patient has completed the intensive phase with the lymphedema therapist and is familiar with the pressures and techniques used in MLD.

Ideally, the self-MLD protocol should be performed at least once a day for about 10 to 15 minutes, directly preceding the exercise program, and should be followed by compression therapy.

The following are basic techniques for unilateral upper and lower extremity lymphedema. These techniques may be changed according to specific requirements and physical limitations of the individual patient. It is important that the patient understands the correct pressure to apply with the strokes, and the self-MLD session should not turn into a kneading/massage session.

Upper Extremity

The stationary circles used in this self-treatment are based on the same principles as those performed by the lymphedema therapist. They should be executed using light pressure in the working phase; during the resting phase of the circle, the hand should relax completely. The amount of pressure is sometimes described as the pressure applied while stroking a newborn's head. The circles should be large enough to stretch the skin, but the hand should not slide over the skin. Self-MLD for the arm is performed best in the sitting position. Each stroke should be repeated five to seven times on the same placement, and, if not noted otherwise, the hand of the unaffected side should be used to perform the strokes.

Note: The self-MLD techniques shown in Figures 5–102 through 5–114 depict the sequence used for a lymphedema on the left arm.

◆ **Pretreatment**

1. Do circles with the fingers lying flat above the collarbone on both sides. The pressure is directed toward the neck. It would be easier for the right hand to manipulate the skin above the left collarbone and vice versa (Fig. 5–102).

2. Do circles in the center of the opposite axilla. Pressure is given with the flat hand of the affected arm and is directed downward (deep) into the axilla (Fig. 5–103).

3. Perform soft effleurage from the affected axilla to the axilla on the other side (Fig. 5–104).

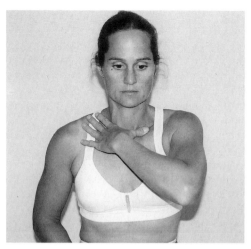

Figure 5–102 Stationary circles above the collar-bone on both sides.

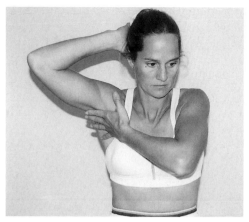

Figure 5–103 Stationary circles in the axilla on the unaffected side.

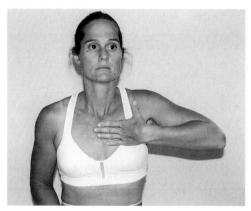

Figure 5–104 Soft effleurage from the affected axilla to the axilla on the other side.

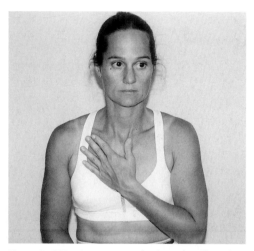

Figure 5–105 Stationary circles from the affected axilla to the axilla on the other side in several placements.

4. Do circles from the affected axilla to the axilla on the other side in several placements. The pressure is directed toward the axilla on the unaffected side (Fig. 5–105).

5. Do circles with the flat hand (use affected arm) in the area of the inguinal lymph nodes on the same side. The hand lies just below the inguinal ligament, and the pressure is directed toward the belly (Fig. 5–106).

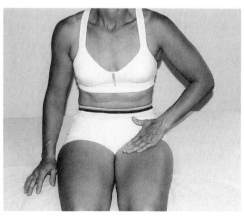

Figure 5–106 Stationary circles in the area of the ▷ inguinal lymph nodes on the same side.

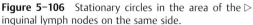

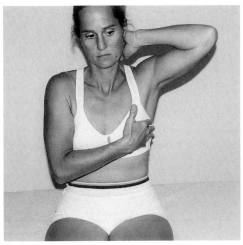

Figure 5–107 Stationary circles with the flat hand from the affected axilla to the inguinal lymph nodes on the same side in several placements.

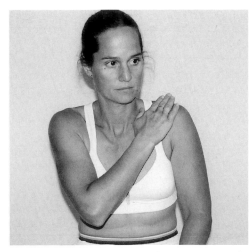

Figure 5–108 Stationary circles on top of the shoulder.

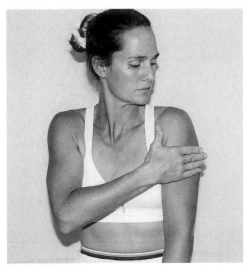

Figure 5–109 – Stationary circles on the lateral upper arm in several placements.

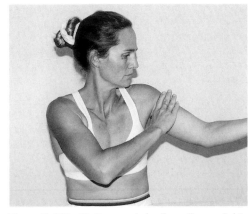

Figure 5–110 Stationary circles from the medial to the lateral upper arm in several placements.

6. Do circles with the flat hand from the affected axilla to the inguinal lymph nodes on the same side in several placements. The pressure is directed toward the inguinal lymph nodes of the same side (Fig. 5–107).

◆ **Arm**

7. Perform soft effleurage strokes covering the entire arm, beginning on the hand and ending on the top of the shoulder.

8. Do circles covering the deltoid and the shoulder of the affected arm; the pressure is directed toward the neck in several placements (Figs. 5–108, 5–109).

9. Do circles with flat fingers from the medial to the lateral upper arm. Work the entire upper arm from the top down to the elbow with this technique. The pressure is directed toward the lateral upper arm (Fig. 5–110).

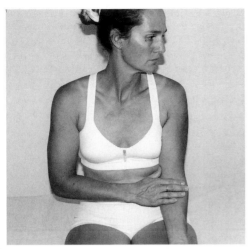

Figure 5–111 Stationary circles in front of the elbow.

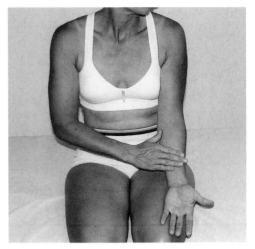

Figure 5–112 Stationary circles on the anterior forearm.

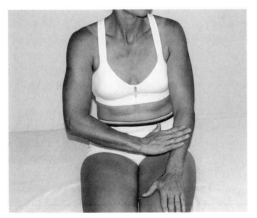

Figure 5–113 Stationary circles on the posterior forearm.

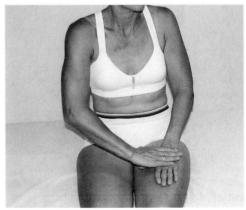

Figure 5–114 Stationary circles on the back of the hand.

10. Rework your lateral upper arm from the elbow to the shoulder with circles. The pressure is directed toward the shoulder.

11. Do circles in the front of the elbow, the forearm, and the hand. Turn your forearm so that you can reach all aspects of it. The pressure is always directed to the upper arm (Figs. 5–111, 5–112, 5–113, 5–114).

12. Rework your upper arm. (You may repeat as many of the hand placements as you wish.)

13. Repeat steps 1, 2, and 5. (You may repeat as many of the hand placements as you wish.)

Lower Extremity

The stationary circles used in this self-treatment are based on the same principles as those performed by the lymphedema therapist. They should be executed using light pressure in the working phase, and the hand should relax

213

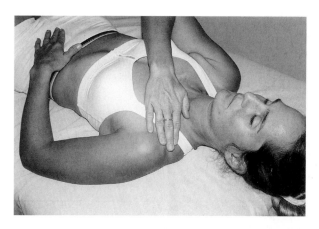

Figure 5–115 Stationary circles above the collarbones on each side.

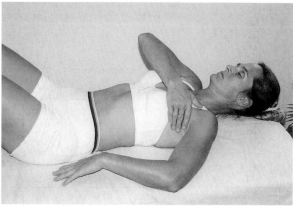

Figure 5–116 Stationary circles in the axilla on the same side.

completely during the resting phase of the circle. The circles should be large enough to stretch the skin, but the hand should not slide over the skin. Self-MLD for the leg should be performed lying in the supine position. Each stroke should be repeated five to seven times on the same placement.

Note: The self-MLD techniques shown in Figures 5–115 through 5–128 depict the sequence used for a lymphedema on the left leg.

◆ **Pretreatment**

1. Do circles with the fingers lying flat above the collarbones on each side. Do each side separately, and use the hand of the opposite side. Switch hands to manipulate the other side. The pressure on both sides is directed toward the neck (Fig. 5–115).

2. Do circles in the center of the axilla on the same side. Pressure is given with the flat hand and is directed downward (deep) into the axilla (Fig. 5–116).

3. Do circles with the flat hand on the side of the trunk, from the waist of the affected side to the axillary lymph nodes on the same side (in several placements). The pressure is directed toward the axillary lymph nodes on the same side (Fig. 5–117).

4. Do circles with the flat hand in the area of the inguinal lymph nodes on the opposite side. The hand lies just below the inguinal ligament, and the pressure is directed toward the belly (Fig. 5–118).

5. Do circles from the inguinal area on the affected side to the inguinal lymph nodes on the other side (in several placements). The

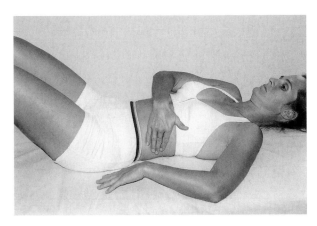

Figure 5–117 Stationary circles from the waist of the affected side to the axillary lymph nodes on the same side in several placements.

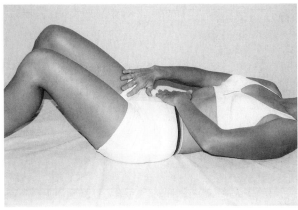

Figure 5–118 Stationary circles on the inguinal lymph nodes of the unaffected side.

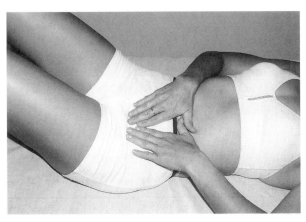

Figure 5–119 Stationary circles from the inguinal area on the affected side to the inguinal lymph nodes on the other side in several placements.

pressure is directed to the inguinal lymph nodes on the unaffected side (Fig. 5–119).

6. Abdominal breathing: Place both hands flat on your belly and inhale against your hands. The hands follow the belly while you exhale; at the end of the exhalation, both hands press downward and upward (into the thorax). Repeat five times (Figs. 5–120, 5–121).

Note: Discuss possible contraindications with your therapist.

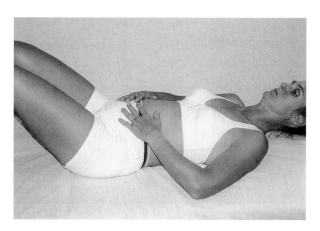

Figure 5–120 Diaphragmatic breathing: inhalation.

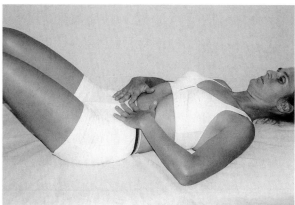

Figure 5–121 Diaphragmatic breathing: exhalation.

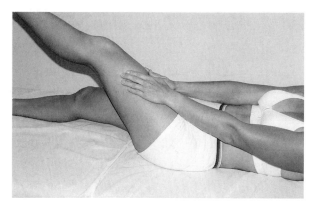

Figure 5–122 Effleurage on the leg.

◆ **Leg**

7. Perform soft effleurage strokes covering the entire leg, beginning at the ankles (or the knee) and ending on the lateral waist (Fig. 5–122).

8. Do circles covering the lateral thigh and the hip in several placements. The pressure is directed toward the trunk (Fig. 5–123).

9. Do circles with both flat hands from the medial to the lateral thigh. Work the entire thigh from the top down to the knee with this technique. The pressure is directed toward the lateral thigh (Fig. 5–124).

10. Do circles with the flat fingers of both hands behind the knee. The pressure is directed toward the thigh (Fig. 5–125).

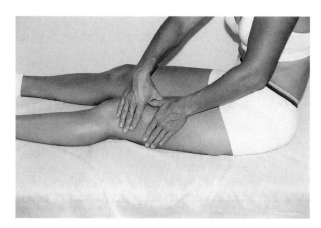

Figure 5–123 Stationary circles covering the lateral thigh and the hip in several placements.

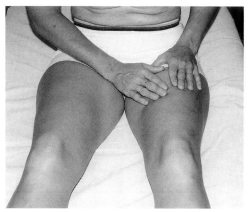

Figure 5–124 Stationary circles from the medial to the lateral thigh.

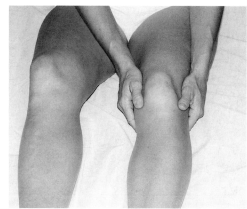

Figure 5–125 Stationary circles behind the knee.

11. Do circles with one or both hands in several placements on the medial lower leg, between the knee and the ankle. The pressure is directed toward the thigh (Figs. 5–126, 5–127).

12. Do circles with the hands lying flat on both sides of the lower leg. The pressure is directed toward the thigh. Do several placements between the knee and the ankles (Fig. 5–128).

13. Do circles with the fingers of one hand lying flat on the back of the foot. The pressure is directed toward the ankles.

14. Rework your leg. (You may repeat as many of the hand placements as you wish.)

15. Repeat steps 2, 4, and 6. (You may repeat as many of the hand placements as you wish.)

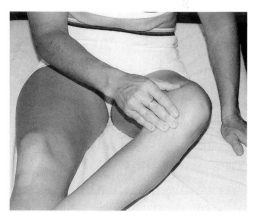

Figure 5–126 Stationary circles below the medial knee.

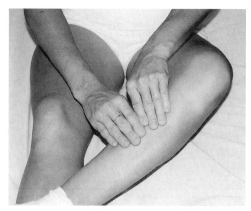

Figure 5–127 Stationary circles in several placements on the medial lower leg.

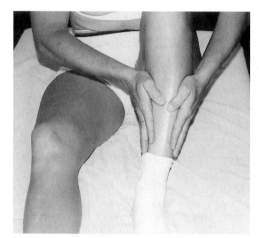

Figure 5–128 Stationary circles on both sides of the lower leg.

Precautions

Anyone who has undergone lymph node excision and/or radiation therapy is at risk of developing lymphedema. The capacity of the lymphatic system to remove fluid and other substances (lymphatic loads) from the tissues has been reduced by these procedures to a certain degree. Lymphedema may occur directly after the surgery/radiation, may develop months or even years following the procedure, or may never evolve.

Certain activities and situations may trigger the onset of lymphedema, or exacerbate the symptoms of existing lymphedema, by further reducing the transport capacity of the lym-

phatic system or by increasing the amount of lymphatic loads. Individuals who are aware of these risk factors know what can be done to avoid the onset of swelling and infections, which are common in patients suffering from lymphedema as well as those at risk. Knowing the necessary precautions helps to prevent aggravation of the symptoms in existing lymphedema.

The following do's and don'ts may have a cumulative effect. Whether one or more of these events or situations will be a triggering element depends on other factors, such as overall health (other conditions) and fitness, the extent of the initial procedure (scarring, number of lymph nodes removed), and obesity.

Patients with lymphedema and those at risk of developing it should observe the following precautionary measures. In many cases, modifications to lifestyle are necessary, but a normal activity level should be maintained. In other words, individuals should not refrain from using the affected extremity for fear of developing lymphedema.

Do's and Don'ts for Upper Extremity Lymphedema

◆ Avoid any injuries to the skin:

1. Gardening: Wear gloves.

2. Pets: Be careful to avoid scratches when playing with animals; wear gloves.

3. Mosquito bites: Use insect repellents, and avoid mosquito-infested areas.

4. Nail care: You should keep your fingernails cut short. Do not use scissors to cut your fingernails, and do not cut the cuticles. Do not apply artificial nails.

5. Shaving: Use an electric razor to remove hair from the axilla; do not use razor blades.

6. Injections: Do not allow injections in the swollen or (at risk) arm. Instead, take injections in the buttocks, the thigh, or the abdominal area.

7. Venapunctures: Do not allow blood to be drawn from the affected (at risk) arm. Have the venapuncture in the other arm, or if both arms are affected, in the lower extremity (certain contraindications may exist). The physician may choose to use

vascular access devices (VADs, ports), if appropriate.

8. To take proper care of minor injuries, always carry an alcohol swab, local antibiotic, and a bandage with you.

9. Should you smoke, do not extinguish the cigarette with your affected hand.

10. No piercing or tattoos on the arm or the upper body quadrants

◆ Do not have blood pressure readings taken on the affected (at risk) arm:

1. Have the clinician use the other arm; if both arms are affected, an oversize pressure cuff may be used on the thigh or calf (blood pressure taken on the leg may produce a higher reading). If you cannot avoid having the blood pressure taken on the affected arm, make sure that the cuff is inflated only 10 mmHg above the systolic pressure (this is the point at which the pulse stops) and that only manual equipment is used (automated equipment generally inflates to a very high pressure, which is held for a prolonged period).

◆ Avoid heat:

1. Avoid hot showers. Dry thoroughly, but avoid scrubbing or rubbing the skin with a towel.

2. Avoid hot packs and/or ice packs on your arm.

3. Avoid saunas or hot tubs and whirlpools; do not sit too close to a working fireplace.

4. Avoid massage (kneading, stroking, etc.) on the arm and the upper thorax. Note: Manual lymph drainage is *not* considered to be a form of massage.

5. Avoid cosmetics that irritate the skin.

6. Avoid getting sunburned. While in the sun, use sunscreen, and cover the affected arm with a long-sleeved shirt or a dry towel.

◆ Clothing/compression sleeve/jewelry:

1. Avoid clothing that is too tight (tight bras, sleeves).

2. You should use a comfortable bra with wide and padded shoulder straps.

3. Do not wear tight jewelry (rings, bracelets); avoid elastic wristbands.

4. Prosthesis: Discuss with your doctor and/or therapist what kind of external breast pros-

thesis is appropriate in your case (heavier silicone or lighter foam).

5. Wear your compression sleeve all day. See your therapist at least every 6 months (or sooner) to check the condition of the sleeve. Use a rubber glove when applying your compression sleeve. If necessary, apply your bandages at night.

◆ Exercises:

1. Always discuss proper exercises and activities with your therapist.

2. Avoid movements that overstrain; should you experience discomfort in the affected arm, reduce the exercise activity and elevate your arm.

3. Avoid heavy lifting.

◆ *Beneficial activities:*

Swimming, lymphedema exercise program, self-MLD, yoga, water aerobics, walking

◆ *Medium-risk activities:*

Jogging/running, biking (use aerobars; minimize gripping), stair exerciser (do not use grips; elevate the arm sometimes), treadmill (use minimal grips), horse riding (hold reins loosely), extreme hiking, mountain climbing

◆ *High-risk activities:*

Gardening (wear gloves), tennis/racquet sports, golf, shoveling snow, moving furniture, carrying luggage, carrying heavy grocery bags, scrubbing, weight lifting with the affected arm (not more that 10–15 lbs), intense horse riding (gripping reins)

If you wish to engage in either medium- or high-risk activities, you should discuss additional precautionary measures (extra compression during the activity) with your therapist or doctor.

◆ Travel:

1. Avoid mosquito-infested regions.

2. Wear an additional bandage or garment on top of your compression sleeve when traveling by car, train, or air (see also Lymphedema and Air Travel later in this chapter as well as Useful Tips for the Airline Traveler). Incorporate frequent stops, or get up from your seat frequently.

- Skin care:
1. Keep your skin meticulously clean.
2. Inspect your skin for any cracks, fungal infections, or rashes.
3. Moisturize your skin daily, especially after taking a shower or bath. Use appropriate ointments or lotions (preferably free of alcohol and fragrance).
4. Dry your skin thoroughly after taking a shower or bath (especially in skin creases and web spaces). Use a soft towel, and do not scrub.
5. If you undergo radiation therapy, apply the ointments recommended by your physician to any radiation redness on your skin. Avoid chlorinated pools and direct exposure to sunlight.

- Nutrition:
1. Obesity may have a negative effect on swelling; therefore, maintain your ideal body weight.
2. There is no special diet for lymphedema. Keep your diet well balanced. Today most nutritionists recommend a low-salt, low-fat, high-fiber diet.
3. Eating too little protein is not recommended and may cause serious health problems. Reducing protein intake will not reduce the protein component in lymphedema.

- See your doctor if you
1. Have any signs of an infection (fever, chills, red and hot skin)
2. Notice any itching, rash, fungal infections, or any other unusual changes on the skin
3. Experience an increase in swelling in your fingers, hand, arm, or chest
4. Experience pain

Do's and Don'ts for Lower Extremity Lymphedema

- Avoid any injuries to the skin:
1. Do not walk barefoot.
2. Pets: Be careful to avoid scratches when playing with animals.
3. Mosquito bites: Use insect repellents, and avoid mosquito-infested areas.

4. Nail care: You should keep your toenails short, but be careful when cutting your toenails; do not cut the cuticles.
5. Shaving: Use an electric razor to remove hair from the leg or lower body quadrant; do not use razor blades.
6. Injections: Do not allow injections in the swollen (at risk) leg, in the buttocks on the affected side, or in the abdominal area.
7. Venapunctures: Do not allow blood to be drawn from the affected (at risk) leg.
8. To take care of minor injuries, always carry an alcohol swab, local antibiotic, and a bandage with you.
9. Wear solid shoes to avoid ankle injuries.
10. No piercing or tattoos on the leg or the lower body quadrants.

- Avoid heat:
1. Do not take hot showers. Dry thoroughly, but avoid scrubbing or rubbing the skin with a towel.
2. Avoid hot packs and/or ice packs on the affected leg.
3. Avoid saunas or hot tubs and whirlpools. Do not sit too close to a working fireplace.
4. Avoid massage (kneading, stroking, etc.) on the affected leg and the lumbar area. Note: Manual lymph drainage is *not* considered to be a form of massage.
5. Avoid cosmetics that irritate the skin.
6. Avoid getting sunburned. While in the sun, use sunscreen, and cover the affected leg with appropriate clothing or a dry towel.

- Clothing/compression stocking/jewelry:
1. Avoid clothing that is too tight (underwear, pants, socks, or stockings that restrict).
2. Do not wear tight jewelry (toe rings); avoid elastic bands around your ankle.
3. Wear your compression stocking/pantyhose all day. Use rubber gloves when applying your compression garment. See your therapist at least every 6 months (or sooner) to check the condition of the garment. If necessary, apply your bandages at night.

- Exercises:
1. Always discuss proper exercises and activities with your therapist.

2. Avoid movements that overstrain. Should you experience discomfort in the affected leg, reduce the exercise activity, and elevate your leg.

3. Elevate your leg as often as possible.

◆ *Beneficial activities:*

Swimming, lymphedema exercise program, self-MLD, yoga, water aerobics, walking, treadmill (10–15 minutes, slow walking speed), easy biking (15–20 minutes; use a wide, comfortable saddle), calf pumps, deep breathing exercises

◆ *Medium-risk activities:*

Light jogging/running, biking (longer than 30 minutes), stair exerciser (longer than 5 minutes), treadmill (longer than 15 minutes), light horse riding, golfing

◆ *High-risk activities:*

Running, tennis/racquet sports, hockey, soccer, wrestling, kickboxing, step aerobics, weight lifting with the affected leg, intense horse riding, sitting or standing over long periods

> If you wish to engage in either medium- or high-risk activities, you should discuss additional precautionary measures (extra compression during the activity) with your therapist or doctor.

◆ Skin care:

1. Keep your skin meticulously clean (use clean undergarments and socks at all times).

2. Inspect your skin for any cracks, fungal infections, or rashes.

3. Moisturize your skin daily, especially after taking a shower or bath. Use appropriate ointments or lotions (preferably free of alcohol and fragrance).

4. Dry your skin thoroughly after taking a shower or bath (especially in skin creases and web spaces). Use a soft towel, and do not scrub.

5. If you undergo radiation therapy, apply the ointments recommended by your physician to any radiation redness on your skin. Avoid chlorinated pools and direct exposure to sunlight.

◆ Nutrition:

1. Obesity may have a negative effect on swelling; therefore, maintain your ideal body weight.

2. There is no special diet for lymphedema. Keep your diet well balanced. Today most nutritionists recommend a low-salt, low-fat, high-fiber diet.

3. Eating too little protein is not recommended and may cause serious health problems. Reducing protein intake will not reduce the protein component in lymphedema.

◆ See your doctor if you

1. Have any signs of an infection (fever, chills, red and hot skin)

2. Notice any itching, rash, fungal infections, or any other unusual changes on the skin

3. Experience an increase in swelling in your toes, foot, leg, or lower body quadrant

4. Experience pain

◆ Travel:

1. Avoid mosquito-infested regions.

2. Wear an additional bandage or stocking on top of your compression garment when traveling by car, train, or air (see also Lymphedema and Air Travel later in this chapter). Incorporate frequent stops, or get up from your seat frequently; elevate your leg(s) as often as possible.

◆ Useful Tips for the Airline Traveler

◆ Plan ahead:

1. Seek the advice of your physician and your lymphedema therapist if there are any questions.

2. Carry medication with you. If your destination is located in hot or mosquito-infested areas, take precautions (sun screen, insect repellents, antibiotics).

3. Bring skin lotion: the air in pressurized cabins is extremely dry.

4. If possible, request an exit seat, which offers more leg room. Definitely request an aisle seat so you can get up periodically without disturbing the person sitting next to you.

5. Allow ample time to check in and reach your departure gate.

6. Wear loose, comfortable clothing and comfortable shoes that have been worn previously. If you have lymphedema of the leg, you should *not* take off your shoes during the flight.

7. Be sure that you can manage your luggage. If you travel with another person or a group, ask someone else to carry the luggage for you. Should you travel on your own, take a smaller suitcase (preferably one with wheels). Do not lift your luggage from the baggage carousel with your affected arm.

8. Check the quality of your compression garment. If you have more than one garment, take the extra one with you as a backup. If your destination is located at high altitudes, you need to take the same precautions as for your flight. Take extra bandages (short stretch) with you.

◆ Inflight:

1. Relax and enjoy your flight.

2. Eat lightly.

3. Drink plenty of water or fruit juices.

4. Do not place anything under the seat in front of you, so you can stretch and exercise your legs.

5. Stand up and walk around the cabin periodically (but observe the fasten seat belt light).

6. Ask somebody else to place your carry-on luggage in the overhead compartment.

7. Be sure to execute some easy-to-remember "muscle pump" exercises (roll your feet, lift the heels and toes in alternating fashion, etc.). Ask your therapist about recommended exercises during the flight.

8. Elevate your arms as often as possible if you have upper extremity lymphedema.

9. Be sure to wear your compression garments.

10. If you have a compression stocking with an open toe, be sure that you apply bandages on your toes and any other part of your foot that may be exposed.

11. It is absolutely necessary to wear a glove (or finger/hand bandage) in addition to your arm sleeve. If you have a gauntlet without finger stubs, you need to bandage your fingers.

12. It is also a good idea to wear an additional short-stretch bandage on top of your compression garment to counter the effects of low cabin pressure; talk to your therapist.

◆ Arrival:

1. Do not remove your compression garment and any additional bandage materials before you reach your final destination.

2. Upon arrival at your hotel or other destination, a rest should be your top priority. Be sure to elevate the affected limb. Doing a few more exercises while wearing your compression garment would be beneficial— use moderation, and remember that rest is more important.

Lymphedema and Air Travel

The aircraft environment and other airline travel–related elements may represent risk factors for the lymphedema patient, as well as individuals at risk to develop lymphedema, that may either exacerbate symptoms in existing lymphedema or cause the onset of lymphedema in those patients at risk (latent lymphedema). Elements in question include the air pressure (and density), cabin pressure, and the cabin environment (air quality, seating).

Air pressure and the effects of altitude: The air pressure is caused by the weight of the air pressing down on the earth, the body, the ocean, and the air below the plane. The pressure value depends on the amount of air above the point where the pressure is measured. Consequently, air pressure decreases as altitude increases. The exact pressure at a particular altitude is also dependent on weather conditions. To understand the general idea of how pressure decreases with altitude, the following approximation can be used: As a rule of thumb, the air pressure drops ~1 inch of mercury for each 1000-foot increase in altitude or ~0.49 pounds per square inch (psi). At sea level, the atmosphere weighs in at ~14.7 psi; the pressure of the atmosphere at 8000 feet is around 10.9 psi.

Cabin pressure: Commercial aircraft are capable of flying at altitudes that are incompatible with human life, yet the passengers and crew are healthy because of the onboard environmental and pressurization systems. Although aircraft cabins are pressurized, while traveling at altitude, the pressure is less than that on the ground. Regulations require that commercial aircraft be capable of maintaining a cabin altitude no higher than 8000 feet at the maximum authorized flight altitude. For most flights, the cabin pressure is the same as that at 5000 to 8000 feet above sea level. In other words, when flying at 18,000 feet, for example, the atmosphere within the aircraft is like that on a 5000- to 8000-foot mountain peak. Referring to the information above, it is apparent that air pressure at 5000 to 8000 feet is lower than that at sea level.

Effects of altitude on air density: In simple terms, density is the mass of anything divided by the volume it occupies. The density of air is directly proportional to the pressure. With increasing altitude, the pressure decreases, and so does the density of air. Because air is a gas, it can be compressed or expanded. When air is compressed (resulting in increased pressure), a greater amount of air occupies a given volume; thus the density of air is increased. When pressure is decreased on a given volume of air, the air expands and occupies a greater space; thus the density of air is decreased. Oxygen accounts for ~21% of the gases in the atmosphere (at sea level as well at altitude), but because air density decreases with altitude, the amount of oxygen inhaled will decrease with every breath taken. Hence less oxygen is absorbed into the blood and circulated throughout the body during flight.

Cabin pressure and the effects on lymphedema: The lower air density with the resulting decrease in oxygen absorbed into the blood does not cause serious problems as long as the traveler, apart from the lymphedema, is in reasonably good health. The decrease in air pressure (the force exerted on the body by the weight of the air), however, may trigger the onset of lymphedema, or it may exacerbate the symptoms in existing lymphedema. This problem is most obvious, but not limited to, flights of 8 hours or more. Many patients report that their extremities had started to swell during air travel. In a 1993 study, 27 of 490 patients reported the onset of lymphedema during aircraft flight (15 legs and 12 arms). Worsening of existing lymphedema was reported by 67 patients (44 legs and 23 arms).

The most reasonable explanation for the onset or worsening of lymphedema (especially on the lower extremity) may be inactivity. Most aircraft are crowded, and passengers, specifically in coach class, are often uncomfortable and unable to stretch or easily leave their seats. It is a well-known fact that even people with an intact lymphatic system develop swollen feet and ankles during long flights. It is apparent that inactivity in combination with a compromised lymphatic drainage may have even more serious consequences. Inactivity, with the legs in a dependent position, coupled with the subsequent pooling of venous blood, will lead to an increase in tissue fluid in the lower extremities. This may be enough to trigger the onset of swelling in those patients with latent lymphedema or worsen already existing lymphedema.

In addition to inactivity, other factors may play a crucial role in those patients traveling with lymphedema. The reduced cabin pressure (10.9 psi vs. 14.7 psi at sea level) does have certain effects on those tissues that are or may be affected by lymphedema (suprafascial tissues). These effects may allow more fluid to leave the blood capillaries, some of which must be removed by the lymphatic system. The increase in the interstitial fluid content may be just enough to trigger the onset of lymphedema in patients with compromised lymphatic drainage or increase the swelling in patients with upper and/or lower extremity lymphedema. It can also be assumed that the lower pressure in cabins allows fibrotic capsules in the tissue to become rounded, causing compression and/or distortion of adjacent structures, such as lymphatic collectors and inlet valves of lymph capillaries. This may result in increased swelling and/or reduced uptake of lymphatic fluid. In many cases, the elastic fibers in the skin are damaged in lymphedema due to the constant stretch caused by the swelling, which may present an additional factor in the worsening of lymphedema in a low cabin pressure environment.

Compression therapy seems to be the most effective measure to counter possible negative effects on lymphedema during air travel. Compression, applied by short-stretch bandages or compression garments (or a combination of), increases the tissue pressure. The elevated tissue pressure effectively reduces the accumulation of fluid in the tissues and promotes lymphatic and venous return.

Air quality and humidity in pressurized cabins: The environmental system in aircraft provides filtration, controls temperature, and is also responsible for keeping humidity at a reasonable level. In modern aircraft, half of the cabin air consists of fresh air drawn from the engine intakes, and the other half is recirculated and filtered air from the cabin. The filtration systems (some aircraft are equipped with high efficiency particulate air filters, or HEPA filters) easily maintain cabin contaminants to low levels. The air is completely exchanged every 2 to 3 minutes, which is far more efficient than environmental systems in a typical home or office building.

Humidity, however, is usually less than 20% in pressurized cabins. This is fairly dry and may cause dehydration, which represents an additional complicating factor in lymphedema. The negative effects of dehydration can be countered by drinking extra water during airplane travel. It must be stressed that alcohol has an additional dehydrating effect and should not be used to replace body fluids.

Recommended Reading

1. Breast Cancer Dig 1984;78
2. Bringezu G, Schreiner O. Die Therapieform Manualle Lymphdrainage. :Verlag Otto Haase; 1987
3. Casley-Smith JR. Lymphedema initiated by aircraft flight. J Aviation Space Environ Med 1996;67(1):52–56
4. FAA Pilot's Handbook of Aeronautical Knowledge. Rev. ed. Chicago: Independent Publishing Group; 1997:AC 61–23C
5. Földi M. Treatment of lymphedema [Editorial]. Lymphology 1994;27:1–5
6. Getz DH. The primary, secondary, and tertiary nursing interventions of lymphedema. Cancer Nurs 1985;8(3):177–184
7. Gleim I. Pilot Handbook. 6th ed. 2000:1092–1141
8. Hocutt JE Jr. Cryotherapy. Am Fam Physician 1981;23(3):141–144
9. Lymphology Association of North America. Certified Lymphedema Therapist Candidate Information Brochure. Available at: http://www.clt-lana.org.
10. Hutzschenreuter P, Ehlers R. The effect of manual lymph drainage on the autonomic nervous system. Zeltschrift fur Lymphologie 1986;19:58–60
11. Nagda NL, Koontz MD. Review of studies on flight attendant health and comfort in airliner cabins. J Aviation Space Environ Med 2003;74:101–109
12. Pendleton L. Staying alive. AOPA Pilot 2002;45(10):121–122
13. Rayman R. Cabin air quality: an overview. J Aviation Space Environ Med 2002;73:211–215
14. Rosenfeld RG, Tesch LG, Rodriguez-Rigau LJ, et al. Recommendations for diagnosis, treatment and management of individuals with Turner syndrome. Endocrinologist 1994;4:351
15. Samant S. Neck dissection, classification. EMedicine
16. Silverstein MD, Heit JA, Mohr DN, et al. Trends in the incidence of deep vein thrombosis and pulmonary embolism: a 25-year population-based study. Arch Intern Med 1998;158:585–593

6

Administration

Health care professionals working in the field of lymphedema management see patients who may suffer from primary or secondary lymphedema, venous insufficiencies, or other conditions that may benefit from complete decongestive therapy. Cases may be relatively simple, or they may involve complicating factors, such as skin alterations, genital involvement, or additional pathologies exacerbating already existing symptoms. Some patients suffer from lymphedema for decades prior to seeing a certified lymphedema therapist, and in many cases the involved extremity has reached proportions so enormous, that it is difficult to comprehend how it was possible for the swelling to get so out of control. However simple or complicated the case may be, best results in lymphedema management are achieved if the patient is seen on a daily basis and treatments are given until the limb is decongested. Treatments furnished two or three times per week may cause more problems than benefit. Compression bandages slide if they are not renewed daily, causing tourniquet effects, or the patient may remove the bandages, leading to reaccumulation of lymph fluid in the extremity. The therapist is forced to spend part of the treatment time to again remove this fluid, which seriously hampers treatment progress.

Reducing the size of a lymphedematous extremity back to a normal or near normal volume is rewarding for both the patient and the therapist. This rewarding and clinically challenging experience is payback for the hardship patients had to endure and any obstacles a health care professional may have to overcome prior to establishing a lymphedema clinic.

This chapter focuses on some key points in the establishment of a lymphedema clinic, whether it is a freestanding treatment center or part of an existing clinic or department.

◆ Setting Up a Lymphedema Clinic

Among the factors influencing the establishment of a well-run lymphedema clinic are the selection of personnel, the determination of required space and equipment, and marketing issues in promoting the clinic.

Personnel

A high level of competency and skill is needed to master all components of complete decongestive therapy and to provide patients with the proper degree of intervention. The quality of training will have a great impact on the level of care the patients receive.

To provide a high standard of care, it is necessary that the therapists are specifically educated and trained in lymphedema management. It is highly recommended that therapists complete a training program in CDT, consisting of 135 classroom hours attained from one training program. The training should consist of one third theoretical instruction and two thirds practical hands-on work.

Successful lymphedema management requires daily treatments in the intensive phase; it is therefore desirable to employ two lymphedema therapists to cover for absence and for professional exchange and support. In a freestanding treatment center, it is also necessary to have at least one more person covering the phone and reception area, as well as dealing with insurance and billing issues.

Required Space

Regulations concerning minimum space and design requirements for health care facilities (health centers, suites, or clinics) may vary from state to state. Regulations can be obtained from professional associations.

It is desirable to have two treatment rooms per therapist, two bathrooms, a shower, an exercise room, a reception area (to include a waiting room), and a storage room.

Treatment room: ~80 to 100 square feet (per room) with the following equipment: treatment table (adjustable in height and able to support patients' weight), chair, clothes hanger, rolling stool, shelf with bandaging and padding materials, and patient education materials

The best patient scheduling is achieved by having two therapy rooms per therapist. If you allow ample time between patients, you may be able to function well with one room per therapist.

Bathroom/shower: ~50 square feet (per bathroom), wheelchair accessible. For appropriate patient hygiene, a shower within the treatment center is desirable. Patients have to wear the compression bandages between the daily treatment sessions and often remove the bandages at home before taking a shower. It is imperative for treatment success that the bandages are not removed at the patient's home (except if they cause pain or numbness in the extremity). Patients taking a shower at their home should protect the bandaged extremity with either a cast shield or a large trash bag. If a shower is not available in the treatment facility, patients should shower at home with the covered bandages in place, remove the bandages in the clinic, and wash the extremity with a washcloth at the clinic's sink.

Exercise room: ~300 to 500 square feet to accommodate exercise mats. For group exercises or support group meetings, a room size of ~1000 square feet is appropriate.

Reception area: ~400 square feet to accommodate patient waiting room, record storage, documentation space, and other materials

If the treatment facility provides twice-a-day treatment, a patient lounge area of ~400 square feet in addition to the reception area, containing a refrigerator, microwave, coffee/tea maker, audiovisual equipment, and comfortable rest area, is desirable.

Storage room: ~50 square feet to accommodate bandaging materials and other items

Equipment

The basic equipment needed for a well-run lymphedema clinic includes the following:

- Furniture for the reception area and treatment rooms

- Adjustable treatment tables
- Compression materials (see Suggested Materials to Start Up a Lymphedema Program later in this chapter)
- Audiovisual equipment and other materials for patient education
- Computer(s) and software (limb measurement program)
- Digital camera(s)
- Measuring tape(s) and documentation forms
- Manual sphygmomanometer(s)
- Exercise equipment (soft balls, sticks, therabands, etc.)
- Basic office supplies

Marketing Issues

Whether the lymphedema treatment center is freestanding or part of an existing clinic or department, referral sources must be developed to ensure success. The following suggestions should be considered to make the clinic's presence known to the lymphedema community and to physicians.

Direct mailings or visits to physicians in the community: The information source should contain a brochure outlining the clinic's services. When designing the brochure, it should be kept in mind that physicians are busy and prefer information that is precise, short, and to the point. A photo depicting a lymphedema patient before and after treatment with manual lymph drainage and complete decongestive therapy on the cover page of the brochure is always helpful to bring the point across.

Certified therapist listing on Web sites: Training centers for CDT generally contain a listing of their graduates on their Web sites, which can be accessed by patients seeking certified therapists.

Certified therapist listings in publications relevant to lymphedema: The National Lymphedema Network distributes a quarterly publication. This publication contains valuable information for lymphedema patients and therapists. For a fee, therapists and clinics may be listed in the resource guide of this publication.

Brochures: Brochures outlining the services provided should be distributed at health fairs and breast cancer/lymphedema–related events and at the offices of oncologists and vascular and plastic surgeons.

In-service presentations: Presentations can be given at local clinics and health care facilities. It is helpful to bring educational materials (posters, slides) to support each presentation.

Advertisements: Local newspapers and other media are appropriate vehicles for advertising services.

Insurance companies: The provider relations department of insurance companies offering coverage in the service area should be contacted and be made aware of the services the facility offers.

◆ Suggested Materials to Start Up a Lymphedema Program

An adequate inventory of supplies should be on hand before the lymphedema program opens. The treatment center should keep a sufficient quantity of compression materials in stock, or the patients themselves should be told to order the materials needed directly from a distributor before the initial treatment. The approximate quantity of compression materials needed for each individual patient during the decongestive phase is determined during the evaluation.

A detailed description of the materials used in lymphedema management and a listing of recommended materials used for upper and lower extremity lymphedema bandaging are given in Chapter 5, Required Materials.

The initial expense to keep a sufficient amount of lymphedema bandaging supply in stock is approximately $2500 to $3000 (this should cover ~10–15 patients).

Short-Stretch Bandages

- 10 rolls of 4 cm
- 20 rolls of 6 cm
- 20 rolls of 8 cm
- 40 rolls of 10 cm
- 5 rolls of 10 cm × 10 m (double length)

- 40 rolls of 12 cm
- 5 rolls of 12 cm × 10 m (double length)

Wide-width short-stretch bandages (white bandages)

- 5 rolls of 15 cm
- 5 rolls of 20 cm

Padding bandages

- 30 rolls of 10 cm
- 40 rolls of 15 cm

Soft foam

- (Best is 0.25 inch and 0.5 inch thickness with a recommended density of ~1.6 pounds per cubic foot, one sheet each)

High-density foam

- 10 pieces small Komprex kidney (size 0)
- 2 pad rolls (8 cm × 2 m × 1 cm)
- 4 sheets (100 cm × 50 cm × 1 cm)

Foam padding rolls (Rosidal Soft)—can be used instead of gray foam

- 30 rolls of 10 cm
- 15 rolls of 15 cm

Gauze Bandages (finger and toe bandages)

- Mollelast: 10 boxes (200 rolls) of 4 cm × 4 m, or 8 bags of Elastomull 1 inch × 4.1 yd
- 10 boxes (200 rolls) of 6 cm × 4 m, or 17 bags of Elastomull 2 inch × 4.1 yd
- Transelast (skin colored): 10 boxes (200 rolls) of 6 cm × 4 m

Stockinettes (tubular gauze)

- 2 boxes for small arms or children's legs (Lohmann size 5 or Tricofix D5)
- 2 boxes for "normal" arms and lower legs (Lohmann size 6 or Tricofix E6)
- 4 boxes for big arms and "normal" legs (Lohmann size 7 or Tricofix E6)
- 5 boxes for very big arms and bigger legs (Lohmann size 9 or Tricofix F7/G9)
- 2 boxes for very big legs, small trunk (Lohmann size K1)
- 2 boxes for extremely large legs and trunk (Lohmann size K2)

Lotion

- 10–15 8-ounce bottles, or 5 16-ounce bottles (Lymphoderm, Eucerin, etc.)

Other

♦ 5 bandage winders

♦ Educational materials (posters, etc.)

Some distributors offer prepacked bandage kits for lymphedema management. These kits are available for either upper or lower extremity lymphedema bandaging and typically contain two complete sets of short-stretch bandages, stockinettes, padding, and gauze bandages. Foam generally is not included and must be ordered separately. Ordering kits instead of separate items may simplify the ordering process, but distributors typically charge an additional amount for the packaging process.

♦ Reimbursements and Billing

If providers work on a private pay basis, a reasonable charge will have to be established, covering all expenses (including bandages, padding materials, etc.), plus profit. A price list detailing all parts of the treatment should be posted in the treatment center.

Health care reimbursement is an ever changing and very complex issue. Lymphedema management services are provided by physical therapists, physical therapist assistants, occupational therapists, occupational therapist assistants, massage therapists, and nurses. Insurance reimbursement may vary depending on providers and practice settings. Providers should confer with insurance companies to inquire about reimbursement policies for their individual professional group. It is also advisable to consult respective professional associations for the most current updates and regulations.

During the past years the Women's Health and Cancer Rights Act of 1998 (WHCRA) had a positive impact on reimbursement for lymphedema management. This federal law, which became effective October 21, 1998, requires group health plans (as well as payers providing individual coverage) that provide coverage for mastectomies, to also cover reconstructive surgery and prostheses following mastectomies. The treatment and management of physical complications resulting from mastectomies, such as lymphedema, are also covered under this act.

Not included in the statutes of this act is the type of treatment that must be provided. This decision is left to the individual insurance provider to determine.

Patients who had problems getting insurance coverage before the WHCRA became effective should contact their insurance company and ask the following questions:

1. Does the Women's Health and Cancer Rights Act of 1998 affect my coverage for lymphedema treatment?

2. Does my insurance policy cover manual lymph drainage and complete decongestive therapy (Current Procedural Terminology [CPT] code 97140) for the treatment of my lymphedema?

3. Is it necessary that a physical therapist perform the manual lymph drainage/complete decongestive therapy to be reimbursed, or can an occupational therapist, registered nurse, or massage therapist administer the therapy?

Patients should also contact their state's insurance department to find out whether the WHCRA will apply to the coverage if they are part of an insured group plan or individual health insurance.

Payers generally do not cover compression bandages and compression garments. Recent improvement has been seen in the coverage for gradient compression garments. Effective October 1, 2003, the Centers for Medicare and Medicaid Services (CMS) approved coverage for compression garments in the treatment of venous stasis ulcerations. Coverage may be provided for garments delivering compression between 30 and 50 mmHg and if the patient has an open venous stasis ulcer that has been treated by a physician or another health care professional.

The CMS article states in part that compression garments that serve a therapeutic or protective function may be covered if certain requirements are met. Because successful long-term lymphedema management depends on gradient compression garments as well, the lymphedema community should advocate for extended coverage to include lymphedema care.

Lymphedema clinics obtain their compression materials from vendors specialized in the distribution of lymphedema management materials. Depending on the individual practice setting, patients may reimburse the providers for materials used or order the necessary supplies directly from vendors.

CPT Codes

Correct coding is one of the most important, and often one of the most frustrating, aspects of successfully operating a practice for lymphedema management. Correct coding is something of a science, made even more complex by frequent changes in the definitions of the codes and the approved methods of combining them.

The five-digit codes apply to medical services or procedures performed by health care providers. The Current Procedural Terminology codes are established by the CPT editorial panel of the American Medical Association and have become the industry's coding standard for reporting.

The following CPT codes are commonly used in billing for lymphedema management; health care providers should be aware that the interpretation of these codes by various payers might vary.

Timed codes
When billing Medicare for any of the timed codes, the providers must follow appropriate CMS guidelines regarding unit of service requirements.

◆ Evaluation codes
◆ 97001: Physical therapy evaluation
◆ 97003: Occupational therapy evaluation

Therapy codes
◆ 97140: Manual therapy techniques (e.g., mobilization/manipulation, manual lymphatic drainage, manual traction), one or more regions. Charge is based on 15-minute increments.
◆ Depending on the condition, the MLD portion of the treatment may last between 30 minutes and 1 hour.
◆ 97530: Therapeutic activities, direct (one-on-one) patient contact by the provider (use of dynamic activities to improve functional performance). Based on 15-minute increments.

◆ Can be used with or without bandages on the affected extremity.
◆ 97110: Therapeutic procedure, one or more areas. Based on 15-minute increments. Therapeutic exercises to develop strength and endurance, range of motion, and flexibility.
◆ Can be used with or without bandages on the affected extremity (theraband, ball, etc.).
◆ 97535: Self-care/home management training. Self-care management, patient education in self-MLD for home program, self-bandaging, do's and don'ts, and appropriate activity guidelines. Charge is based on 15-minute increments.
◆ 97750: Physical performance test, measurements. Circumferential and/or volumetric measurements, with written report (measurement forms, volume programs). Charge is based on 15-minute increments.
◆ 97504: Orthotics fitting and training. Pressure garment measurements for upper or lower extremity and trunk
◆ 97039: Unlisted therapeutic procedure. Skin care, breathing exercises, deep abdominal techniques, therapist's application of low-pH skin lotion, antibiotic ointment or other skin treatments on the affected limb prior to bandaging
◆ ICD-9 codes

ICD-9 codes describe medical procedures performed by physicians and other health providers. The ICD-9 codes were developed by the Health Care Financing Administration (now the CMS) to assist in the assignment of reimbursement amounts to providers by Medicare carriers. A large number of managed care and other insurance companies, however, base their reimbursements on the values established by the CMS.

◆ 457.0 Postmastectomy lymphedema
◆ 457.1 Other lymphedema
◆ 757.0 Chronic hereditary lymphedema
◆ 729.81 Swelling of limb (upper and lower extremity)
◆ 629.8 Swelling of female genital organ
◆ 608.86 Swelling of male genital organ
◆ 607.83 Swelling of penis

Recommended Reading

1. American Medical Association. CPT Look Up Page. Available at:
   https://webstore.ama-assn.org/search/CptLookup.jhtml
2. Centers for Medicare and Medicaid Services. Medicare Newsletter Aug. 1, 2003. Available at:
   http://www.mutualmedicare.com/pdf/newsletters/2003080100s.pdf
3. Centers for Medicare and Medicaid Services. The Women's Health and Cancer Rights Act. Available at:
   http://www.cms.hhs.gov/hipaa/hipaa1/content/whcra.asp
4. Electronic Code of Federal Regulations 14 CFR, chapter 1, part 25, section 25–831
5. Electronic Code of Federal Regulations 14 CFR, chapter 1, part 25, section 25–841
6. Lymphology Association of North America Certified Lymphedema Therapist Candidate information brochure. Available at: http://www.clt-lana.org

Sample Forms and Templates

The following is a compilation of sample forms that may be helpful in the process of establishing a lymphedema clinic.

Patient Information

Date: _____

Patient's Name: _____

Address: _____

City: _____ State: _____ Zip Code: _____

Date of Birth: _____

Phone: (_____) _____ (Res.)

(_____) _____ ext. _____ (Business)

Marital Status: (M)   (S)   (O)ther

Social Security No.: _____

Patient's Employer: _____

Address: _____

City: _____ State: _____ Zip Code: _____

Phone: (_____) _____

Name of Spouse/Parent/Significant Other: _____

Address (if different than patient): _____

City: _____ State: _____ Zip Code: _____ Phone: _____

PLEASE HAVE INSURANCE CARD(S) AVAILABLE TO BE COPIED

Insurance Company: _____

Policy Holder's Name: _____ Policy Holder's Date of Birth: _____

Primary Care Physician: _____

Physician's Address: _____

Phone: (_____) _____ UPIN#: _____

How did you hear about our facility?: _____

Did you receive our brochure by mail? _____ YES _____ NO

I HAVE RECEIVED A COPY OF THE NOTICE OF PRIVACY PRACTICES _____ Yes _____ No

Figure 6–1 Patient information form.

Lymphedema Evaluation

Name: _____ Date: _____

1. For how long have you had lymphedema? _____

2. Have you ever had any lymphedema infections? _____

3. Do you ever leak fluid? _____

4. Do you take prophylactic antibiotics? _____

5. Do you take diuretics for lymphedema? _____

6. Do you take benzopyrones for lymphedema? _____

7. Do you take any other drugs for lymphedema? _____

8. Does anyone in your family have lymphedema? _____

9. Which extremity has lymphedema?
   (check all that apply)   Left Arm _____ Right Arm _____
                             Left Leg _____ Right Leg _____

10. Have you had prior treatment for lymphedema?
    (check all that apply)   Surgery _____ Compression Garment _____
                             Antibiotics _____ Pneumatic Pump _____
                             Manual Lymph Drainage _____

11. Do you have bronchial asthma? _____

12. Do you have hypertension? _____

13. Do you have diabetes? _____

14. Do you have allergies? _____

15. Do you have any cardiac problems? _____

16. Do you have any kidney problems? _____

17. Do you have any circulatory problems? _____

18. What medication(s) are you currently taking? _____

19. Have you ever had radiation therapy? _____

20. Have you ever received chemotherapy? _____

21. What operation(s) have you had? _____

(over)

Figure 6–2 Lymphedema evaluation, page 1.

Lymphedema Evaluation

(continued)

22. Which physician referred you to our facility? _____

    Name: _____

    Address: _____

    Phone: (   ) _____

23. Can we write to or discuss your lymphedema problem with this physician?
    YES _____ NO _____

24. If you are treated at this office, you will then be asked to follow a maintenance program at
    home.
    This consists of:
    a) Elastic sleeve or stocking worn during the day.
    b) Bandaging of limb overnight.
    c) Meticulous skin care to avoid infections.
    d) Remedial exercises to accelerate lymph flow.

    Are you prepared to follow such a program? _____

Figure 6-2 Lymphedema evaluation, page 2.

Physical Examination

Patient's Name: _____ Date: _____

D.O.B. _____

General Appearance: _____   Genitalia: _____

_____   _____

_____   _____

_____   _____

_____   Musculo/Skeletal: _____

Skin: _____   _____

_____   _____

_____   _____

HEENT: Head- _____   _____

        Ears- _____   Neurological: _____

        Eyes- _____   _____

        Nose- _____   _____

        Throat- _____   _____

Neck: _____   _____

_____   Other: _____

_____   _____

Chest/Lungs: _____   _____

_____   _____

_____

Cardiac: _____   Right Left   Left Right

_____

_____

Abdomen/Back: _____

_____

_____

_____

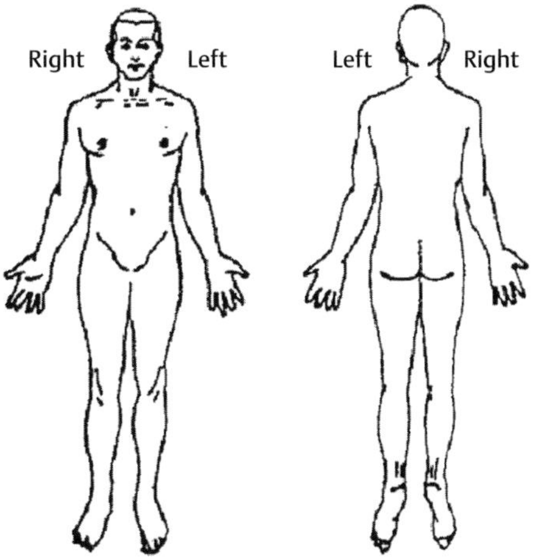

Figure 6–3 Physical evaluation form.

PATIENT: _____ DIAGNOSIS: _____

PRETREATMENT AFFECTED LIMB RIGHT ( ) LEFT ( ) BOTH ( )

DATE MEASURED

MEASUREMENTS

RIGHT	LEFT							

MEASUREMENTS ARE TAKEN IN CENTIMETERS cm 2.54 cm = 1 in.

WEIGHT

DATE WEIGHT

Lbs.	

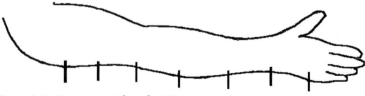

Figure 6–4 Measurement form for UE.

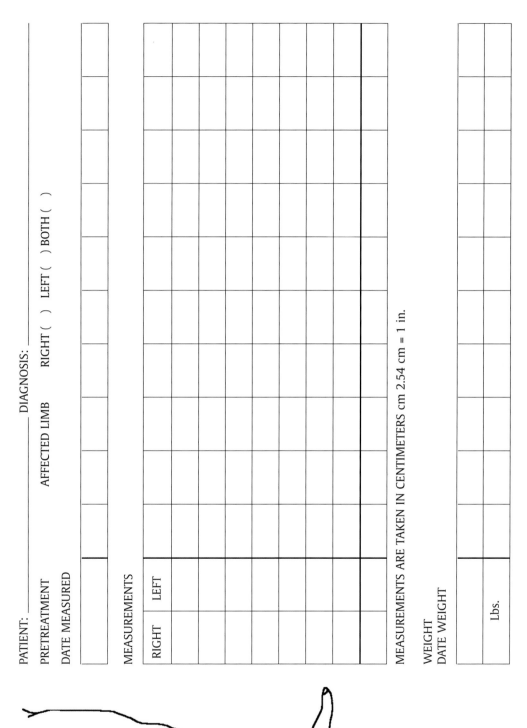

PATIENT: _____ DIAGNOSIS: _____

PRETREATMENT   AFFECTED LIMB   RIGHT ( )   LEFT ( )   BOTH ( )

DATE MEASURED

MEASUREMENTS

RIGHT	LEFT										

MEASUREMENTS ARE TAKEN IN CENTIMETERS cm 2.54 cm = 1 in.

WEIGHT

DATE WEIGHT

Lbs.

Figure 6–5 Measurement form for LE.

Progress Notes

PATIENT: _____

D.O.B.: _____

Date	

Figure 6–6 Progress notes form.

Photography Release Form

I _____ hereby give the
Facility's Name and Address the absolute and irrevocable right to take and permission to use photographs of me, or in which I may be included with others.

a) To copyright the same in said organization's own name or any name that they choose, and/or

b) To use re-use, publish and republish the same in whole or in parts, individually or in conjunction with other photographs, in any medium and for the purpose of medical information of the public, medical staff of clinic employees, including (but not by the way of limitation) illustration, promotion, and advertising and trade, and/or

c) To use my name in connection therewith if they so choose Yes _____ No _____

d) Restrictions: _____ No facial photographs _____ Other _____
_____

I hereby release and discharge the Academy of Lymphatic Studies from any and all claims and demands arising out of or in conjunction with the use of photographs, including but not limited to any and all claims of libel, invasion of privacy, etc.

This authorization and release shall also ensure to the benefit of the legal representatives, licensees and assigns of the Academy of Lymphatic Studies.

I am over the age of eighteen, have read the foregoing and fully understand the contents thereof.

ADULT RELEASE   MINOR RELEASE

_____   _____
(Subject's Name)   (Minor's Name)

_____   _____
(Signature)   (Signature – Parent, Guardian)

                                         _____
                                              (Relationship to Subject)

_____   _____
(Witness)   (Date)

Figure 6–7   Photography release form.

Notice of Privacy Practices
Patient Consent Form

Name of Practice: _____

The Department of Health and Human Services has established a "Privacy Rule" to help insure that personal health care information is protected for privacy. The Privacy Rule was also created in order to provide a standard for certain health care providers to obtain their patients' consent for uses and disclosures of health information about the patient to carry out treatment, payment or health care operations. As our patient we want you to know that we respect the privacy of your personal medical records and that we will do all we can to secure and protect that privacy. We strive to always take reasonable precautions to protect your privacy. When it is appropriate and necessary, we provide the minimum necessary information to only those we feel are in need of your health care information and information about treatment, payment or health care operations, in order to provide health care that is in your best interest.

We also want you to know that we support your full access to your personal medical records. We may have indirect treatment relationships with you (such as laboratories that only interact with physicians and not patients), and may have to disclose personal health information for purposes of treatment, payment or health care operations. These entities are most often not required to obtain patient consent.

You may refuse to consent to the use or disclosure of your personal health information, but this must be in writing.

Receipt of Notice of Privacy Practices
Written Acknowledgment Form

I, (Patient's Name) _____, have received and

reviewed a copy of (Name of Practice) _____ 's Notice of Privacy Practices.

Signature of the patient or the patient's guardian: _____

Date: _____

Figure 6–8 Privacy rules consent form.

Patient Authorization for Use and Disclosures of Protected Health Information to Third Parties

Name of Practice: _____

Section A: Must be completed for all authorizations

I hereby authorize the use of disclosure of my individually identifiable health information as described below. I understand that this authorization is voluntary. I understand that if the organization authorized to receive the information is not a health plan or health care provider, the released information may no longer be protected by federal privacy regulations

Patient's Name: _____ ID Number: _____

Persons/organizations providing information:

_____

Persons/organizations receiving the information:

_____

Specific description of information (including date(s)):

_____

_____

Section B: Must be completed only if a health plan or health care provider has requested the authorization

1. The provider must complete the following statement:
   will the healthcare provider requesting the authorization receive financial or in-kind compensation in exchange for using or disclosing the health information described above?
   Yes _____ No _____

2. The patient must read and initial the following statement:
   I understand that I will receive a copy of this form once I have signed it. Patient's initials: _____

Section C: Must be completed for all authorizations

The patient or the patient's representative must read and initial the following statements:
1. I understand that this authorization will expire on _____/_____/_____ (DD/MM/YYYY)
   Initials: _____

2. I understand that I may revoke this authorization at any time by notifying the practice in writing. I understand that this revocation will not have any effect on any actions they took before they received the revocation. Initials: _____

Signature of the patient or the patient's representative: _____

Printed name of the patient or the patient's representative: _____

Relationship to the patient: _____

Figure 6–9 Health information consent form.

Letter of Medical Necessity

Date:

RE:

To Whom It May Concern:

I had the pleasure of seeing Mr./Mrs. _____ on _____

He/she was found to have Primary/Secondary Lymphedema of the _____ following

_____

I believe he/she will benefit from _____ treatments of Complete Decongestive Therapy, given daily for a total of _____ weeks.

Complete Decongestive Therapy:

Each CDT treatment consists of four steps –

1. Meticulous skin and nail care, including the eradication of any infection

2. Manual Lymph Drainage, a manual treatment technique that stimulates lymph vessels to contract more frequently and that channels lymph and edema fluid toward adjacent, functioning lymph systems. Manual Lymph Drainage begins with stimulation of the lymph vessels and nodes in adjacent basins (neck, contralateral/ipsilateral axilla and/or groin), which is followed by manual decongestion, in segmental order, of the involved trunk, upper part, lower part of the extremity, wrist (ankle) and hand (foot). Edema fluid and obstructed lymphatics are made to drain toward the venous angle, toward functioning lymph basins across the mid-line of the body, down toward the groin, over the top of the shoulder, around the back and so forth.

3. Compression Bandaging is done immediately after Manual Lymph Drainage. Bandages are applied from the distal to the proximal aspect of the extremity with maximal pressure distally and minimal pressure proximally. This is done by using several layers of cotton bandages or foam materials to ensure uniform pressure distribution or to increase pressure in areas that are particularly fibrotic. The bandages do not constrict blood flow but increase diminished skin and interstitial pressures. This prevents any re-accumulation of excavated edema fluid and also prevents the ultrafiltration of additional fluid into the interstitial space.

4. The bandaged patient is next guided through a series of decongestive exercises with the muscles and joints functioning within closed space. The exercises increase lymph flow in all available lymph channels and in collateral pathways that are used to make the passage to the venous angle.

This should reduce his/her swelling and stabilize his/her condition. Without this therapy, his/her swelling can be expected to progress and lead to complications.

The patient will also be instructed in a home maintenance program so that he/she can continue treatment on his/her own at home.

Sincerely,

Figure 6–10 Example of letter of medical necessity.

Information on Lymphedema

What Is Lymphedema?

Lymphedema is a swelling of a body part, most often the extremities. It may also occur in the face, the trunk, the abdomen or the genital area. Lymphedema is the result of an accumulation of protein-rich fluid in the superficial tissues, which can have significant pathological and clinical consequences for the patient if left untreated. Once present, this chronic and progressive condition will not disappear again.

Causes of Lymphedema

Lymphedema is classified as either primary or secondary. Primary lymphedema is caused by congenital malformations of the lymphatic system and may be present at birth or develop later in life, often in puberty or during pregnancy. Primary forms usually affect the lower extremities but may also be present in upper extremities.

Secondary lymphedema is more common and often the result of surgery or radiation therapy for cancer. Surgical procedures in combination with the removal of lymph nodes, such as mastectomies or lumpectomies with the removal and/or radiation of axillary lymph nodes, are a very common reason for the onset of secondary lymphedema in the United States. Other causes include trauma or infection of the lymphatic system. Severe venous insufficiencies may also contribute to the onset of lymphedema (phlebolymphostatic edema).

Primary and secondary lymphedema may affect the upper or lower extremity. In general it can be said that the legs are more often involved in primary lymphedema whereas secondary forms are more commonly found in the upper extremities.

Symptoms of Lymphedema

Early stages of lymphedema (stage I) may be temporarily reduced by simple elevation of the limb. Without proper treatment, however, the protein-rich swelling causes a progressive hardening of the affected tissues; this condition is known as lymphostatic fibrosis and is present in stage II lymphedema. Other complications such as fungal infections, additional hardening and very often an extreme increase in volume of the swollen extremity are typical for stage III lymphedema.

Primary and secondary lymphedema usually affects one extremity only; if both extremities, for example, both legs, are involved, the swelling appears asymmetrically.

Treatment Methods

Medication: Diuretics are often prescribed in order to control lymphedema but are proven to have very poor long-term results in the treatment of this condition. Diuretics decrease the water content of the swelling while the protein molecules remain in the tissues. As soon as the diuretic loses its effectiveness, these proteins continue to draw water to the edematous area.

Surgery: Several surgical procedures for lymphedema are described. It is safe to say that not a single one of these surgeries performed during the past century showed consistent results.

Pneumatic Compression Pumps: This mechanical device works with sleeves containing compressed air, which are applied to the patients swollen extremity. Inappropriate use of these devices can cause serious complications in lymphedema patients. In some cases pumps may be applied under the supervision of specially trained therapists and in combination with other treatment modalities (see below).

Complete Decongestive Therapy (CDT): Since there is no cure for lymphedema, the goal of the therapy is to reduce the swelling and to maintain the reduction. For the majority of the patients this can be achieved by the skillful application of this therapy, which is safe, reliable and non-invasive. CDT shows good long-term results in both primary and secondary lymphedema; it consists of two phases and the following combined modalities –

Manual Lymph Drainage (MLD): this gentle manual treatment technique increases the activity of certain lymph vessels and manually moves interstitial fluid. Applied correctly, a series of MLD treatments decreases the volume of the affected extremity to a normal or near normal size and is applied daily in the first phase of the therapy.

Compression Therapy: the elastic fibers in the skin are damaged in lymphedema. In order to prevent reaccumulation of fluid it is necessary to apply sufficient compression to the affected extremity.

Figure 6–11 Information on lymphedema for patients.

Compression therapy also improves the function of the muscle pumps, helps to reduce fibrotic tissue and promotes venous and lymphatic return.

In the first phase of CDT compression therapy is achieved with the application of special short-stretch bandages. These bandage materials are used between MLD treatments and prevent the reaccumulation of lymph fluid, which has been moved out of the extremity during the MLD session. Once the extremity is decongested, the patient wears compression garments during the day. In some cases it may be necessary for the patient to additionally apply bandages during nighttime. In order to achieve best results, specially trained personnel should take measurements for these elastic support garments; incorrectly fitted sleeves or stockings will have negative effects. The type of garments (round or flat-knit style) and the compression class depend on many factors such as the patient's age and the severity of the swelling. For upper extremity lymphedema, compression classes I (20–30 mmHg) or II (30–40 mmHg); for lymphedema of the lower extremities, compression classes II, III (40–50 mmHg) or IV (>50 mmHg) are suitable. In some cases it may be necessary to apply compression class III to an upper extremity or an even greater compression than class IV to a lower extremity lymphedema. This can be achieved by wearing two stockings on top of each other, or by the application of bandages on top of a stocking.

To have the maximum effect, garments must be worn every day and replaced after six months.

Exercises: a customized exercise program is designed by the therapist for each patient. These decongestive exercises aid the effects of the joint and muscle pumps and should be performed by the patient wearing the compression bandage or garment. Vigorous movements or exercises causing pain must be avoided. Exercises should be performed slowly and with both, the affected and non-affected extremity.

Skin care: the skin in lymphedema is very susceptible to infections and usually dry. A low-pH lotion, free of alcohol and fragrances should be used to maintain the moisture of the skin and to avoid infections. You should consult your physician if there are any fungal infections present in your affected extremity.

Do's and Don'ts

Your lymphedema therapist will explain to you in detail how to avoid infections and other conditions, which could lead to a worsening of your lymphedema. Listed below are just a few general guidelines:

Avoid any injuries to the skin – be careful working in the garden, playing with your pets or doing housework. Avoid the use of scissors to cut your nails and don't cut your cuticles. Injuries, even small ones may cause infections.

Avoid mosquito bites – wear insect repellents when outdoors. A single mosquito bite can cause an infection.

Use caution when exercising – avoid movements that overstrain, discuss proper exercises and activities with your therapist

Avoid heat – very hot showers, hot packs on your extremity, sunbathing and the use of saunas could have a negative effect on your lymphedema. Avoid extreme changes in temperature (hot/cold), massages ("Swedish") on your affected extremity or any cosmetics that irritate the skin.

Inform all health care personnel that you have lymphedema – injections or acupuncture in your affected extremity should be avoided. Blood pressure should be taken on the extremity free of lymphedema.

Nutrition is important – there is no special diet for lymphedema. Today most nutritionists recommend a low salt, low fat diet. Obesity may have a negative effect on your swelling.

Travel – avoid mosquito-infected areas; when traveling by airplane apply an additional bandage on top of your garment.

Clothing – clothing that is too tight may restrict the proper flow of lymph. Avoid tight bras, panties or socks and make sure your jewelry fits loosely.

See your doctor – if you have any signs of an infection (fever, chills, red and hot skin), fungal infections or if you notice any other unusual changes that may be related to your lymphedema.

General Tips – always wear your compression garments during the day and if necessary your bandages at night; elevate your extremity as often as possible during the daytime; perform your exercises daily and always consult your doctor or therapist should you have any questions about your lymphedema.

GLOSSARY

Anastomosis

1. A natural communication between two vessels; may be direct or by means of connecting channels. 2. The surgical or pathological connection of two tubular structures.

Plural: *anastomoses*

Venes DJ, ed. Anastomosis. In: Taber's Cyclopedic Medical Dictionary. 19th ed. Philadelphia: FA Davis Co; 2001:93

Angiography

1. A description of blood vessels and lymphatics. 2. Diagnostic or therapeutic radiography of the heart and blood vessels using a radiopaque contrast medium. Types include magnetic resonance imaging, interventional radiology, and computed tomography. 3. Recording of arterial pulse movements by use of a sphygmograph.

Venes DJ, ed. Angiography. In: Taber's Cyclopedic Medical Dictionary. 19th ed. Philadelphia: FA Davis Co; 2001:106

Angioma

A form of tumor, usually benign, consisting principally of blood vessels (hemangioma) or lymph vessels (lymphangioma). It is considered to be remnants of fetal tissue misplaced or undergoing disordered development.

Venes DJ, ed. Angioma. In: Taber's Cyclopedic Medical Dictionary. 19th ed. Philadelphia: FA Davis Co; 2001:106

Angiosarcoma

Malignant neoplasm originating from blood vessels.

Synonym: *hemangiosarcoma*

Venes DJ, ed. Angiosarcoma. In: Taber's Cyclopedic Medical Dictionary. 19th ed. Philadelphia: FA Davis Co; 2001:108

Ankle–Brachial Index (ABI)

The ankle–brachial index is used to identify the presence of peripheral arterial disease (PAD) in the lower extremities. Instead of a stethoscope, a Doppler device (usually a 5 or 7 mHz hand-held Doppler) is used to listen to the systolic blood pressure on the arms and ankles; the ABI is measured in the resting position. To calculate the ABI, the systolic pressures of the ankles are divided by the systolic pressure of the arm on the same side; i.e. left ankle pressure divided by left brachial pressure determines the ABI on the left side. ABI values above 0.9 are generally normal; values below 0.9 indicate angiographic arterial disease.

Baker's Cyst

(William M. Baker, Brit. surgeon, 1839–1896) A synovial cyst (pouch) arising from the synovial lining of the knee. It occurs in the popliteal fossa.

Venes DJ, ed. Baker's cyst. In: Taber's Cyclopedic Medical Dictionary. 19th ed. Philadelphia: FA Davis Co; 2001:192

Bioburden

The number of contaminating microbes on a certain amount of material prior to that material being sterilized.

OMD Online Medical Dictionary. Bioburden. Available at: http://cancerweb.ncl.ac.uk/cgi-bin/omd?query=bioburden&action=Search+OMD (2001). Accessed February 2004

Bulla

A large blister or skin vesicle filled with fluid; a bleb.

Plural: *bullae*

Venes DJ, ed. Bulla. In: Taber's Cyclopedic Medical Dictionary. 19th ed. Philadelphia: FA Davis Co; 2001:276

Cardiac Edema

A: An accumulation of serum fluid from blood plasma in the interstitial tissues as a result of congestive heart failure. In severe cases, the fluid may also accumulate in serous cavities.

Anderson K, Anderson L, Glanze W. Cardiac edema. In: Mosby's Medical Dictionary. 5th ed. St. Louis, MO: Mosby; 1998:268

B: Accumulation of fluid due to congestive heart failure. It is most apparent in the dependent portion of the body.

Venes DJ, ed. Cardiac e. In: Taber's Cyclopedic Medical Dictionary. 19th ed. Philadelphia: FA Davis Co; 2001:604

Cellulitis

A: A diffuse, acute infection of the skin and subcutaneous tissue characterized most commonly by local heat, redness, pain, and swelling, and occasionally by fever, malaise, chills, and headache. Abscess and tissue destruction usually follow if antibiotics are not taken. The infection is more likely to develop in the presence of damaged skin, poor circulation, or diabetes mellitus. In addition to appropriate antibiotics, treatment includes warm soaks, elevation, and avoidance of pressure to the affected areas.

Anderson K, Anderson L, Glanze W. Cellulitis. In: Mosby's Medical Dictionary. 5th ed. St. Louis, MO: Mosby; 1998:290

B: A spreading bacterial infection of the skin, usually caused by streptococcal or staphylococcal infections, that results in severe inflammation with erythema, warmth, and localized edema. The extremities, esp. the lower legs, are the most common sites. Adjacent soft tissue may be involved, esp. in patients with diabetes mellitus. Cellulitis involving the face is called erysipelas. When it affects the lower extremities, cellulitis must be differentiated from stasis dermatitis, which is associated most commonly with bilateral chronic dependant edema, and occasionally with deep venous thrombosis. Patients with diabetes mellitus are at increased risk for cellulitis because of the peripheral vascular disease, neuropathy and decreased immune function associated with diabetes.

ETIOLOGY: Bacteria gain access through breaks in the skin and spread rapidly; lesions between the toes from athlete's foot are common entry sites.

TREATMENT: For mild cases of cellulitis, oral dicloxacillin or cefazolin is effective. For severe cases, intravenous penicillinase-resistant penicillins are used; imipenem and surgical debridement to obtain cultures and to rule out fasciitis are recommended for patients with diabetes.

Venes DJ, ed. Cellulitis. In: Taber's Cyclopedic Medical Dictionary. 19th ed. Philadelphia: FA Davis Co; 2001:343

Chyle

A: The cloudy liquid products of digestion taken up by the small intestine. Consisting mainly of emulsified fats, chyle passes through fingerlike projections in the small intestine, called lacteals, and into the lymphatic system for transport to the venous circulation at the thoracic duct in the neck. Also called chylus. –chylous, *adj.*

Anderson K, Anderson L, Glanze W. Chyle. In: Mosby's Medical Dictionary. 5th ed. St. Louis, MO: Mosby; 1998:339

B: The milklike, alkaline contents of the lacteals and lymphatic vessels of the intestine, consisting of digestive products and principally absorbed fats. It is carried by the lymphatic vessels to the cisterna chyli, then through the thoracic duct to the left subclavian vein, where it enters the bloodstream. A large amount forms in 24 hours.

Venes DJ, ed. Chyle. In: Taber's Cyclopedic Medical Dictionary. 19th ed. Philadephia: FA Davis Co; 2001:385

Colloid

1. A gluelike substance, such as a protein or starch, whose particles (molecules or aggregates of molecules), when dispersed as much as possible in a solvent, remain uniformly distributed and do not form a true solution. 2. The size of a microscopic colloid; particles ranging from 10^{-9} to 10^{-11} meters (1 to 100 nm). 3. A homogeneous gelatinous substance found within the follicles of the thyroid gland and containing the thyroid hormones.

colloidal, *adj.*

Venes DJ, ed. Colloid. In: Taber's Cyclopedic Medical Dictionary. 19th ed. Philadelphia: FA Davis Co; 2001:412

Comorbidity (comorbid disease)

A disease that worsens or impacts the primary disease (e.g., the primary disease could be cancer and the comorbid disease emphysema).

Venes DJ, ed. Comorbid disease. In: Taber's Cyclopedic Medical Dictionary. 19th ed. Philadelphia: FA Davis Co; 2001:421

Congenital

Present at birth.

Venes DJ, ed. Congenital. In: Taber's Cyclopedic Medical Dictionary. 19th ed. Philadelphia: FA Davis Co; 2001:431

Congestive Heart Failure (CHF)

A: An abnormal condition that reflects impaired cardiac pumping, caused by myocardial infarction, ischemic heart disease, or cardiomyopathy. Failure of the ventricle to eject blood efficiently results in volume overload, chamber dilatation, and elevated intracardiac pressure. Retrograde transmission of increased hydrostatic pressure from the left heart causes pulmonary congestion; elevated right heart pressure causes systemic venous congestion and peripheral edema.

Anderson K, Anderson L, Glanze W. Congestive heart failure (CHF). In: Mosby's Medical Dictionary. 5th ed. St. Louis, MO: Mosby; 1998:386

Contralateral

Pertaining to the opposite side. The opposite of *ipsilateral.*

Coracoid Process

A long, curved projection from the neck of the scapula overhanging the glenoid cavity; it gives attachment to the short head of the biceps, the coracobrachialis, and the pectoralis minor muscles, and the conoid and coracoacromial ligaments.

Synonym: *processus coracoideus*

OMD Online Medical Dictionary. Coracoid process. Available at: http://cancerweb.ncl.ac.uk/cgi-bin/omd?query=coracoid+process (2000). Accessed February 2004

Deep Venous Thrombosis (DVT)

A blood clot in one or more of the deep veins in the legs (the most common site), arms, pelvis, neck axilla, or chest. The clot may damage the vein or may embolize to other organs (e.g. the heart or lungs). Such emboli are occasionally fatal.

ETIOLOGY: DVT results from one or more of the following conditions: blood stasis (e.g. bedrest); endothelial injury (e.g., after surgery or trauma); hypercoagulability (e.g., factor V Leiden, or deficiencies of antithrombin III, protein C or protein S); congestive heart failure; estrogen use; malignancy; nephrotic syndrome; obesity; pregnancy; thrombocytosis; or many other conditions). DVT is a common occurrence among hospitalized patients, many of whom cannot walk or have one or more of the other risk factors just mentioned.

SYMPTOMS: The patient may report a dull ache or heaviness in the limb, and swelling or redness may be present, but just as often patients have vague symptoms, making clinical diagnosis unreliable.

DIAGNOSIS: Compression ultrasonography is commonly used to diagnose DVT (failure of a vein to compress is evidence of a clot within its walls). Other diagnostic techniques include impedance phlethysmography and venography.

TREATMENT: Unfractionated heparin or low molecular weight heparin (LMWH) is given initially, followed by several months of therapy with an oral anticoagulant such as warfarin.

COMPLICATIONS: Pulmonary emboli are common and may compromise oxygenation or result in frank cardiac arrest. Postphlebitic syndrome, a chronic swelling and aching of the affected limb, also occurs often.

PREVENTION: In hospitalized patients and other immobilized persons, early ambulation, pneumatic compression stockings, or low doses of unfractionated heparin, LMWH, or warfarin may be given to reduce the risk of DVT.

Venes DJ, ed. Thrombosis—deep venous t. In: Taber's Cyclopedic Medical Dictionary. 19th ed. Philadephia: FA Davis Co; 2001:1948

Dehiscence

1. A bursting open, as of a graafian follicle or a wound, especially a surgical abdominal wound. 2. In dentistry, an isolated area in which the tooth root is denuded of bone from the margin nearly to the apex. It occurs more often in anterior than posterior teeth, and more on the vestibular than the oral surface.

Venes DJ, ed. Dehiscence. In: Taber's Cyclopedic Medical Dictionary. 19th ed. Philadelphia: FA Davis Co; 2001:500

Desiccation

The process of drying up.

Diffusion

1. The tendency of molecules of a substance (gaseous, liquid, or solid) to move from a region of high concentration to one of lower concentration. 2. Absorption of a liquid, such as the absorption by cells of water from lymph when the percentage of salt is less in the lymph than in the cells. When the percentage is greater in the lymph, water is withdrawn from the cells. SEE: *osmosis.* 3. A process whereby various gases interpenetrate and become mixed through the incessant motion of their molecules. Similarly, if aqueous solutions of different materials stand in contact, mixing occurs on standing even if the solutions are separated by thin membranes.

Venes DJ, ed. Diffusion. In: Taber's Cyclopedic Medical Dictionary. 19th edition. Philadelphia: FA Davis Co; 2001:541

Diuretic

1. Increasing urine secretion. 2. An agent that increases urine output. Diuretics are used to treat hypertension, congestive heart failure, and edema. Common side effects of these agents are potassium depletion, low blood pressure, dehydration, and hyponatremia.

Venes DJ, ed. Diuretic. In: Taber's Cyclopedic Medical Dictionary. 19th ed. Philadelphia: FA Davis Co; 2001:564

Diverticulitis

Inflammation of a diverticulum or diverticula in the intestinal tract, especially in the colon, causing pain, anorexia, fevers, and occasionally peritonitis.

Venes DJ, ed. Diverticulitis. In: Taber's Cyclopedic Medical Dictionary. 19th ed. Philadelphia: FA Davis Co; 2001:564

Diverticulosis

Diverticula in the colon without inflammation or symptoms. Only a small percentage of persons with diverticulosis develop diverticulitis.

Venes DJ, ed. Diverticulosis. In: Taber's Cyclopedic Medical Dictionary. 19th ed. Philadelphia: FA Davis Co; 2001:564

Ecchymosis

A bruise, that is, superficial bleeding under the skin or a mucous membrane.

Plural: *ecchymoses*
ecchymotic, *adj.*

Venes DJ, ed. Ecchymosis. In: Taber's Cyclopedic Medical Dictionary. 19th ed. Philadelphia: FA Davis Co; 2001:596

Endothelium

A form of squamous epithelium consisting of flat cells that line the blood and lymphatic vessels, the heart, and various other body cavities. It is derived from mesoderm. Endothelial cells are metabolically active and produce several compounds that affect the vascular lumen and platelets. Included are endothelium-derived relaxing factor (EDRF), prostacyclin, endothelium-derived contracting factors 1 and 2 (EDCF1, EDCF2), endothelium-derived hyperpolarizing factor (EDHF), and thrombomodulin.

Venes DJ, ed. Endothelium. In: Taber's Cyclopedic Medical Dictionary. 19th ed. Philadelphia: FA Davis Co; 2001:642

Erysipelas

A: An infectious skin disease characterized by redness, swelling, vesicles, bullae, fever, pain, and lymphadenopathy. It is caused by a species of group A, β-hemolytic streptococci. Treatment includes antibiotics, analgesics, and packs or dressings applied locally to the lesions.

Anderson K, Anderson L, Glanze W. Erysipelas. In: Mosby's Medical Dictionary. 5th ed. St. Louis: Mosby; 1998:583

B: An infection of the skin (usually caused by a group of streptococci) that is marked by a bright red, sharply defined rash on the face or the legs. Systemic symptoms such as fevers, chills, sweats, or vomiting may occur; local tissue swelling and tenderness are common,. A toxin released into the skin by *Streptococcus pyogenes* creates many of the signs and symptoms of the infection.

TREATMENT: Penicillins, erythromycin, first-generation cephalosporins, vancomycin, or clindamycin may effectively eradicate the responsible bacteria. Analgesic and antipyretic drugs, such as acetaminophen or ibuprofen, provide comfort.

Venes DJ, ed. Erysipelas. In: Taber's Cyclopedic Medical Dictionary. 19th ed. Philadelphia: FA Davis Co; 2001:667

Eschar

This is a dry scab that forms on skin that has been burned or exposed to corrosive agents.

OMD Online Medical Dictionary. Coracoid process. Available at: http://cancer-web.ncl.ac.uk/cgi-bin/omd?query=eschar&action=Search+OMD (2001). Accessed February 2004

Fascia

A fibrous membrane covering, supporting, and separating muscles.

Plural: *fasciae*

fascial, *adj.*

Venes DJ, ed. Fascia. In: Taber's Cyclopedic Medical Dictionary. 19th ed. Philadelphia: FA Davis Co; 2001:706

Filaria

A long thread-shaped nematode belonging to the superfamily Filarioidea. The adults live in vertebrates. In humans, they may infect the lymphatic vessels and lymphatic organs, circulatory system, connective tissues, subcutaneous tissues, and serous cavities. Typically, the female produces larvae called microfilariae, which may be sheathed or sheathless. They reach the peripheral blood or lymphatic vessels, where they may be ingested by a blood-sucking arthropod (a mosquito, gnat, or fly). In the intermediate host, they transform into rhabditoid larvae that metamorphose into infective filariform larvae. These migrate to the proboscis and

are deposited in or on the skin of the vertebrate host.

Plural: *filariae*

filarial, *adj.*

Venes DJ, ed. Filaria. In: Taber's Cyclopedic Medical Dictionary. 19th ed. Philadelphia: FA Davis Co; 2001:726

Filariasis

A chronic disease caused by the parasitic nematode worm *Wuchereria bancrofti* or *Brugi malayi*.

Gate-Control Theory (Gate-Control Hypothesis)

A: A theory to explain the mechanism of pain; small fiber afferent stimuli, particularly pain, entering the substantia gelatinosa can be modulated by large fiber afferent stimuli and descending spinal pathways so that their transmission to ascending spinal pathways is blocked (gated).

Synonym: *gate-control hypothesis*

OMD Online Medical Dictionary. Gate-control theory. Available at: http://cancer-web.ncl.ac.uk/cgi-bin/omd?gate-control+theory (2000). Accessed February 2004

B: The hypothesis that painful stimuli may be prevented from reaching higher levels of the central nervous system by stimulation of larger sensory nerves. This is one of the proposed explanations of the action of acupuncture.

Venes DJ, ed. Gate theory. In: Taber's Cyclopedic Medical Dictionary. 19th ed. Philadelphia: FA Davis Co; 2001:782

Hereditary

Pertaining to a genetic characteristic transmitted from parent to offspring.

Venes DJ, eEd. Hereditary. In: Taber's Cyclopedic Medical Dictionary. 19th ed. Philadelphia: FA Davis Co; 2001:888

Hilum (Hilus)

1. A depression or recess at the exit or entrance of a duct into a gland or of nerves and vessels into an organ. 2. The root of the lungs at the level of the fourth and fifth dorsal vertebrae.

Plural: *hila*

Venes DJ, ed. Hilum. In: Taber's Cyclopedic Medical Dictionary. 19th ed. Philadelphia: FA Davis Co; 2001:901

Homeostasis

The state of dynamic equilibrium of the internal environment of the body that is maintained by the ever changing processes of feedback and regulation in response to internal and external changes.

homeostatic, *adj.*

Venes DJ, ed. Homeostasis. In: Taber's Cyclopedic Medical Dictionary. 19th ed. Philadelphia: FA Davis Co; 2001:909

Hyperkeratosis

1. An overgrowth of the cornea. 2. An overgrowth of the horny layer of the epidermis.

Venes DJ, ed. Hyperkeratosis. In: Taber's Cyclopedic Medical Dictionary. 19th ed. Philadelphia: FA Davis Co; 2001:934

Hypoproteinemia

A decrease in the amount of protein in the blood.

Venes DJ, ed. Hypoproteinemia. In: Taber's Cyclopedic Medical Dictionary. 19th ed. Philadelphia: FA Davis Co; 2001:950

Hysterectomy

Surgical removal of the uterus. Each year, about 500,000 women undergo hysterectomies. Indications for the surgery include benign or malignant changes in the uterine wall or cavity and cervical abnormalities (including endometrial cancer, cervical cancer, severe dysfunctional bleeding, large or bleeding fibroid tumors, prolapse of the uterus, or severe endometriosis). The approach to excision may be either abdominal or vaginal. The abdominal approach is used most commonly to remove large tumors; when the ovaries and the fallopian tubes also will be removed; and when there is need to examine adjacent pelvis structures, such as the regional lymph nodes. Vaginal hysterectomy is appropriate when uterine size is less than that in 12 week gestation, no

other abdominal pathology is suspected, and when surgical plans include cystocele, enterocele, or rectocele repair.

Venes DJ, ed. Hysterectomy. In: Taber's Cyclopedic Medical Dictionary. 19th ed. Philadelphia: FA Davis Co; 2001:953

Ileus

An intestinal obstruction. The term originally meant colic due to intestinal obstruction. It is characterized by loss of the forward flow of intestinal contents, often accompanied by abdominal cramps; constipation; fecal vomiting; abdominal distention; and collapse.

Venes DJ, ed. Ileus. In: Taber's Cyclopedic Medical Dictionary. 19th ed. Philadelphia: FA Davis Co; 2001:962

Ipsilateral

Pertaining to the same side. The opposite of *contralateral* or *crossed* side.

Lipectomy

Excision of fatty tissues.

Lipedema

A condition in which fat deposits accumulate in the lower extremities, from the hips to the ankles, accompanied by symptoms of tenderness in the affected areas.

Anderson K, Anderson L, Glanze W. Lipedema. In: Mosby's Medical Dictionary. 5th ed. St. Louis, MO: Mosby; 1998:946

Liposuction

The removal of subcutaneous fat tissue with a blunt-tipped cannula introduced into the fatty area through a small incision. Suction is then applied and fat tissue removed. Liposuction is a form of plastic surgery intended to remove adipose tissue from localized areas of fat accumulation as on the hips, knees, buttocks, thighs, face, arms, or neck. To be cosmetically successful, the skin should be elastic enough to contract after the underlying fat has been removed Liposuction will not benefit dimpled or sagging skin or flabby muscles. There are no health benefits to liposuction, and as with any surgery there may be risks such as infection, severe postoperative pain, cardiac arrhythmias, shock, and even death. There is also the possibility that the results will be unsatisfactory to the patient.

Synonym: *suction lipectomy*

Venes DJ, ed. Liposuction. In: Taber's Cyclopedic Medical Dictionary. 19th ed. Philadelphia: FA Davis Co; 2001:1120

Lymph

A: A thin watery fluid originating in organs and tissues of the body that circulates through the lymphatic vessels and is filtered by the lymph nodes. Lymph enters the bloodstream at the junction of the internal jugular and subclavian veins. It contains chyle, erythrocytes, and leukocytes, most of which are lymphocytes.

Anderson K, Anderson L, Glanze W. Lymph. In: Mosby's Medical Dictionary. 5th ed. St. Louis, MO: Mosby; 1998:966

B: The name given to tissue fluid that has entered lymph capillaries and is found in larger lymph vessels. It is alkaline, clear and colorless, although lymph vessels from the small intestines appear milky from the absorbed fats (chyle). The protein content of the lymph is lower than that of plasma, osmotic pressure is slightly higher, and viscosity slightly less. Specific gravity is 1.016 to 1.023. Lymph is mostly water, and contains albumin, globulins, salts, urea, neutral fats, and glucose. Its cells are mainly lymphocytes and monocytes, formed in the lymph nodes and nodules. Lymph capillaries, found in most tissue spaces, collect tissue fluid, which is then called lymph. Lymph from the lower body flows to the cisterna chyli in the abdomen and continues upward through the thoracic duct, which receives intercostal lymph vessels, the left subclavian trunk from the left arm, and the left jugular trunk from the left side of the head. The thoracic duct empties lymph into the blood in the left subclavian vain near its junction with the left jugular vein. The right lymphatic duct drains lymph from the upper right quadrant of the body and empties into the right subclavian vein. As the lymph flows through the lymph vessels toward the subclavian veins, it passes through lymph nodes, which contain macrophages to phagocytize bacteria or other pathogens that may be present.

Venes DJ, ed. Lymph. In: Taber's Cyclopedic Medical Dictionary. 19th ed. Philadelphia: FA Davis Co; 2001:1138 (excerpt)

Lymphadenitis

An inflammation of the lymph nodes.

Lymphangiectasia

Dilatation of the lymphatic vessels (megalymphatics).

Lymphangiogram

A radiograph of the lymphatic vessels and nodes.

Synonym: *lymphogram*

Venes DJ, ed. Lymphangiogram. In: Taber's Cyclopedic Medical Dictionary. 19th ed. Philadelphia: FA Davis Co; 2001:1140

Lymphangiography

A: The x-ray examination of lymph nodes and lymphatic vessels after an injection of contrast medium.

B: Immediate radiological investigation of the lymphatic vessels after injection of a contrast medium via cutdown, usually on the dorsum of the hand or foot. Delayed films are taken to visualize the nodes. This technique has been replaced by computed tomography and magnetic resonance imaging.

Synonym: *lymphography*

Venes DJ, Ed. Lymphangiography. In: Taber's Cyclopedic Medical Dictionary. 19th ed. Philadelphia: FA Davis Co; 2001:1140

Lymphangioma

A: A benign, yellowish tan tumor on the skin composed of a mass of dilated lymph vessels. The tumor is removed by excision or electrocoagulation for cosmetic reasons. Also called angioma lymphaticum.

Plural: *lymphangiomas, lymphangiomata*

Anderson K, Anderson L, Glanze W. Lymphangioma. In: Mosby's Medical Dictionary. 5th ed. St. Louis, MO: Mosby; 1998:966

B: A tumor composed of lymphatic vessels.

Venes DJ, ed. Lymphangioma. In: Taber's Cyclopedic Medical Dictionary. 19th ed. Philadelphia: FA Davis Co; 2001:1140

Lymphangitis

An inflammation of one or more of the lymphatic vessels, usually resulting from an acute streptococcal infection of one of the extremities. It is characterized by fine red streaks extending from the infected area to the axilla or groin, and by fever, chills, headache, and myalgia. The infection may spread to the bloodstream. Penicillin and hot soaks are usually prescribed; aseptic technique is important to avoid contagion.

Anderson K, Anderson L, Glanze W. Lymphangitis. In: Mosby's Medical Dictionary. 5th ed. St. Louis, MO: Mosby; 1998:966–967

Lymphatic System

A: A vast, complex network of capillaries, thin vessels, valves, ducts, nodes, and organisms that help protect and maintain the internal fluid environment of the entire body by producing, filtering, and conveying lymph and by producing various blood cells. The lymphatic network also transports fats, proteins, and other substances to the blood system and restores 60% of the fluid that filters out of the capillaries into the interstitial spaces during normal metabolism. The peripheral parts of the lymphatic complex do not directly communicate with venous system into which the lymph flows, but the endothelium of the veins at the junction of the blood and the lymphatic network is continuous with the endothelium of the lymphatic vessels. Small semilunar valves throughout the lymphatic network help to control the flow of lymph and, at the junction with the venous system, prevent venous blood from flowing into the lymphatic vessels. The lymph collected from throughout the body drains into the blood through two ducts situated in the neck. Various body dynamics as respiratory pressure changes, muscular contractions, and movements of organs surrounding lymphatic vessels combine to pump the lymph through the lymphatic system. The thoracic duct that rises into the left side of the neck is the major vessel of the lymphatic system and conveys lymph from the whole body, except for the right quadrant, which is served by the right lymphatic duct. Lymph flows into the general circulation through the thoracic duct at a rate of ~125 mL per hour during routine exertion. Various body dynamics, such as respiratory pressure changes, muscular contractions, and movements of organs surrounding lymphatic vessels combine to pump the lymph through the lymphatic system. The lymphatic capillaries, which are the beginning of the system, abound in the dermis of the skin, forming a continuous network over the entire body, except for the cornea. The system also includes specialized lymphatic organs, as the tonsils, the thymus, and the spleen.

Anderson K, Anderson L, Glanze W. Lymphatic system. In: Mosby's Medical Dictionary. 5th ed. St. Louis, MO: Mosby; 1998:967

B: The system that includes all the lymph vessels that collect tissue fluid and return it to the blood (lymph capillaries, lacteals, larger vessels, the thoracic duct, and the right lymphatic duct), and the organs made of lymphatic tissue (lymph nodes and nodules, the spleen, and the thymus) that produce lymphocytes and monocytes, defend against pathogens, and provide immunity.

Venes DJ, ed. L. system. In: Taber's Cyclopedic Medical Dictionary. 19th ed. Philadelphia: FA Davis Co; 2001:1141

Lymphedema

An abnormal accumulation of tissue fluid (potential lymph) in the interstitial spaces. The mechanism for this is either impairment of normal uptake of lymph by the lymphatic vessels or excessive production of lymph caused by venous obstruction that increases capillary blood pressure. Stagnant flow of tissue fluid through body structures may make them prone to infections that are difficult to treat; as a result lymphedematous limbs should be protected from cuts, scratches, burns, and blood drawing. Common causes of lymphedema include neoplastic obstruction of lymphatic flow (e.g., in the axilla, in metastatic breast cancer); postoperative interference with lymphatic flow (e.g., in filariasis); radiation damage to lymphatics (e.g., after treatment of pelvic or lung cancers). *Congenital lymphedema:* Chronic pitting edema of the lower extremities.

Synonym: *Milroy's disease*

Venes DJ, ed. Lymphedema. In: Taber's Cyclopedic Medical Dictionary. 19th ed. Philadelphia: FA Davis Co; 2001:1141–1142

Lymph Node

A: One of the many small oval structures that filter the lymph and fight infection and in which lymphocytes, monocytes, and plasma cells are formed. The lymph nodes are different sizes, some as small as pinheads, others as large as lima beans. Each node is enclosed in a capsule, is composed of a lighter colored cortical portion and a darker medullar portion, and consists of closely packed lymphocytes, reticular connective tissue laced by trabeculae, and three kinds of sinuses, subcapsular, cortical, and medullar. Lymph flows into the node through afferent lymphatic vessels that open into the subcapsular sinuses. Most lymph nodes are clustered in areas such as the mouth, the neck, the lower arm, the axilla, and the groin. The lymphatic network and nodes of the breast are especially crucial in the diagnosis and treatment of breast cancer. Also called lymph gland.

Anderson K, Anderson L, Glanze W. Lymph node. In: Mosby's Medical Dictionary. 5th ed. St. Louis, MO: Mosby; 1998:968

B: A: One of the many small oval structures that filter the lymph and fight infection and in which lymphocytes, monocytes, and plasma cells are formed. The lymph nodes are different sizes, some as small as pinheads, others as large as lima beans. Each node is enclosed in a capsule, is composed of a lighter colored cortical portion and a darker medullar portion, and consists of closely packed lymphocytes, reticular connective tissue laced by trabeculae, and three kinds of sinuses, subcapsular, cortical, and medullar. Lymph flows into the node through afferent lymphatic vessels that open into the subcapsular sinuses. Most lymph nodes are clustered in areas such as the mouth, the neck, the lower arm, the axilla, and the groin. The lymphatic network and nodes of the breast are especially crucial

in the diagnosis and treatment of breast cancer. Also called lymph gland.

Venes DJ, ed. L. node. In: Taber's Cyclopedic Medical Dictionary. 19th ed. Philadelphia: FA Davis Co; 2001:1138

Lymphocele

A cyst that contains lymph.

Venes DJ, ed. Lymphocele. In: Taber's Cyclopedic Medical Dictionary. 19th ed. Philadelphia: FA Davis Co; 2001:1143

Lymphocyte

A white blood cell responsible for much of the body's immune protection. Fewer than 1% are present in the circulating blood; the rest lie in the lymph nodes, spleen and other lymphoid organs, where they can maximize contact with foreign antigens. Lymphocytes vary from 5 to 12 μm in diameter; subpopulations may be identified by unique protein groups on the cell surface called clusters of differentiation. T cells, derived from the thymus, make up approximately 75% of all lymphocytes; B cells, derived from the bone marrow, 10%. A third classification is natural killer cells. In the blood, 20 to 40% of the white cells are lymphocytes.

Venes DJ, ed. Lymphocyte. In: Taber's Cyclopedic Medical Dictionary. 19th ed. Philadelphia: FA Davis Co; 2001:1143

Lymphoma

A: A type of neoplasm of lymphoid tissue that originates in the reticuloendothelial and lymphatic systems. It is usually malignant but in rare cases may be benign. It usually responds to treatment. Two main kinds of lymphomas are Hodgkin's disease and non-Hodgkin's lymphoma (NHL). A third form, Burkitt's lymphoma, is rare in North America but relatively common in Central Africa. A rare form of lymphoma is mycosis fungoides, a chronic T cell variation of the disease affecting the skin and internal organs. It is an insidious disorder, beginning as a plaquelike pruritic rash that spreads through the skin and becomes nodular and systemic. The various lymphomas differ in degree of cellular differentiation and content, but the manifestations are similar in all types. Hodgkin's disease lymphomas tend to affect young adults but usually respond to recently developed types of therapy. The NHL usually strikes patients around middle age and can be more difficult to treat. Characteristically, the appearance of a painless, enlarged lymph node or nodes is followed by weakness, fever, weight loss, and anemia. With widespread involvement of lymphoid tissue, the spleen and liver usually enlarge, and gastrointestinal disturbances, malabsorption, and bone lesions frequently develop. Men are more likely than women to develop lymphoid tumors. There has been a dramatic increase in the incidence of acquired immunodeficiency syndrome (AIDS)–related NHL, which is attributed to prolonged survival of AIDS patients related to the availability of antiretroviral agents. Treatment for lymphoma includes intensive radiotherapy, chemotherapy and biologic therapies. Kinds of lymphoma include Burkitt's lymphoma, giant follicular lymphoma, histiocytic malignant lymphoma, Hodgkin's disease, and mixed cell malignant lymphoma. Formerly called leukosarcoma.

Plural: *lymphomas, lymphomata*
lymphomatoid, *adj.*

Anderson K, Anderson L, Glanze W. Lymphoma. In: Mosby's Medical Dictionary. 5th ed. St. Louis, MO: Mosby; 1998:970

B: A malignant neoplasm originating from lymphocytes.

Burkitt's lymphoma: A form of malignant, non-Hodgkin's lymphoma that causes bone-destroying lesions of the jaw. The Epstein-Barr virus is the causative agent. It was initially reported in Central Africa.

Cutaneous T cell lymphoma (CTCL): A malignant non-Hodgkin's lymphoma with a predilection for infiltrating the skin. In its earliest stages, it often is mistaken for a mild, chronic dermatitis because it appears as itchy macules and patches, often in the chest or trunk. Later, the lesions may thicken, become nodular, or spread throughout the entire surface of the skin, the internal organs, or the bloodstream.

Non-Hodgkin's lymphoma (NHL): A group of malignant solid tumors of B or T lymphocytes that are newly diagnosed in about 45,000 Americans annually.

SYMPTOMS: Painless lymphadenopathy in two thirds of patients is the most frequent presenting symptom. Others have fever, night sweats, loss of 10% or more of body weight in the 6 months before presenting with symptoms of infiltration into non lymphoid tissue. Additional involvement is in the peripheral areas such as epitrochlear nodes, the tonsillar area, and bone marrow. NHL is 50% more frequent in men than in women of similar age. In most cases the cause of NHL is unknown, but patients who have received immunosuppressive agents have a more than 100 times greater chance of developing NHL, probably owing to the immunosuppressive agents activating tumor viruses.

TREATMENT: Specific therapy depends on the type, grade, and stage of the lymphoma. Combination chemotherapies, bone marrow transplantation, radiation therapy, and photochemotherapy may be given, depending on the specific diagnosis.

Venes DJ, ed. Lymphoma. In: Taber's Cyclopedic Medical Dictionary. 19th ed. Philadelphia: FA Davis Co; 2001:1144

Lymphorrhea

Flow of lymph from ruptured lymph vessels onto the surface of the skin.

Venes DJ, ed. Lymphorrhagia. In: Taber's Cyclopedic Medical Dictionary. 19th ed. Philadelphia: FA Davis Co; 2001:1145

Lymphostasis

Stoppage of the flow of lymph fluid.

Macromolecule

A large molecule such as a protein, polymer, or polysaccharide.

Venes DJ, ed. Macromolecule. In: Taber's Cyclopedic Medical Dictionary. 19th ed. Philadelphia: FA Davis Co; 2001:1148

Macrophage

A monocyte that has left the circulation and settled and matured in a tissue. Macrophages are found in large quantities in the spleen, lymph nodes, alveoli, and tonsils. About 50% of all macrophages are found in the liver as Kupffer's cells. They are also present in the brain as microglia, in the skin as Langerhans' cells, in bone as osteoclasts, as well as in serous cavities and breast and placental tissue. Along with neutrophils, macrophages are the major phagocytic cells of the immune system. They have the ability to recognize and ingest all foreign antigens through receptors on the surface of their cell membranes; these antigens are then destroyed by lysosomes. Their placement in the peripheral lymphoid tissues enables macrophages to serve as the major scavengers of the blood, clearing it of abnormal or old cells and cellular debris as well as pathogenic organisms. Macrophages also serve a vital role by processing antigens and presenting them to T cells, activating the specific immune response. They also release many substances that participate in inflammation, including chemokines and cytokines, lytic enzymes, oxygen radicals, coagulation factors, and growth factors.

Venes DJ, ed. Macrophage, macrophagus. In: Taber's Cyclopedic Medical Dictionary. 19th ed. Philadelphia: FA Davis Co; 2001:1148–1149

Melanoma

A: Any of a group of malignant neoplasms, primarily of the skin, that are composed of melanocytes. A melanocytic nevus may be acquired or congenital. The congenital nevus is regarded as more likely to develop into a malignant melanoma, primarily because of its larger size. Smaller melanomas tend to develop from a pigmented nevus over a period of several months or years. They may be sporadic and occur most commonly in fair-skinned people having light-colored eyes. A previous sunburn also increases a person's risk. Any black or brown spot having an irregular border; pigment appearing to radiate beyond that border; a red, black, and blue coloration observable on close examination; or a nodular surface is suggestive of melanoma and is usually excised for biopsy. Melanomas may metastasize and are among the most malignant of all skin cancers. Prognosis depends on the kind of melanoma, its size, depth of invasion, and location, and the age and condition of the patient. Because of

the occurrence of melanomas and melanocytic nevi in certain families, a familial atypical mole and melanoma syndrome (FAM-M) has been designated. It is defined by the occurrence of melanoma in one or more first- or second-degree relatives, a large number of moles, and moles that demonstrate certain cellular features. Patients with the syndrome have a high lifetime risk of development of melanoma. Kinds of melanoma are amelanotic melanoma, benign juvenile melanoma, lentigo maligna melanoma, nodular melanoma, primary cutaneous melanoma, and superficial spreading melanoma.

Anderson K, Anderson L, Glanze W. Melanoma. In: Mosby's Medical Dictionary. 5th ed. St. Louis, MO: Mosby; 1998:1007

B: A malignant tumor of melanocytes that often begins in a darkly pigmented mole and can metastasize widely. The incidence of melanoma is rising more rapidly than that of any other cancer. In the U.S. in 1997, approximately 40,000 new cases of melanoma were diagnosed; in the year 2000, the disease affects 1 in 75 Americans. In 1999 the American Cancer Society estimated there would be 44,200 new cases of the disease. More than 90% of melanomas develop in the skin; about 5% occur in the eye, and 2.5% occur on mucous membranes. The likelihood of long-term survival depends on the depth of the lesion at diagnosis (thicker lesions are more hazardous), the histological type (nodular and acral lentiginous melanomas are worse than superficial spreading or lentigo malignant melanomas), and the patient's age (older patients do more poorly) and gender (men tend to have a worse prognosis than women).

ETIOLOGY: Excessive exposure to ultraviolet light, especially sunlight, causes melanoma. It is more common in whites than blacks, and it appears as a genetic illness in some families.

SYMPTOMS: Melanomas are marked by their asymmetry, irregular border, and varied color. The diameter is usually greater than 6 mm (about 1/4 in.). A change in surface appearance or size of a mole often brings the lesion to medical attention.

PREVENTION: Suntanning should be discouraged. Persons spending considerable time outside should wear protective clothing to shield against ultraviolet radiation and use sunscreens on exposed skin.

TREATMENT: Melanomas are treated with surgery, to remove the primary cancer, along with adjuvant therapies to reduce the risk of metastasis. Interferon alpha and levamisole have been used as immunotherapeutics. Vaccines have been developed against melanoma; they appear to improve prognosis in affected patients.

Venes DJ, ed. Melanoma. In: Taber's Cyclopedic Medical Dictionary. 19th ed. Philadelphia: FA Davis Co; 2001:1181–1182

Monocyte

A mononuclear phagocytic white blood cell derived from myeloid stem cells. Monocytes circulate in the bloodstream for ~24 hours and then move into tissues, at which point they mature into macrophages, which are long lived. Monocytes and macrophages are one of the first lines of defense in the inflammatory process. This network of fixed and mobile phagocytes that engulf foreign antigens and cell debris is commonly called the macrophage system.

Venes DJ, Ed. Monocyte. In: Taber's Cyclopedic Medical Dictionary. 19th ed. Philadelphia: FA Davis Co; 2001:1227

Nephrotic Syndrome

A condition marked by increased glomerular permeability to proteins, resulting in massive loss of proteins in the urine, edema and hypoalbuminemia, hyperlipidemia, and hypercoagulability. Several different types of glomerular injury can cause the syndrome, including membranous glomerulopathy, minimal-change disease, focal segmental glomerulosclerosis, and membranoproliferative glomerulonephritis. These pathological findings in the kidney result from a broad array of diseases such as diabetic injury to the glomerulus, amyloidosis, immune-complex deposition disease, vasculitis, systemic lupus erythematosus, and toxic injury to the kidneys by drugs. The disease's prognosis depends on the cause. For example, if the cause is exposure to a drug or toxin, the removal of that substance may be curative. When the disease results from glomerulosclerosis caused by AIDS, death may occur within months. Renal biopsy usually is needed to determine the precise histological cause, treatment, and prognosis. Idiopathic NS is diagnosed when the known causes of NS have been excluded. It is usually diagnosed in adults by use of renal biopsy. Causes are classified according to the changes found in the capillaries of the glomerulus when examined by use of electron microscopy.

SYMPTOMS: Patients with nephrotic syndrome may initially present with fluid retention in the legs or symptoms caused by blood clotting (e.g., in the renal vein). The hyperlipidemia that often accompanies the syndrome may lead to symptoms caused by atherosclerosis.

TREATMENT: Diuretics are used to treat symptomatic edema. Anticoagulants may be used to treat and prevent clotting. Lipid-lowering medications are used to prevent atherosclerosis. Renally, tailored diets, with defined quantities of sodium, potassium, and protein, often are recommended. Corticosteroids and immunosuppressive drugs (e.g., cyclophosphamide) are used to manage nephrosis caused by some histological subtypes. When renal failure accompanies nephrotic syndrome, dialysis may be required.

Venes DJ, ed. Nephrotic syndrome. In: Taber's Cyclopedic Medical Dictionary. 19th ed. Philadelphia: FA Davis Co; 2001:1279 (excerpt)

Osmosis

The passage of solvent through a semipermeable membrane that separates solutions of different concentrations. The solvent, usually water, passes through the membrane from the region of lower concentration of solute to that of a higher concentration of solute, thus tending to equalize the concentrations of the two solutions. The rate of osmosis is dependent primarily upon the difference in osmotic pressures of the solutions on the two sides of a membrane, the permeability of the membrane, and the electric potential across the membrane and the charge upon the walls of the pores in it.

osmotic, *adj.*

Venes DJ, ed. Osmosis. In: Taber's Cyclopedic Medical Dictionary. 19th ed. Philadelphia: FA Davis Co; 2001:1361–1362

Palliative

1. Relieving or alleviating certain symptoms without curing. 2. An agent (therapeutic procedure, medication) that alleviates or eases a painful or uncomfortable condition.

Venes DJ, ed. Palliative. In: Taber's Cyclopedic Medical Dictionary. 19th ed. Philadelphia: FA Davis Co; 2001:1392

Papilloma

1. A benign epithelial tumor. 2. Epithelial tumor of skin or mucous membrane consisting of hypertrophied papillae covered by a layer of epithelium. Included in this group are warts, condylomas, and polyps.

Venes DJ, ed. Papilloma. In: Taber's Cyclopedic Medical Dictionary. 19th ed. Philadelphia: FA Davis Co; 2001:1401

Protein (Blood Protein)

One of a class of complex nitrogenous compounds that are synthesized by all living organisms and yield amino acids when hydrolyzed. Proteins provide the amino acids essential for the growth and repair of animal tissue.

COMPOSITION: All amino acids contain carbon, hydrogen, oxygen, and nitrogen. Some also contain sulfur. About 20 different amino acids make up human proteins, which may contain other minerals, such as iron or copper. A protein consists of from 50 to thousands of amino acids arranged in a very specific sequence. The essential amino acids are those the liver cannot synthesize (tryptophan, lysine, methionine, valine, leucine, isoleucine, phenylalanine, threonine, arginine, and hsititine); they are essential in the diet, and a protein containing all of them is called a complete protein. An incomplete protein lacks one or more of the essential amino acids. The nonessential amino acids are synthesized by the liver.

SOURCES: Milk, eggs, cheese, meat, fish, and some vegetables such as soybeans are the best sources. Proteins are found in both vegetable and animal sources of food. Many incomplete proteins are found in vegetables; they contain some of the essential amino acids. A vegetarian diet can make up for this by combining vegetable groups that complement each other in their basic amino acid groups. This provides the body with complete protein. Principal animal proteins are lactalbumin and lactoglobulin in milk; ovalbumin and ovoglobulin in eggs; serum albumin in serum; myosin and actin in striated muscle tissue; fibrinogen in blood; serum globulin in serum; thyroglobulin in thyroid; globin in blood; thymus histones in thymus; collagen and gelatin in connective tissue; collagen and elastin in connective tissue; and keratin in the epidermis. Chondroprotein is found in tendons and cartilage; mucin and mucoids are found in various secreting glands and animal mucilaginous substances; caseinogen in milk; vitellin in egg yolk; hemoglobin in red blood cells; and lecithoprotein in the blood, brain, and bile.

FUNCTION: Ingested proteins are a source of amino acids needed to synthesize the body's own proteins, which are essential for the growth of new tissue or the repair of damaged tissue; proteins are part of all cell membranes. Excess amino acids in the diet may be changed to simple carbohydrates and oxidized to produce adenosine triphosphate and heat; 1 g supplies 4 kcal of heat. Infants and children require from 2 to 2.2 g of protein per kilogram of body weight per day. This should be calculated on the basis of the ideal, rather than the actual, weight of the child. Age also is a factor in determining protein requirements, the amount decreasing with age. Physical work, menstruation, pregnancy, lactation, and convalescence require increased protein intakes. Excess protein in the diet results in increased nitrogen excretion in the uri.

Blood protein: A broad term encompassing numerous proteins, including hemoglobin, albumin, globulins, the acute-phase reactants, transporter molecules, and many others. Normal values are hemoglobin, 13 to 18 g/dl in men and 12 to 16 g/dl in women; albumin, 3.5 to 5.0 g/dl of serum; globulin, 2.3 to 3.5 g/dl of serum. The amount of albumin in relation to the amount of globulin is referred to as the albumin-globulin (A/G) ratio, which is normally 1.5:1 to 2.5:1.

Venes DJ, ed. Protein. In: Taber's Cyclopedic Medical Dictionary. 19th ed. Philadelphia: FA Davis Co; 2001:1577–1578 (excerpt)

Pulmonary Edema

A: The accumulation of extravascular fluid in lung tissues and alveoli, caused most commonly by congestive heart failure. Serous fluid is pushed back through the pulmonary capillaries into alveoli and quickly enters bronchioles and bronchi. The condition also may occur in barbiturate and opiate poisoning, diffuse infections, hemorrhagic pancreatitis, and renal failure and after a stroke, skull fracture, near drowning, inhalation of irritating gases, and rapid administration of whole blood, plasma, serum albumin, or intravenous fluids. Observations: Signs and symptoms of pulmonary edema include tachypnea, labored shallow respirations, restlessness, apprehensiveness, air hunger, or cyanosis and blood tinged or frothy pink sputum. The peripheral and neck veins are usually engorged; the blood pressure and heart rate are increased; and the pulse may be full and pounding or weak and thready. There may be edema of the extremities, crackles in the lungs, respiratory acidosis, and profuse diaphoresis. Interventions: Acute pulmonary edema is an emergency requiring prompt treatment. The patient is placed in bed in a high Fowler's position, and the immediate administration of intravenous morphine sulfate is usually ordered to relieve pain, to quiet breathing, and to allay apprehension. A cardiotonic, such as digitalis, a fast-acting diuretic, such as furosemide or ethacrynic acid, and a bronchodilator, such as aminophylline, may be given; oxygen may be ordered. While the patient is acutely ill, the blood pressure, respiration, apical pulse, and breath sounds are checked every hour or continually monitored. Parenteral fluids, if indicated, are infused slowly in limited quantities; a low-sodium diet is served; and the patient's intake and output of fluids are measured. The patient is weighed daily, and any sudden gain is noted and reported. In addition to receiving continued care and emotional support, the patient exercises to tolerance, plans frequent rest periods, reports any symptoms, avoids smoking, and follows the regimen ordered for medication, diet, and return checkups.

Anderson K, Anderson L, Glanze W. Pulmonary edema. In: Mosby's Medical Dictionary. 5th ed. St. Louis, MO: Mosby;, 1998:1354–1355

B: Effusion of serous fluid into the alveoli and interstitial tissue of the lungs. The cause is weakening or failure of the left ventricle, which allows blood to back up and increase filtration pressure in the pulmonary capillaries. This is life threatening. Acute pulmonary edema may be a sign of severe pulmonary or heart disease. The outcome will depend upon the success of treating the primary illness.

Synonym: *acute edema of lung*

Venes DJ, ed. Pulmonary e. In: Taber's Cyclopedic Medical Dictionary. 19th ed. Philadelphia: FA Davis Co; 2001:604 (excerpt)

Reflex Sympathetic Dystrophy

A: A syndrome characterized by severe burning pain in an extremity accompanied by sudomotor, vasomotor, and trophic changes in bone without an associated specific nerve injury. This condition is most often precipitated by trauma to soft tissue or nerve complexes. The skin over the affected region is usually erythematous and demonstrates hypersensitivity to tactile stimuli and erythema.

B: An abnormal response of the nerves of the face or an extremity, marked by pain, autonomic dysfunction, vasomotor instability, and tissue swelling. Although the precise cause of the syndrome is unknown, it often follows trauma, stroke, neuropathy, or radiculopathy. In about one third of all patients, the onset is insidious. Affected patients often complain of burning pain with any movement of an affected body part, excessive sensitivity to light touch or minor stimulation, temperature changes (heat or cold) in the affected limb, localized sweating, localized changes of the skin color, or atrophic changes in the skin, nails, or musculature.

SYN: *Shoulder-hand syndrome; Sudeck's atrophy*

TREATMENT: Early mobilization of the body part, with multimodality therapy, may improve the symptoms of RSD. Drug therapies often include prednisone or other Corticosteroids and narcotic analgesics; transcutaneous electrical stimulation, physical therapy, or nerve blocks may also prove helpful.

Venes DJ, ed. Reflex sympathetic dystrophy. In: Taber's Cyclopedic Medical Dictionary. 19th ed. Philadelphia: FA Davis Co; 2001:1651

Sebaceous

Containing, or pertaining to, sebum, an oily, fatty matter secreted by the sebaceous glands.

Venes DJ, ed. Sebaceous. In: Taber's Cyclopedic Medical Dictionary. 19th ed. Philadelphia: FA Davis Co; 2001:1731

Serum Sickness

An adverse (type III hypersensitivity) immune response following administration of foreign antigens, esp. antiserum obtained from horses or other animals. Animal serum was previously used for passive immunization against rabies. Serum sickness can also occur following administration of penicillin and many other drugs. Antigen-antibody complexes form and deposit on the walls of small blood vessels, stimulating an inflammatory response that produces a pruritic rash, fever, joint pain and swelling, myalgias and enlarged lymph nodes 7 to 14 days after exposure. Treatment consists of salicylates (such as aspirin) and antihistamines to minimize inflammation; corticosteroids may be given for severe symptoms.

Venes DJ, ed. Serum sickness. In: Taber's Cyclopedic Medical Dictionary. 19th ed. Philadelphia: FA Davis Co; 2001:1746

Stent

(Charles R. Stent, Brit. dentist, 1845–1901) 1. Originally a compound used in making dental molds. 2. Any material or device used to hold tissue in place or to provide support for a graft or anastomosis while healing takes place.

Venes DJ, ed). Stent. In: Taber's Cyclopedic Medical Dictionary. 19th ed. Philadelphia: FA Davis Co; 2001:1829 (excerpt)

Stewart-Treves Syndrome (see Angiosarcoma)

Thrombophlebitis

Inflammation of a vein in conjunction with the formation of a thrombus. It usually occurs in an extremity, most frequently a leg. Treatment: The therapeutic goal is to prevent a thrombus from becoming an embolus that may reach the lung. The anticoagulant heparin is used but requires careful monitoring of the patient's response. Therapy may also include ligation of the vein proximal to the thrombus to prevent pulmonary embolism.

Venes DJ, ed. Thrombophlebitis. In: Taber's Cyclopedic Medical Dictionary. 19th ed. Philadelphia: FA Davis Co; 2001:1946–1947 (excerpt)

Thymus

A lymphoid organ located in the mediastinal cavity anterior to and above the heart, composed of two fused lobes each containing multiple lobules, which are roughly divided into an outer cortex and inner medulla. Immature T cells (thymocytes) make up most of the cortex and some of the medulla. The remaining cells are epithelial cells, with some macrophages. Epithelial cells in some areas of the medulla develop hard cores and are known as Hassall's corpuscules; their purpose is unknown. The thymus is the primary site for T-lymphocyte differentiation. During the prenatal period, lymphoid stem cells migrate from the bone marrow to the thymus. They fill and expand the intestinal spaces between epithelial cells and proliferate rapidly. Almost all of these immature thymocytes are destroyed, to eliminate those that would attack self-antigens. Approx. 1% of the thymocytes mature into T cells, with either a CD4 or a CD8 protein marker and receptors capable of binding with specific antigens. The mature T lymphocytes leave the thymus and migrate to the spleen, lymph nodes, and other lymphoid tissue, where they control cell-mediated immune responses. The thymus weighs 15 g to 35 g at birth and continues to grow until puberty, when it begins to shrink and the lymphoid tissue is replaced by fibrotic tissue; only about 5 g of thymic tissue remains in adulthood. The reason for involution may be that the organ has produced enough T lymphocytes to seed the tissues of the immune system and is no longer necessary. Removal of the thymus in an adult does not cause the decrease in immune function seen when the gland is removed from children.

Venes DJ, ed. Thymus. In: Taber's Cyclopedic Medical Dictionary. 19th ed. Philadelphia: FA Davis Co; 2001:1950 (excerpt)

Trophic

Of or pertaining to nutrition.

OMD Online Medical Dictionary. Coracoid process. Available at: http://cancerweb.ncl.ac.uk/cgi-bin/omd?query=trophic&action=Search+OMD (2001). Accessed February 2004

Ultrafiltration

Filtration of a colloidal substance in which the dispersed particles, but not the liquid, are held back.

Venes DJ, ed. Ultrafiltration. In: Taber's Cyclopedic Medical Dictionary. 19th ed. Philadelphia: FA Davis Co; 2001:2024

Urticaria

Multiple swollen raised areas on the skin that are intensely itchy and last up to 24 hr; they may appear primarily on the chest, back, extremities, face, or scalp. SYN: *hives, nettle rash*

ETIOLOGY: Urticaria is caused by vasodilation and increased permeability of capillaries of the skin as the result of mast cell release of vasoactive mediators. The mast cell degranulation is the result of an immunoglobulin E-mediated reaction to allergens (e.g., foods, drugs, or drug additives), heat cold and, rarely, infections or emotions. Urticaria is a primary sign of local and systemic anaphylactic reactions. It affects people of all ages but is most common between 20 and 40 years of age. Urticaria is closely related to angioedema, which causes edema in deeper regions of the skin and subcutaneous tissue.

TREATMENT: Drugs that block histamin-1 (H_1) receptors (antihistamines) are the primary treatment for urticaria. The use of both H_1 and H_2 receptor blockers has been recommended but has not been proven more effective. Patients should avoid identified allergens. Corticosteroids are not usually used.

Venes DJ, ed. Urticaria. In: Taber's Cyclopedic Medical Dictionary. 19th ed. Philadelphia: FA Davis Co; 2001:2044

Index

Italic numbers refer to figures

Hyperkeratosis
  defined, 251
  lymphedema and, 60
Hyperplasia, primary lymphedema and, 47
Hypolasia, primary lymphedema and, 47
Hypoproteinemia, 251
Hysterectomy, 251

I

ICD-9 codes, lymphedema clinic guidelines, 230
Ileus, 251
Immune function, lymph nodes, 12
Indirect lymphography, lymphedema diagnosis, 68
Infection
  lymphedema and, 60, 61
  secondary lymphedema and, 50, 51
Inflammation, traumatic edema, 90–91
Inflammatory rheumatism. See Rheumatoid arthritis
Information resources, lymphedema clinics, 227–228
Inguinal lymph nodes, 25
Inguinal lymph node fibrosis, 48
Initial lymph vessel plexus, 5
Injury, lymphedema risk and, 57
Insufficiencies, lymphatic system, 41
Intensive phase, 123
Internal jugular lymph nodes, anatomy, 10, 18–19, 19
Interstitial fluid colloid osmotic pressure (COP$_{IP}$), filtration and reabsorption, 37–38
Interstitial fluid pressure (IP), filtration and reabsorption, 37–38
Intraterritorial lympho-lymphatic anastomoses
  anatomy, 16
  bilateral primary lymphedema, lower extremity, 158–159
  bilateral secondary lymphedema, lower extremity, 155–156
  lipolymphedema, 163–164
  lymph collectors, 7
  unilateral primary lymphedema, lower extremity, 156–157
Invasive therapy, lipedema management, 89
Ipsilateral, defined, 251

J

Joint capsule, inflammatory rheumatism, 92–93
Jugular lymphatic trunk, anatomy, 9, 9–10
Jugular lymph nodes, 18
Jugular trunk, 9
Jugular vein, 9

K

Kunke, E., 102–103
Klippel-Trénaunay-Weber syndrome, 167

L

Laplace's law, compression therapy, 113
Latency stage, lymphedema, 54
Lateral arm territory, 24
Lateral thigh territory, 26

Lateral neck/submandibular area, manual lymph drainage techniques, 135–136, 135–136
Leg, self-managed manual lymph drainage, 216–218, 216–218
Letter of medical necessity sample, 242
Lipectomy, defined, 251
Lipedema
  defined, 251
  definite, 87
  etiology and natural history, 87
  evaluation, 88, 88
  hemorrhages, 87–88
  pathology and pathophysiology, 87–88
  stages, 88
  therapeutic approach, 88–89
Lipodermatosclerosis, lymphedema, 77
Lipolymphedema, treatment sequence, 163–164
Liposuction
  defined, 251–252
  lymphedema management, 73
Long-stretch bandages, compression therapy, 113–114
Lotions
  compression therapy, 168–169
  lymphedema clinic supply requirements, 228–229
Lower back, decongestive therapy, 209–210
Lower extremity
  bilateral primary lymphedema, 157–159
  bilateral secondary lymphedema, 154, 154–156
  compression bandaging, 178–187, 179–187
    hip attachments, 184, 186, 187
  decongestive exercises, 208–210
  lymphatic drainage, 8, 24–28, 24–28
  lymphedema in, 65
  manual lymph drainage, 145–146, 145–147
    do's and don'ts, 220–221
    self-managed techniques, 213–218, 215–218
  self-bandaging techniques, 202–206, 203–206
  unilateral primary lymphedema, treatment sequence, 156–157
  unilateral secondary lymphedema, treatment sequence, 151–153, 152
  venous dynamics, chronic venous insufficiency, 74, 74–75
Low-volume insufficiency, lymphatic physiology, 42–43, 43
Lumbar area, manual lymph drainage, 139–140, 140
Lumbar lymphatic trunks, 7–8, 7–9
Lumpectomy, secondary lymphedema and, 49, 49
Lymph, defined, 252
Lymphadenitis, defined, 252
Lymphangiectasia
  defined, 252
  primary lymphedema and, 47
Lymphangiogram, 252
Lymphangiography, 252
Lymphangioma, 252–253
Lymphangiomotoricity
  lymph collectors, 6, 6
  manual lymph drainage, 104
Lymph angion, 6, 6
Lymphangiopathy, lymphedema staging, 54
Lymphangitis, 253
Lymphatic cysts, 59, 96, 246
Lymphatic drainage
  complete decongestive therapy, 103
  components, 16–28, 17
  lower extremity, 8, 24–28, 24–28
  mammary gland, 8, 20–23, 20–23
  trunk, 13–14, 19–20, 20
  upper extremity, 14, 23–28, 23–28
Lymphatic fistulas, 59